Praise for *Practice a*

Matthew Remski was one of the first teachers to speak out on social media about physical and emotional injury and trauma in yoga. In doing so, he created a safe space for people to connect with each other over shared experiences and ultimately heal their own trauma. *Practice and All is Coming: Abuse, Cult Dynamics, and Healing in Yoga and Beyond* sheds light on the sexual and physical assault that has taken place in the yoga community, while providing a resource that helps teachers and students recognize when they may be in an unsafe situation and empowers them to protect themselves. This book should be required reading for every yoga teacher training.

Trina Altman, BA, E-RYT 500, PMA-CPT
Creator of Yoga Deconstructed© and Pilates Deconstructed.©

This is a horrifying and necessary tale that all current yoga practitioners and teachers need to know and reckon with. Jois and Ashtanga had a significant influence on what yoga is today in the U.S. and worldwide—from the ethics practices of teachers, to the way we pedestal (and isolate) teachers, to assists, to studio culture. This centers Ashtanga yoga, but as Remski suggests, it is relevant to every yoga lineage, and of course we know that it's culture-wide. Remski recognizes the qualities of isolation, lack of agency, victim-blaming, and silencing present in these survivors' accounts as implicit in rape culture. The responsibility therefore extends beyond the "perpetrators", and falls on all of our shoulders as bystanders and participants in "yoga community". We need to face and discuss this history and that of any harm in order to move into the true promise of living out yogic teachings — harmlessness, integrity, generosity, non-attachment, and the wise use of sexual energies.

Jacoby Ballard, *Yoga Teacher and Social Justice Educator.*

Packed with interviews of horrific abuse and real stories of recovery, Remski presents us an authoritative guide on the effects of sexual abuse, misconduct and trauma in the modern, globalized yoga world as well as analysis that invites the possibility of change to this culture of abuse. The struggle and resilience of the interviewees make for an intense and powerful read. It is in the context of colonial, plundering and appropriation of yoga culture that yoga has come bearing the scars of its violent impacts with the West. Remski does not pretend to separate himself in some false veneer of objectivity. He reflects on and owns his privilege as a cis white man and speaks to his learning curve in becoming an ally and even accomplice to those more often targeted for abuse. In fact, this is what makes the book so powerful: Remski himself is committed to unpacking and transforming the cult dynamics and cultures that surround such abuse and in doing so, shows us how we can do our part as well. *Practice and All is Coming* offers hope and practical solutions for those who seek — and I do hope this is all of us — an end to the cycle of trauma, abuse of power and sexual violence in yoga culture today.

Susanna Barkataki, *Founder & Director of Education, Ignite | Yoga and Wellness Institute.*

Matthew Remski opens a window into a part of the yoga world most people have never seen — a world where trusting seekers with open minds and full hearts are cruelly betrayed. He explores how this happens, what the sometimes debilitating and pervasive after-effects can be, and how to heal from it all. By interviewing many former followers and experts in the field, Matthew offers the reader a wonderfully rich and up-to-date synthesis of data and practical information. His book is unique, as it provides a significant amount of hard-hitting personal stories and facts while simultaneously being infused with sensitivity and an awareness of the impact these can have on those reading the book who have been through trauma. I will certainly be recommending this book to my clients and colleagues.

Rachel Bernstein, *LMFT, Educator and Therapist, Cult Specialist, Host of the "IndoctriNation" podcast.*

Matthew Remski has written a painstaking and unflinching book that details multiple women's first person accounts of sexual abuse at the hands of Ashtanga yoga founder K. Pattabhi Jois, and the subsequent denial and cover up within his community. This is a vital read that highlights the courage of the women who came forward within a culture of cognitive dissonance, unquestioning obedience, and magical thinking, in which pain is re-labeled as healing, injury as opening, and isolation as enlightenment. At the same time, Remski thoughtfully navigates how yoga teachers and practitioners can continue to practice yoga today in all forms, while acknowledging the darker side of its origins. A heartbreaking and illuminating read.

Sarah Court*, PT, DPT, e-RYT.*

I welcome the powerful voices of the courageous, truth-speaking women that are heard so clearly in this valuable study. I applaud Matthew's sensitive and subtle exposure of power imbalance, and his impeccable intentions to bring the voices from the margins to the centre. I give thanks that his moral compass guided him to reveal a crucial issue at the heart of modern yoga, and I hope that everyone who has ever shown up to a yoga class reads this book. I recommend it as required reading for every yoga teacher training course on the planet.

Uma Dinsmore-Tuli, Ph.D., Ph.D., *Author of Yoni Shakti: A Woman's Guide to Power and Freedom Through Yoga and Tantra.*

For those of us who consider ourselves yoga teachers it may be especially important to scrutinize ourselves and our community with clarity and honesty, in particular when to comes to the issue of power. Yoga, with all of its promise, is as susceptible as any other human institution to becoming an environment for the abuse of power and all the suffering this engenders. With *Practice and All is Coming*, Matthew Remski has done us a great service by applying intellectual rigor to help us see how destructive power dynamics can set in and fester, and then by suggesting how we can make yoga practice a safe, respectful, and empowering experience for all who show up.

David Emerson, *YACEP, TCTSY-F | He/Him/His, Director: The Center for Trauma and Embodiment at JRI, author Trauma-Sensitive Yoga in Therapy and co-author Overcoming Trauma through Yoga.*

Amongst the responses to the revelations of sexual abuse that have marred a number of yoga communities, *Practice and All Is Coming* is unparalleled. Of immense value to both practitioners and academics, the text centers the voices of the female victims of serial abuser Pattabhi Jois and illuminates the wider psychoanalytic and structural conditions that enabled such abuse. Practitioners will be gifted a demystification of transnational yoga and a way to both understand and prevent the toxic dynamics that have produced abuse. Academics will find a strong case for the utility—and even ethical necessity—for bringing cultic studies back into the field of New Religious Movements. With this ambitious and well-executed text, Remski has established himself as one of the most perspicacious and important scholar-practitioners of contemporary transnational yoga.

Ann Gleig, *Associate Professor of Religion and Cultural Studies, University of Central Florida.*

The future of yoga depends on our ability to reconcile a past fraught with abuse and injury. If we ignore the pain that was caused in the name of yoga, our communal body will never heal. Yoga will go the way of step aerobics and the power of the teachings will evaporate into the history books. The first step in healing is acknowledging that there is a problem, and that is what Matthew Remski so powerfully demonstrates in *Practice and All is Coming: Abuse, Cult Dynamics, and Healing in Yoga and Beyond.* This is a text that can heal the wounds of yoga and allow us to re-imagine it as a safe practice for everyone, free from abuse and injury.

Jivana Heyman*, Founder and Director of Accessible Yoga.*

This is a potent treatise, bringing well-needed thoughtful and measured scrutiny to a controversial subject. Remski provides a thorough exposition of one of the icons of modern yoga - not to simply critique or discredit, but more to examine possible solutions to the unveiled issues. The book itself is part of the solution, in that it provides a platform enabling previously-muted voices to be heard. In response to these voices, he goes on to construct a research-grounded framework that elevates safety and inclusivity. This could be the means to propel the field of yoga forward with more integrity, and indeed, more authenticity. This book should be considered required reading for all those involved in yoga therapy training, and I strongly recommend it to all yoga professionals as well.

Cassi Kit*, Director, Faculty, and Administrative Coordinator, School of Embodied Yoga TherapyYoga, Therapist (C-IAYT, PYT).*

Starting with the first principle of yoga which is non-harming (ahimsa), and applying the clear seeing of meditation (dhyana), Remski offers us a framework for understanding how confusion and messiness around lineage and power has led to so much pain and suffering inside the world of yoga. This is also a guidebook in the yogic principle of self-study (svadyaya) helping us all look honestly at ourselves and our community. I am so grateful that finally, Remski offers us a way forward — with both practical means and inspiration - to remind us that yoga is a living practice and in the end, always about relationship.

Cyndi Lee*, author of Yoga Body, Buddha Mind; OM yoga Today; OM yoga, A Guide to Daily Practice; OM at Home, A Yoga Journal; and the OM Yoga in a Box series.*

As globalized convert yoga finally recovers from the drunken honeymoon of orientalist cultural appropriation it enjoyed for a century or so, it finds itself sober and shocked, #MeToo revelations toppling school after school. Matthew Remski's deep reporting here on just one of these tragedies offers not a simple indictment of Pattabhi Jois's person or teaching, but a broad-reaching call for the best of Western theory and activism to be brought to a problem created by colonial encounter and resolvable only by changing the terms of that encounter. The book, like the yoga it deconstructs, unfolds "a vinyasa of meanings," moving between the psychodynamic implications of the guru-student tradition and the harm-reduction practices that could both preserve and irrevocably change it. Most importantly, Remski centers the voices of women, using his position to witness and amplify their narratives in their own words. Few other books from within the convert yoga community ask so fluently and humbly how sincere non-Indian practitioners might be in wise relationship with the ancient lineages of Yoga, and the culture that developed them. Few outside it describe a tragedy of the modern colonial encounter with such an intimate and heart-rending precision.

Sean Feit Oakes, *PhD.*

Matthew Remski has authored a remarkable book. His fair examination of some of the cultish and dogmatic elements in yogic culture —and the impact they've had on women, in particular—is erudite, well-researched and engaging. But what's of particular note in his work is the empathy, sensitivity and respect he takes in addressing the abuse inherent in authoritarian systems. In doing so, he's created a testament to those whose lives have been directly impacted by such abuses of power.

Carrie Owerko, *Senior Level Iyengar Yoga Teacher, Laban Movement Analyst, Functional Range Conditioning Mobility Specialist.*

This book is the result of a herculean effort by Matthew Remski in giving a voice to and unearthing the rampant, darkest, dirtiest, disturbing open secret in the yoga world. The painstaking research and interviews, all of which have helped open the floodgates, is truly commendable, and will serve as a foundation for setting better mechanisms for prevention of abuse in the name of spiritual practices and even in other walks of life.

Dr. Nivedita Pingle, *M.B.B.S. Yoga Vidnyan Visharad.*

Thank you Matthew Remski and the courageous women who have stepped forward to offer this pivotal work. *Practice and All is Coming* is a service to humanity, to the yoga world at-large, to long-time practitioners and future generations so that we can evolve into cultivating a safe space that all beings deserve. This incredibly thorough, sensitive and somatically sophisticated work is ESSENTIAL to the evolution of yoga for the maturity to unpack the shadow of abuse, body-image distortion and power-dynamics effecting many without conscious awareness of these undercurrents, while also recommending best practices and a PRISM method to move forward so that we may work towards ending abuse of all forms and transforming dominance-structures so that all beings are respected, safe and empowered in their journey of embodiment.

Shiva Rea*, author, Tending the Heart Fire and founder Samudra Global School for Living Yoga.*

While Matthew Remski is the courageous, insightful, and compassionate author of this informative, challenging, and thought-provoking book, this book is clearly a group effort. Equal parts theory, training manual, expose, and memoir, *Practice and All is Coming: Abuse, Cult Dynamics, and Healing in Yoga and Beyond* is a foray into the difficult topics of personal agency, spirituality authority, and cult dynamics. In addition to his clearly articulated understanding of the problems inherent in many spiritual schools, Remski provides hope for healing the confusion and anguish that arise in the heart of sincere practitioners when they are betrayed by the revered powers in which they have placed their trust. If you practice or teach yoga, please consider this book an essential companion on your path.

Christina Sell*, author of Yoga From the Inside Out: Making Peace with Your Body Through Yoga, My Body is a Temple: Yoga as a Path to Wholeness, and A Deeper Yoga: Beyond Body Image to Freedom.*

In this illuminating book Matthew Remski brings light to the often-bypassed toxic dynamics and deception that occur in the yoga subculture and new-age spirituality. Through compassionate inquiry, Remski provides a platform for honest discourse into cult dynamics, power imbalances, and why as humans we might trade autonomy and authenticity for acceptance under the guise of healing and community. To practice compassion, we must first acknowledge suffering and yet victims' voices continue to be silenced and edited in order to protect images in the Ashtanga community and beyond. As more abuse and manipulation is uncovered and exposed many schools, studios, and practitioners are reluctant to "throw the baby out with the bathwater". However, Remski challenges us to examine who is the baby and what is the bathwater, separating our own healing and self-awareness practices from branding and systems of power. In addition to providing insight into the psychology of attachment and contemporary distortions of the guru model, this book provides reflections on how to move forward and ensure that these shadows do not continue to undermine equality, empowerment, and healing in the yoga community. To the women who courageously shared your stories: may you continue to feel heard, respected, and supported.

Michele Theoret, *MACP; President and lead facilitator Empowered Yoga, Mindfulness & Lifestyle, Director BEology Project Foundation.*

Trouble in yoga paradise . . . In this lucid, measured, incisive and compassionate book, Matthew Remski lays bare the toxic dynamic of manipulation, indoctrination, negation, and deception that oftentimes undergirds guru worship in such complex social systems as the yoga subculture. As he demonstrates, when enabled by their cult followers, mulabandha-adjusting spiritual autocrats posing as enlightened beings can prove just as toxic to the broader culture as pussy-grabbing political demagogues posing as successful real estate developers. More than an expose of the sexual predations of a renowned guru figure, Remski has also provided the yoga community with a road map to self-healing and closure.

David Gordon White, *Distinguished Professor of Religious Studies, emeritus, University of California, Santa Barbara.*

PRACTICE

AND ALL IS COMING

ABUSE, CULT DYNAMICS, AND HEALING IN YOGA AND BEYOND

BY

MATTHEW REMSKI

VOLUME 1 OF THE WAWADIA PROJECT

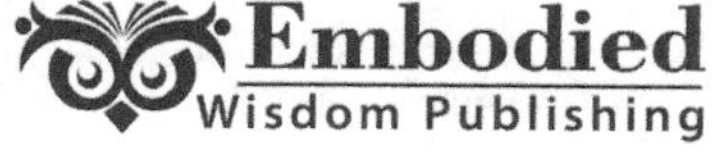

2019

PRACTICE AND ALL IS COMING:
Abuse, Cult Dynamics, and Healing in Yoga and Beyond

Embodied Wisdom Publishing Ltd
140 Ashworth Bush Road
RD7 Rangiora 7477 New Zealand

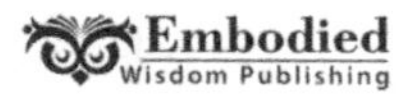

Editor:	Maitripushpa Bois
Illustrator:	Sonya Rooney, Christchurch, New Zealand
Cover and text design:	James Dissette
Printed by:	IngramSpark
ISBN	978-0-473-47207-8 (pb)/ 978-0-473-46771-5 (ePub) 978-0-473-46772-2 (Kindle)/ 978-0-473-46773-9 (PDF)
Title	Practice and All Is Coming: Abuse, Cult Dynamics, and Healing in Yoga and Beyond
Author	Matthew Remski
Format	Hardcover/softcover/eBooks
Publication Date	03/2019

Environmental Responsibility: To ensure we minimise our environment impact we ensure the printers we contract have current chain-of-custody certification for fiber used throughout the production process. This includes the following European or Americacertifications:

- The Forest Stewardship Council™ (FSC®)
- Programme for the Endorsement of Forest Certification™ (PEFC™)
- The Sustainable Forestry Initiative® (SFI®).

Dedication and Thanks

Dedicated to the women harmed by K. Pattabhi Jois, and to everyone working for a culture of care and justice in the yoga world and beyond.

SPECIAL THANKS TO...

The ever-patient WAWADIA contributors. Especially Studio Patron Empowered Yoga in Edmonton (Michele Theoret), and Patrons Linda McGrath, Joseph Goodman, and Clemens Schumacher.

And to Galen Tromble, for his generous and unconditional financial support of the project. You can find Galen's work, which applies the teachings and practices of yoga to the challenge of climate change at climateyogi.org.

For support, wisdom, and encouragement: Donna Farhi, Lauren McKeon (my editor at The Walrus), Theodora Wildcroft, Carol Horton, Be Scofield, Tiffany Rose, Jamie Mathieson, Yvonne Werkman, Steve McGrath, Frank Jude Boccio, Andrew Tanner, Shannon Roche, Elizabeth Kadetsky, Kathryn Bruni-Young, J. Brown, Cassi Kit, Anne Pitman, Jivana Heyman, Leena Miller Cressman, Emma Dines, Laurel Beversdorf, Jill Miller, Jules Mitchell, Ted Grand, Christine Wushke, Sarah Holmes de Castro, Asia Nelson, Susanna Barkataki, Teo Drake, Jacoby Ballard, Rachel Brathen, Danielle Kinahan, Ariana Rabinowitz, David Rendall, Miranda Leitsinger, Linda Malone, Natalie Miller, Carly Budhram, Chris Calarco, Daniel Clement, Tamar Samir, Ann Gleig, Jason Birch, Jacqui Hargreaves, Jim Mallinson, Mark Singleton, Christopher Wallis, Alexandra Stein, Jennifer Freyd, Dan Shaw, Andrew McDuffee, Ruth Warner, Sean Feit Oakes, Leslie Hayes, Colin Hall, Elizabeth Emberly, Jason Sharpe, Uma Dinsmore-Tuli, Nirlipta Tuli, Tatjana Mesar, Dimi Currey, Norman Blair, Birgitte Gorm Hansen, Ann-Charlotte Monrad, Kalli Anderson,

Pam Rubin, David Remski, Jill Remski, Cathleen Hoskins, John Bemrose, Danielle Rousseau, Christi-an Slomka, and The Yoga Service Council.

Thank you to Maitripushpa Bois, my editor, for helping me find the pathway from criticism to empowerment.

And to Alix Bemrose for your insight, support, weathering the backlash and abuse alongside me, and for being you.

In fact, it is in the nature of the Indian tradition that the student should strive to understand the teacher, for in striving, and not from being spoon-fed, is knowledge revealed.

—Eddie Stern, *Preface to Guruji: A Portrait of Sri K. Pattabhi Jois Through the Eyes of His Students*[1]

Table of Contents

Read, Reflect, Participate

Would you like to help build safer communities by contributing to a shared understanding of toxic group dynamics? There's an online opportunity to do just that in conjunction with the conclusion of this book.

Part Six summarizes the analytical principles used in this book to examine the context and enablement of abuse within yoga and spiritual communities. In addition, it offers over 50 study questions for teachers, trainees, and group administrators to help foster communities of transparency and care.

An online service has been built for members, teachers, and trainees in yoga and other spiritual organizations to respond to, collate and submit their study questions as part of their ongoing personal and professional development.

With the consent of participants, we will collate, proof, and publish some of this material to a dedicated blog for broader discussion. Through this initiative, the ideas in this book may stimulate ongoing research, discussion, examination, and accountability that nurture community health and safety.

The URL below will lead you to the book's endnotes with live links, embedded video and podcast resources, and research articles cited.

You can access those resources and gain access to the online workbook here: https://embodiedwisdom.pub/paaic-resources/

Content Warning

This book records the graphic testimonies of women who describe being sexually assaulted by an acclaimed yoga master while practicing in his classes. It also documents the ways in which their experiences were denied, rationalized, or spiritualized by fellow practitioners, some of whom knew full well what was occurring. The testimonies are arranged to preserve accuracy while minimizing gratuitous detail and repetition. There are also several graphic descriptions of video and pictorial evidence that depict assault.

This material is presented here with context, analysis, and calls-to-action, in the hope of building safer spaces for the practice of yoga, Buddhism, mindfulness, eco-spirituality, and other forms of self-help, self-inquiry, and healing.

For some thoughts on self-care while reading, please go to page 30.

"I'm not even sure he knew my name."

—Interview with "T.M."* 3/30/2018.
Full transcript in Appendix 1 (*see* p. 293).

Let's see. I was a very adventurous, spirited young woman with a desire to connect and belong. I know many people reframe that as some kind of pathology or ego-seeking something, but I think it's a desire that all humans share, to have meaningful connection.

I had encountered Ashtanga. I thought it was great. I was a little bit of an extreme personality. I like to push things all the way to their limit to see if the ideas and the promises worked. In my mid-twenties, I went to Mysore for eight months.**

I was one of Pattabhi Jois's favorites. He basically dry humped me every day for eight months in multiple positions. His infamous "adjustments" of sticking his crotch in your ass or your crotch, and then just pumping. Like it literally was dry humping. People think that that's a funny term that I'm using, but it's actually descriptive.

Immediately, I was told...

[laughing]

I'm sorry I have to laugh on some of this—even at the time, I was laughing, even though I found it deeply confusing and went along with it during that eight months—

I was told that "It was not sexual." I was told *immediately* that this was not sexual.

* T.M. has chosen to remain anonymous.

**Mysore, now known by its pre-colonial name Mysuru, was home to Pattabhi Jois (1915–2009) from the age of twelve. It is also the home of the Krishna Pattabhi Jois Ashtanga Yoga Institute (KPJAYI), which remains highly influential in the global Ashtanga yoga community. This book will generally use "Mysore" because most of the interviewees use it, as do the vast majority of Ashtanga practitioners who either travel there or take part in daily "Mysore-style" classes in their local *shalas*, or studios.

I was like: "Really? Because a guy's crotch in your ass or your own crotch, pumping in the early morning, that's not sexual? What is it?"

They would develop very elaborate ideologies and rationalizations for what this was. This was some kind of *Shakti* whatever.* I was like, "Yeah, but isn't *that* sexual?" In what definition of *Shakti* do you have that there's not something sexual happening?

Jois was quite fixated on me in these behaviors. I was there, in a foreign country with very thin social ties. It makes complete sense to me that I was quite confused and didn't really know how to respond, particularly since people got strangely jealous of the fact that I was one of his favorites and were wondering why they weren't getting that attention. As though this were some kind of lauded place for a person to be.

Of course, no one would admit openly to being jealous.

I'm not even sure he knew my name. I didn't get any sense that I was an important student that he was transmitting something to. That was not the experience. It was more like I was a piece of ass in an open position that he could dry hump. That's what it felt like to be the receiver, and then the chorus of interpretations of that morphing it into something else, as a special thing, was just incredibly confusing for me.

* *Shakti* is a Sanskrit term for the female-coded energy that some physical yoga practices are said to unlock.

Introduction

om
may grace protect us
may grace nourish us
may our studies be vigorous and radiant
may we not hate each other
om
as we nurture peace in ourselves
for others
and for the world

—Adapted from Taittirya Upanishad, this is a mantra traditionally chanted at the beginning of studies.

WHAT THIS BOOK WILL DO

This book presents a case study of abuse, institutional betrayal, and healing as it has occurred and is unfolding within diverse parts of the late Pattabhi Jois's Ashtanga yoga community. It more fully documents the testimony from women who Jois sexually assaulted than has been previously covered. It will report on intergenerational echoes of harm within that part of the Ashtanga world that has remained professionally and emotionally identified with Jois and his teaching style. Analysis will show that the Jois event resonates with imbalanced and gendered power dynamics between teachers and students in the wider yoga world.

The reporting will track how the globalized,* now-instantly-connected, and diverse Ashtanga network has responded to the abuse revelations in both defensive and progressive ways. This will provide an instructive example of how the mechanisms of in-group social control and even society-wide rape culture operate—but can also begin to dissolve—as a yoga community moves through crisis and towards new growth. The conclusion will center upon action items for personal and collective awareness and accountability, offered with the intention of helping to foster safer spaces for not only yoga practice, but also any spiritual or wellness endeavor centered on group activity.

This book will center voices like that of T.M. while offering cultural, social, and psychological contexts and resources for understanding how the assault and betrayal of care happened, and was allowed to happen, for almost three decades. It will cover how the abuse was hidden from members implicitly, through the idealization of Jois as "Guruji"** in everyday conversation, and explicitly, through published media that presented Jois as a purely wholesome figure. Uncovering these dynamics will help explain why—even though Jois's behavior had been an open secret—T.M. and other women didn't know about it before they practiced with him, and were still encouraged to go study with

* The terms "global" and "globalized" will also be used in a historical sense in this book, indicating the era of rapid transcultural spread and commodification of yoga practice from the 1960s onwards. The term "modern" will often refer to the period directly preceding, in which mainly Indian teachers synthesized new forms of physical practice from both indigenous medieval sources and European physical culture influences.

**In this book, I'll use the term "Guruji" when used by his disciples, or in the case of the book with that title. I'll use "guru" only when quoting another source. These terms are problematic on two counts. Given that Jois has been shown to have been a sexual offender, the first term can be triggering to his victims. Additionally, there is controversy over whether "guru" is an appropriate term for an offender, and whether it was ever appropriate to begin with, given the strict guidelines for a guru's behavior and responsibilities in a traditional or premodern Indian context. Using the term uncritically to refer to Jois may contribute to the continuing appropriation and degradation of what is properly a sacred concept and role.

him. It will help to explain why, when they questioned the behavior, it was rationalized and even made out to be a sign of Jois's spiritual power.

Tools from the literature of cult analysis will be useful in unpacking the mechanisms at play in recruiting, retaining, and deploying members who wind up both participating in and being victimized by abusive dynamics. The central task here will be to show how interpersonal and group forms of *deception*—the first of all cultic mechanisms—can be used to manipulate the beliefs and behaviors of group members, while also covering over the harm a group commits. The most important cult-studies resource used here is the work of Alexandra Stein, which will help to show how the power dynamics at play between an abusive leader and their students can show signs of "disorganized attachment" patterning.[2] This is seen when the students are caught up in a cycle of running towards the very person who harms them, in an anxious search for love.

Invoking a concept like "deception" in the opening pages necessitates a disclaimer: this book is not about evil or intentional malice. The deceptive notions explored here—that Pattabhi Jois was a spiritual master, that his technique was ancient, that his touch was healing, and that injuries were signs of positive advancement—might have been consciously or unconsciously held by practitioners. They might have been communicated through earnest attempts at care. It's impossible to say. We won't be examining people's *intentions*. Rather, we'll focus on *impacts* by peering into the gap between what was said and believed about Jois and his method, and the reality of what was experienced. We'll explore how this gap allowed the abuse to be initiated through social grooming, escalated through somatic dominance framed as love and intimacy, and allowed to continue for so long.

Because deception and disorganized attachment patterning are by no means unique to the Jois story, the frameworks of Stein and others can shed helpful light on what seems to be a pandemic of institutional failure of care within large yoga communities and other spiritual and self-help organizations. The field of cult studies is famous for its internal disagreements, but consensus stands firm around one idea: *education about toxic group dynamics makes us all less susceptible to them.*

It would be both unjust and counter-productive for the reader to come away from this book associating the term "Ashtanga yoga" with an airtight, uniform, all-abusive organization. The community inspired by Jois's yoga is far too diverse for that. Researchers point out that a "cult can be either a *sharply bounded social group* or a *diffusely bounded social movement* held together through a shared commitment to a charismatic leader."[3]

Today's Ashtanga yoga practitioners orient themselves along a broad spectrum of commitment to that leader. Some are dyed-in-the-wool devotees to Jois, even after his death in 2009, and endow his method with supernatural value. They may be few in number, but they can hold social positions with broad influence. Less committed or professionally enmeshed practitioners simply love the meditative sensuality of the movements and breathing. They don't center their emotional lives around their yoga mats, and would never think of making a pilgrimage to Mysore or lighting candles in front of Jois's portrait.

Within this spectrum, but usually closer to the "sharply bounded" center of a group, cultic harm can emerge whenever the charismatic spark of leaders and their high-profile followers meets the dry wood of members' aspirations. Add the winds of cross-cultural mystique, misunderstanding, misogyny, greed, ambition, and the sunken costs of devotion, and this contact can ignite a firestorm of full-blown exploitation. It can burn individuals like T.M. in ways that change the course of entire lives, while causing smoke damage to the wider industry.

There are countless tragic elements in this story. But it is not, overall, a tragedy. The fact that the global Ashtanga community is diverse and the fires of its harm are localized means that it has a natural resilience and capacity for reform. So while it is useful to identify cultic dynamics where they burn in order to promote safer yoga practice generally, this book also includes the voices of Ashtanga leaders who have begun to analyze and deconstruct the power dynamics that have been harmful. They also practice along a spectrum of experience and commitment. Among them are those who have struggled to put out the cultic fire within themselves, as well as those who were only barely singed. Following a close examination of what the *abuse* was and how *cult dynamics* enabled it, these reformers provide the basis for the ultimate theme of this book's subtitle: *healing*.

A MAP (BEGINNING WITH WHERE I'M COMING FROM)

Now we can lay out the priorities and challenges of this endeavor, and introduce the voices at the heart of the story.

The first task involves clarifying both *methodological* issues (*how* we talk about things) and *positionality* issues (*why* we talk about them, through points of view that are influenced by experience or privilege).

Providing a basic account of my own cultic experience in two yoga-type groups, for instance, will both ground my presentation of the relevance of Stein and other researchers, while also making my personal and activist investments in this history more transparent.

In a similar vein, briefly describing my embodied experience in the broader "cult" of toxic masculinity and male violence—and their impacts on people's agency in learning environments—will shed light on why I zero in on this neglected theme in the history of modern yoga. It will strengthen an examination of how the male-dominated leadership of Ashtanga yoga suppressed stories like T.M.'s for so long.

But it will also reveal a weakness: I participated in this suppression, simply by being invested in the patronizing (and patriarchal) marketing narrative of yoga culture. There was a time when I, like many others, wanted to believe that yoga spaces by definition were *safe* spaces, and that a good student should interpret the offenses of yoga masters (often rationalized as "skillful means" or "crazy wisdom") as beneficial spiritual challenges, instead of reporting them to the police.

My blind spots and learning curves will become clear as the Introduction merges into **Part One: Learning to Listen**, which recounts how I initially sidelined the abuse story of my friend Diane Bruni while ignoring the video evidence of Jois's assaults for years. I feel it's important to show how my own fear and shame thickened a potent barrier to safety and justice in this arena: the dominant culture's unwillingness to face its shadows. As a professional, English-speaking, white male yoga teacher, I'm part of that dominant culture. I had to learn how *not* to defend it from its shadier realities. By showing how I was educated by my interviewees about abuse, victimization, truth-telling, and recovery, I hope to provide a small example of how listening is hard for a beneficiary of the dominant culture—which is dominant in part because it is set up to not listen—yet still is learnable.

That learning is complicated by the personal and group tension between recognition and denial that vibrates as abuse stories come to light. Almost all of the women who share their stories in this book describe some degree of internal splitting between knowing that what was happening to them was wrong, and a socially conditioned response that told them to ignore or deny it. By examining how the yoga world responded to the video evidence for Jois's behavior **(p. 46)**, we'll see how this tension scaled up into a group phenomenon, in which many people felt that what they were seeing was wrong, but simultaneously found ways to minimize, deflect, or deny that feeling. **Part One** will conclude by introducing a best-practices tool called **PRISM**. This was designed to ease this tension between the recognition and denial of abuse in the yoga and other spiritual worlds, provide a pathway towards resilience, and hopefully help end intergenerational harm.

Part Two: Two Survivor Stories, will delve into the testimony of two women—Karen Rain and Tracy Hodgeman—to give an immersive experience of what abuse in some parts of Ashtanga yoga felt like, the interpersonal betrayals that rationalized their suffering, and some of the processes by which they gained clarity about what happened. The interviews with Karen and Tracy unfolded over many meetings and several years. Their words, and the process by which they became able to speak, form the groundwork for an alternative history of Ashtanga yoga, and a community in transformation.

Part Three: Developing Discernment, will expand outwards into the social betrayals that can result from a yoga group's value claims. We'll see how a blend of Ashtanga literature and advertising covered over the abuse at the root of the community, while building its market value globally. This literature scaled the interpersonal deception experienced by women like T.M. upwards into a form of propaganda.

Central to this literature has been the 2010 book *Guruji: A Portrait of Sri K. Pattabhi Jois Through the Eyes of His Students*, edited by Jois disciples Guy Donahaye and Eddie Stern. Nine months after the Jois abuse revelations erupted in November 2017, Donahaye wrote the following.

> Since his death, Guruji has been elevated to a position of sainthood. Part of this promotion has been due to the book of interviews I collected and published with Eddie Stern… which paints a positive picture of his life and avoids exploring the issues of injury and sexual assault. In emphasizing only positive stories it has done more to cement the idea that he was a perfect yogi, which he clearly was not. By burnishing his image, we make it unassailable—it makes us doubt the testimony of those he abused. This causes further harm to those whose testimony we deny and to ourselves.[4]

A large focus of **Part Three** will be on the "loaded language" that some Ashtanga content providers have employed, and how it can be used to both establish authority and inhibit questions. This close reading of Ashtanga-specific terms and ideas can be applied to the claims of any yoga or spiritual group.

According to cultic studies pioneer Robert Jay Lifton, loaded language is audible in any "thought-terminating cliché", which compresses complex problems into "brief, highly reductive, definitive-sounding phrases, easily memorized and expressed." Not only can this jargon defend against scholarly investigation and victim-centered accounts of experiences within a community, it can also begin to constrict the imaginations of those who use it, year in and year out.[5] This will be important to remember in **Part Five: A Long Shadow, Brightening**, where we witness some Jois disciples struggle to let go of the idealizing language they used for decades to assert and reaffirm who he was.

Part Four: Disorganized Attachments, will present the heart of Stein's work in relation to examples from Ashtanga literature and interview data. Stein's work is approachable and applicable to every relationship a yoga, spiritual, or eco-spirituality practitioner might have to any teacher or group. It's particularly applicable to the language of devotion in certain Ashtanga circles, where, as we'll see, Jois was explicitly presented as a safe and protective father figure. In this section, I'll interject a brief account of my daily experience in one yoga-related cult that exemplifies Stein's description of the highly aroused state generated by the confusion of love and harm. I believe that this is an important set of sensations to understand, because spiritual groups can easily interpret the hypervigilant awareness of intense shared practice—which feels so alive and on the edge of something, but may also be tangled up with uncertainty and fear—as a sign of spiritual awakening.

Part Five: will open with evidence that the enabling of Jois's sexual assaults in the Ashtanga community is not isolated: it's an intergenerational problem. We'll look at two public allegations. The first is of sexual assault by a Jois-certified teacher, and the other an allegation of rape against a teacher authorized by Sharath Rangaswamy, now also known as Sharath Jois. Rangaswamy is the grandson of Pattabhi Jois, and the current director of the Krishna Pattabhi Jois Ashtanga Yoga Institute (KPJAYI) in Mysore. Also included is a brief review of documents from a lawsuit against a Jois disciple and senior teacher in New York's Jivamukti Yoga School who used her experience of intimate cuddling with Jois after classes to rationalize sexually harassing her female apprentice.

Although it has recently begun to adopt consent policies for physical touch by its teachers, the Jivamukti Yoga School contributed historically to the popularization of Jois's *implied consent* context for touch. This was one of the key factors that permitted Jois's assaults, and inhibited his victims from resisting them. Another factor is the gender imbalances and normalized sexuality of some parts of Ashtanga adjustment culture, as we'll see in a promotional video made for certified Ashtanga teacher Tim Miller, and an essay published by authorized teacher Ty Landrum.

As senior Jois disciples began to grapple with increasing public awareness of Jois's assaults in the winter of 2017–2018, several released statements of deep regret, but only partial acknowledgment and limited accountability. **Part 5** will continue with a brief survey of some of these statements to show how the loaded language, "self-sealing", and victim-blaming processes characteristic of high-demand groups can both hide institutional abuse and hamper even well-meaning attempts at reform. Yet all is not negative. This part closes with a focus on the voices of Ashtanga teachers who have stepped into leadership roles as the culture finds its resilience. Some are starting to organize structures outside of KPJAYI, as we'll see from the mission statement of the Amayu Community, recently formed to foster "excellence in Ashtanga yoga training, mentoring and development, driven by *consent and student empowerment*."[6]

The **ultimate goal** of this book is for the reader—especially any student, teacher, or trainer within a spiritual community—to come away with:

1. memorable and practical information on the basic energies and patterns of toxic group dynamics that permit abuse, and

2. personal and collective strategies for being able to intuit signs of that toxicity, and to let those who have been most impacted by it lead the discussion of remedies.

Part Six: Better Practices and Safer Spaces: Conclusion and Workbook is written as a resource for practitioners dedicated to understanding and mitigating toxic group dynamics in yoga and beyond. It provides a list of the critical feeling and thinking skills that can help to shield individuals against the deceptions of toxic groups. It will then introduce some best practices for leaders and organizations in the field. Central among them is the **PRISM** model for promoting transparency, accountability, and harm reduction for future practitioners and group members. Its five steps are summarized here.

1. **Pause** to reflect on the idea that each yoga/spiritual method and community carries value, but also, potentially, a history of abuse.

2. **Research** the literature on the method to find and understand that history.

3. **Investigate** whether the harm has been acknowledged and addressed.

4. **Show** how you will embody the virtues and not bypass the wounds of the community.

5. **Model** transparent power sharing and engaged ethics for future practitioners.

A further tool offered is a scope of practice for the study of yoga humanities, designed to help students and teacher trainees interrogate the sources they learn from. With books like *Guruji* on the market providing advertising for an unregulated industry that up to this point has been dominated by charismatic men, they need it. **Part Six** is also a workbook. Each section contains a series of educational essay/reflection questions that will help students, trainees, and trainers become clear on how the principles and strategies are applicable to their inner lives, relationships and communities.

USING THE LANGUAGE OF CULTIC STUDIES, CAREFULLY

I am not an Ashtanga yoga practitioner. For some Jois disciples, this means I fail a basic litmus test of credibility. They regularly ask me questions like: "If you don't do the practice, how can you presume to know anything about what's happening between Jois and his students?" The short answer is that I asked many of them what was happening, and listened to them answer in their own words.

Questions from outsiders, however, don't always work. Timing and trust is everything. Larry Gallagher, a journalist on assignment to Mysore with *Details* magazine in 1995, asked Karen Rain (whose story is featured in **Part Two**) pointed questions about Jois's "adjustments", which Rain has now gone on to define as assaults. Rain remembers brushing the questions aside. She wanted it to seem like everything was okay. "I was in total denial at the time," she says.

For different reasons than those of victims, many interviewees who witnessed Jois's assaults struggled with questions of how much to say, whether to say it openly, whether to go on record, whether I was the right person to talk to, and whether my motivations were safe or positive or productive. They worried about friendships they have nurtured over the years, about betraying and being betrayed. Some were worried about whether speaking would destroy their careers within the culture. Nobody said outright that they were worried about the potential legal liability involved in admitting they knew that Jois was a sexual predator and did little or nothing to stop him, but this may have been a silencing factor as well.

Many interviewees seemed to exhibit what the late clinical psychologist Margaret Singer described as the "fishbowl effect", reported by people who leave or are leaving highly charged groups. Singer uses the term to describe how former group members feel around friends and family as they readjust to life apart from the group. They can feel as though they are being constantly watched—both by group members wondering if they'll be staying and what they'll say if they leave, and non-group members, wondering if they are alright.[7] Singer was writing in 1979, decades before social media began to compound this claustrophobic and shame-generating surveillance problem.

Some of the most high-profile Jois students and witnesses to the assaults who were eventually willing to speak out publicly are those who found success outside of the group long ago. Beryl Bender Birch and Bryan Kest, for example, both studied intensely with Jois but then peeled away from Jois's Ashtanga to innovate forms of Power Yoga. They have both spoken out in acknowledgment of Jois's abuse. People who still identify with Jois's spiritual mastery have a much harder time. It's very hard to remain within the fold and speak to an outsider or the media about one's doubts, fears, or complicities without fear of social or financial repercussions, or deepening one's own internal conflicts. This is an important clue to understanding the broader dynamics at play.

WHAT DOES "CULT" REALLY MEAN?

Those broader dynamics are often referred to with a popular but problematic term. The word "cult" is not only imprecise; it can be inflammatory and marginalizing. Even lifelong cultic studies researchers are conflicted about using it. "Even though we have each studied cults and educated people about this subject for more than 20 years, neither of us has ever felt completely comfortable with the term 'cult.'"[8] In certain quarters, it might itself be classified as a form of "loaded language", employed to dismiss entire religious or political groups out of hand.

Janja Lalich and Madeleine Tobias provide a list of helpful synonyms for "cult". They use terms like "high-demand", "high-control", "totalistic", "totalitarian", "closed charismatic", "ultra-authoritarian", and "self-sealed".[9] The term "self-sealed" is related to Lalich's work on "bounded choice", which she uses to describe an environment in which every occurrence is interpreted to suit the needs of the group or its leader.

> When the process works, leaders and members alike are locked into what I call a "bounded reality"—that is, a self-sealing social system in which every aspect and every activity reconfirms the validity of the system. There is no place for disconfirming information or other ways of thinking or being.[10]

The notion of "undue influence" is another useful framework. Undue influence is a legal concept dating back over 500 years, applied to assess whether a contract formed between a person with more power and a person with less power is truly consensual.[11] As we'll see, non-consent is a core feature of the Jois landscape. Throughout this book, I'll alternate synonyms for "cult" to soften any impression that we're speaking about a precise phenomenon. We're not. We're talking about patterns and relationships.

Terms aside, the most widely accepted definition for what this book addresses as it explores how Jois's abuse was enabled and obscured for years was first presented in 1986 by psychiatrist Louis Jolyon West and counseling psychologist Michael Langone. They write that a cult is:

> a group or movement exhibiting great or excessive devotion or dedication to some person, idea, or thing, and employing unethical manipulative or coercive techniques of persuasion and control (e.g., isolation from former friends and family, debilitation, use of special methods to heighten suggestibility and subservience, powerful group pressures, information management, suspension of individuality or critical judgment, promotion of total dependency on the group and fear of leaving it), designed to advance

> the goals of the group's leaders, to the actual or possible detriment of members, their families, or the community.[12]

A POTENTIALLY HARMFUL TERM

It's a stark definition. There's no doubt that it can be felt as degrading for members of groups to which it is applied. This problem is of great concern to scholars in religious studies, especially those who study movements like Ashtanga yoga professionally. To the consternation of some cult researchers, many religious studies researchers have sidestepped the labeling problem by using the term "New Religious Movement" to describe communities that they say meet the spiritual and social needs of their members in ways that resemble how older and more organized religions meet the needs of their constituents. They privilege the internal descriptions by which a group gives itself meaning. Their tendency is to value what a group says about itself, to understand its ways and longings according to the terms it uses. They do not apply analytical frameworks that alienate group members.

It makes sense. Nobody affiliated with any spiritual group wants to refer to themselves or hear themselves referred to as being cult members. Researchers of all stripes know that if they use the term, or allow its premises to influence their fieldwork, they may immediately lose interview access. Suspicious or threatened group members may not trust them. This could silence the most intimate and tender things the group would want to share about its experience. The entire research project—to understand why and how a group values what it does—may lack the input of the very people who live these values.

In my own experience, when I was "on the inside", I would have angrily rejected the language of cult analysis as applied to my lived experience. I was lucky to have a dear friend who used a softer, more personal language to question my behaviors and convictions.[13] It was only after withdrawing from these groups and re-establishing a safe haven of relationships outside of them—where I could recognize that I had been harmed and may have harmed other people within them—that I was able to hear and metabolize that language. At some point, the terms that had once sounded poisonous and shameful to me crossed a subtle line to become central to my own healing. Or perhaps it was I who crossed that line, into a world in which my thoughts were not so systematically controlled.

Insiders, outsiders, and scholars of all persuasions can argue *ad nauseam* whether "Ashtanga yoga" fits the technical definitions of "cult".

As you move through the evidence of this book, you might recognize some or all of the elements that West and Langone list at play. "Great or excessive devotion or dedication to some person, idea, or thing." "Unethical manipulative or coercive techniques of persuasion and control." "Use of special methods to heighten suggestibility and subservience, powerful group pressures, information management, suspension of individuality or critical judgment." But how systemic are these elements in Ashtanga yoga today? How do we even define the boundaries of Ashtanga yoga, as a practice or community? The short answer is that it's complicated, but it is also crucial to get this right.

The possibility that cult language might not only feel discriminatory but also be used to discriminate against earnest practitioners is not lost on those who seek to exonerate groups that have harbored abuse. In a blog post that claimed Jois's "mistakes" had been "largely accounted for and removed from the Ashtanga yoga system", Ashtanga celebrity Kino MacGregor wrote that "references to Ashtanga yoga as a 'cult' that perpetuates sexual assault are simply a gross mischaracterization of the spiritual lineage of yoga and defames the hundreds of thousands of practitioners who have benefited from the practice and numerous teachers who have given their lives to the teaching yoga [sic]."[14] Here, MacGregor exposes the Achilles' heel of cult analysis discourse—*if* it is used like a blunt knife. She does it, however, by conflating that portion of the Ashtanga world that abused and enabled abuse with the "spiritual lineage of yoga" in general. In response to such defenses, a discussion of cultic dynamics in the Ashtanga world has to pinpoint where and how those dynamics in fact *did* perpetuate sexual abuse, without tarring the entire community with the same brush. A survey of the community's diversity is a good place to start.

FINDING THE "CULTIC" WHILE HONORING A DIVERSE COMMUNITY

If there's an inner core to the global Ashtanga movement, it consists of senior teachers, now roughly between 50 and 70 years of age, who started practicing with Jois directly 30 years ago or more. Some were *certified* to teach the full method by Jois himself—the highest qualification the community recognizes. Some framed their certificates, hand-written by the master on now-yellowing paper. Some didn't. Some maintained their status and relationship to the Jois family; some didn't.

Downstream from the old-timers are teachers who have been

authorized by the Jois family through KPJAYI. They have earned the right to instruct the method through their dedicated study pilgrimages to Mysore, where they now practice under Rangaswamy's supervision. Certified and authorized teachers share the professional and social distinction of being "listed" on Rangaswamy's official website.*[15] Most teachers of this rank have dedicated assistants who work with them every morning, back in their home shalas all over the world. Some assistants are on the KPJAYI track, while others are not. Some may develop dysfunctional relationships with their bosses that echo aspects of the relationships their bosses had with Jois. Some may not.

But beyond these pathways that lead away from and back to Mysore and the direct Jois legacy, there are parallel expressions of Ashtanga culture, only barely affiliated with Jois, his method, or even India. There's Scott Johnson, who teaches every morning close to London Bridge. His class is called "Mysore Style", but he's never been to Mysore. Never saw the need to go. Norman Blair, also in London, practices and teaches "Ashtanga with Love and Props" at the shala of a colleague. ("Props" are blocks, straps, bricks, and other devices used to help practitioners get into postures. They are typically frowned upon by "traditional" Ashtanga teachers. Although, as we'll see, "traditional" is a loaded-language term.) Norman originally learned Ashtanga from one of Jois's certified teachers, but he never bought into the hierarchy. He's not one for groups.

Alison Ulan in Montreal, who studied under Jois personally and has taught the method since the mid-1990s, never received formal authorization to do so. Kiran Bouquet, who was assaulted by Jois in 1983, still teaches Ashtanga yoga in her rural community in Australia. She too has never held any professional status in the world governed by Jois's list. Finally, there are countless Ashtanga practitioners around the world who have become teachers through non-Ashtanga training programs, but whose teaching transmits the core principles of Jois's method.

Then there are the students. There is no solid data on the levels of commitment and involvement amongst rank-and-file Ashtanga practitioners. Anecdotally, the demographic is diverse. There are people who are intrigued

* This is the list used by KPJAYI to verify and recommend certified and authorized teachers, but it is contested within the global community. An older list, assembled by referrals from senior teachers and maintained at "Ashtanga Yoga Teachers" (*see* note 15) does not label teachers as either certified or authorized. While some teachers are listed in both places, those who appear only on the older list are generally understood to be "original" disciples of Jois who did not shift their studentship to Rangaswamy after his grandfather's death in 2009, and no longer return to Mysore for training.

by the method alone, and have no interest in its leadership or even any community beyond those who show up on the same mornings they do. Then there are those who year by year wade deeper into the lifestyle, diet, ideology, and devotions that can lead to being on Jois's list. Some visit their local shala six mornings per week, others twice, and still others practice only at home.

Bottom line: Jois's legacy is now diffuse enough that Ashtanga communities around the world vary in size and can feel quite different from each other. There are hundreds of shalas, and many of them may quietly provide safe space for the business of yogic self-inquiry, largely independent of the somatic and psychosocial influence of the late master and his most dedicated inheritors.

Any community with cultural power will radiate the heat of an internal fire of passion, creativity, and highly charged relationships. This fire can burn members who are in the wrong place at the wrong time. The question for practitioners is not so much whether they should or shouldn't engage with a loose global community such as Ashtanga yoga, but whether they can ask the right questions about where that heat is coming from, what it's doing, and how close they really want to get to it. The study questions in **Part Six** are designed to help distinguish the cultic from the communal, to help feel when an initially inspirational fire swells into a destructive force.

MALE VIOLENCE IN MODERN YOGA

I grew up in an all-male Catholic school environment in which corporal punishment was one of the primary ways in which the social hierarchy was organized. On a daily basis, I was either receiving corporal punishment, or watching it being administered to boys like me. As I researched the histories of the men who brought yoga to the non-Indian world from the 1960s onwards—Pattabhi Jois, B.K.S. Iyengar (1918–2014), Bikram Choudhury (1944–), and others—it became clear that this was a formative experience in their boyhoods as well.* *They all describe being physically abused while learning to do yoga.*

When I began to connect my schoolboy years with my later experience of being forcefully and non-consensually adjusted by yoga teachers, I could feel in my bones a shared intergenerational pattern that had nothing to do with wellness or spirituality. In some communities, "yoga culture" can be a delivery device for what the broader culture, for good or ill, is already passing down.

Sixteen women in this book have accused Pattabhi Jois of sexual assault

* My experience in the 1970s and 1980s in Toronto was not compounded by the colonial violence that early modern Indian yoga innovators were resisting. There is rich research yet to be done on the intersections between violence in pre-colonial and colonial Indian schooling, and how corporal punishment in places like the Mysore Palace may have intensified through the influence of the European teaching method.

or digital rape. There is also photographic evidence that Jois sexually assaulted men, as well, although no male victims have publicly disclosed to date. Sexual assault and rape are not about sex; they are about power. My experience with male violence is that it is expressed early and abused often through dominance hierarchies set up between men. The normalcy with which men assault women's bodies overflows from the violence that often forms a basic economy between men. One senior Jois student who wanted to remain off-record said it succinctly: Jois physically assaulted the men and sexually assaulted the women. It's not rocket science to figure out which of those two targets was more familiar to him. You only have to skim Jois's own account of being beaten by his teacher, Tirumalai Krishnamacharya, from the age of twelve.

"By the time he taught us ten asanas," Jois once told his senior student Eddie Stern, "sometimes we couldn't do them… he would beat us. And the beating was unbearable, that's how it was. We were about ten or fifteen boys who didn't care. We carried on unmindful of the beatings we got from him."[16] In later years, Jois repeatedly remembered Krishnamacharya as a "dangerous man". Krishnamacharya himself described his own teacher in resonant, but less explicit terms. "Every slackening of effort was punished," he recalled about what it was like to study with him, "every emotion banished."[18]

So far, historians of modern yoga have seemed as reluctant to explore the influence and trauma of male violence upon its interpersonal and intergenerational relationships as they have been to use cult analysis to explore its structural dynamics. The groundbreaking scholarship that studies the role of Krishnamacharya in what has been called the "Mysore asana revival" of the 1930s, for instance, only glances at the fact that he was a harsh taskmaster.[19] Reports of Jois and Iyengar being beaten by their teacher are available, and sometimes cited, but there has so far been no extended discussion of what this violence might have felt like in their bodies, every single day. How it influenced their somatic concerns, even as they were developing somatic skills. How it might have filled them with a double message that had a profound impact upon their embodied selves: *protect yourself against assault*, but also *surrender to correction*. Available scholarship offers no discussion of the disorganized attachments possible within such scenarios, exemplified most clearly in the young life of Iyengar, who was not only beaten by Krishnamacharya, but also relied on him for food, shelter, and later, livelihood, when he provided a crucial referral to Iyengar's first employer.[20] There's almost no discussion of how violence may have impacted these men over the long term, or influenced their teaching, or been discharged in turn onto their own students.[21]

This is an understandable omission in a discipline that studies the history of yoga instead of patterns of intergenerational violence. Also, daring to approach this line of thought can cause vertigo: one might begin to feel that the yoga techniques passed down from Krishnamacharya were not only vehicles for self-inquiry, but also vehicles for the expression of male domination over men and women alike, spiritualized through ancient references to yoga as mastery over material nature.

ABOUT THE TITLE

Many yoga enthusiasts will recognize the aphorism in the title of this book, even if they're not part of the Ashtanga world. Jois was famous for this and other curt sayings. The second-best-known among these is "Yoga is 99% practice, and 1% theory."

Jois's appeal to his disciples involved, in part, his apparent ability to preach a gospel of pragmatic spirituality and no-nonsense action. This echoed some of the ethos of the medieval *hathayoga* that was repackaged by his own teacher, Krishnamacharya, in the 1930s to serve an emergent nationalist gym culture that positioned yoga as pathway to invigorating a population oppressed by centuries of colonial rule.[22] The medieval traditions that inspired this modern movement were renowned for eschewing bookishness in favor of the experiential and mystic. They viewed practice as a private communion, not to be mediated by philosophizing or weakened by gossip. The yogi who talked about practice not only wasn't doing it; he was wasting the energy it demands.

Interviews with older Jois students indicated that this mystical anti-intellectualism was often attractive to many of the college-graduated-and-dropped-out yoga seekers of the late hippie era. It got them out of the endless talk of changing the *world*, and into contemplating how to change the *self*. It located moral and spiritual meaning in bodily discipline, and gave structure to lives deconstructed by rebellion and drug trips. "The modernity of the 1970s," as historian Sam Binkley writes, "expressed a search for something solid to hold on to in the ether of vaporized foundations."[23] Students spoke of Jois's postures like they were life-preservers in that ether. The sequences, which Jois counted out in prayer-like rhythms, seemed to offer a faithful heartbeat amidst so much acid rock.

But this same silent work ethic, disinterested in conversation and reinforced through Jois's own limited English, was also a key factor in the silencing of those who would have complained about his abuse. The idea was that the practice, its leader, and the culture that surrounded both would be misunderstood through analysis, and desecrated through criticism.

That silencing was embodied. One student who wanted to remain nameless said the trance-like breathing rhythm in the room, mingled with Jois's counting or commands, made it feel as though it would be impossible to speak. She said she felt she would be breaking a spell if she had a question about something, let alone an objection. The discipline could merge with a bodily training to see and hear and speak not only no evil, but nothing external at all. The command was to stay inside yourself, because the teacher would meet you there.

The title of this book reclaims "Practice and All Is Coming" for several reasons. First, it honors the students who were silenced by the phrase. How do you un-silence a silencing phrase? You print it large, and against its hackneyed meaning. The irony of this gesture expresses solidarity with other ways in which Jois's aphorism was used against itself by disenchanted students. Tracy Hodgeman, who describes Jois assaulting her in Mysore in 1997 (p. 79), told me that her Seattle community used to metabolize the pervasive injuries caused by Ashtanga yoga with a joke: "Do your practice, and all is coming *APART!*" was what Jois really meant to say.

A second reading of the title is a criticism of how such aphorisms are so often used by high-demand groups to present a manipulative fallback position in times of institutional crisis. When evidence for Jois's behavior finally went mainstream in the fall of 2017, devoted group members would regularly face the controversy, uncertainty, and shame by suggesting that Ashtanga practice itself was the answer to the group's problems. They would repeat this very "loaded language" phrase in conversations and social media threads to quell dissent, to soothe each other, and support the premise that the master's teaching content could be separated from his actions. People would say things like: "Didn't Guruji always tell us—'Practice and all is coming'? Isn't that what his advice would be now?" It didn't seem to register that they were quoting from the source of the problem.

I recognized the strategy. When in 2003 and 2012 scandals rocked the high-demand Buddhist group I had been part of, I watched my former group colleagues use the disgraced leader's own sayings to defend him, as though the "truth" of what he taught could somehow erase his deceptive or even abusive behavior.

The drive to save some part of a beloved leader's legacy amidst his own self-destruction is a very human response. But in these cases, it also reflects an educational deficit. While all South Asian wisdom traditions emphasize ethical behavior as the foundation of spiritual maturity, neither yoga nor Buddhism in their modern and globalized forms have developed explicit and consistent tools for understanding and preventing institutional harm. Further, the good intentions behind any desire to preserve the teaching content of an organization where abuse has been revealed can be compromised by the motivations of those whose social and professional identities are often reliant upon that same content. It can make good career sense to tell the rank-and-file to keep practicing, especially if one is rising into a leadership role within the practice community.[24]

Despite its apparent simplicity as a "one-size-fits-all" motto, the aphorism "practice and all is coming" did not prevent abuse. It did not prevent the enabling. It did not prevent the high-demand group dynamics that allowed Jois's influence to grow even as he escalated his assaults over the years. If Ashtanga practice offered answers to these material problems in the postures and breathing, members would have already found them. They'll find answers, rather, by studying rape culture, the effects of trauma, and the mechanisms of group control. Yes: practice has helped many people with many challenges on an individual level. But it has not worked to stop, understand, or prevent institutional abuse.

Nevertheless, we can also imagine that the dogged determination carried in the phrase "Practice and all is coming" has done its work to produce good in Ashtanga culture. Which is why the title finally hints at the fact that, regardless of how Jois may have meant the aphorism or how his disciples used it, those who have engaged with the Jois tragedy on their paths to becoming reformers in the Ashtanga world and beyond have given the phrase a new meaning. As they recognized the abuse in their community and experienced a combination of trauma, disillusionment, and outrage, they had to broaden their definition of what "practice" meant in order to get by. Some of them kept going with the sacred morning ritual of breath and movement they inherited from Jois. Others found therapy, dance, art, or social activism. Karen Rain learned to ride a unicycle, which helped to stabilize her spine. And then she began to write searing critiques of rape culture, which helped to strengthen her voice.[25]

For all of them, practice could no longer be just about postures, or daily discipline, or the subtleties of internal sensation. It couldn't be about private bliss, or the narcissism of "all is coming" to some isolated self. It had to expand to reveal yoga as an inquiry into the relationships that actually form the self through both harm and healing.

VOICES THAT SPOKE OUT

This book is built on interviews with well over a hundred people: Ashtanga practitioners current and past, scholars of medieval and modern forms of yoga, and journalists who cover similar territory. But the heart of what this book has to offer beats in the voices of interviewees who were willing to speak out about their negative or traumatizing experiences. Many went further than simply speaking out. They had enough patience to consider my often-difficult questions about how they became ensnared by toxic dynamics, what it all felt like in granular detail, and how they recovered. Many of those voices belong to women who describe being assaulted or digitally raped by Pattabhi Jois, either at his home-base shala in Mysore, or in locations around the world as he toured.

These voices will echo throughout the book, multiple times, as elements of the stories they tell help to build broader themes. They form a bedrock of evidence for Jois's abuses being consistent from at least 1983 to 2003. This forces us to look at the event as systemic: no one gets away with criminal activity for decades without organized—if unconscious—support. This is not a story about bad apples, but about damage at the roots of an orchard.

The stories of the women in this book are all highly individual, but they share many similarities. Those similarities are crucial for showing the social patterns at play. However, repetition, or the feeling of it, carries risks like compassion fatigue. The challenge has been to strike two types of balance: between the voices and their contexts, and between including enough of each story to show the pervasion of the problems at Mysore, but not so much as to create a sense of despairing voyeurism. Also, some story elements have been broken up for easier digestion.

Some voices are given more space, as the natural outcome of how much time the person spent with Jois and the inner Ashtanga world, and therefore how much they have to describe. In others, it's the outcome of how deeply the assault resonated with prior personal events, or informed the subject's professional life afterwards. Women like Anneke Lucas and Marisa Sullivan, for example, have continued to work in the yoga industry. They've done a lot of work—some quiet, some explicit—to process what occurred, and help heal themselves and others.

Most of **Part Two** is reserved for a deep dive into the narratives of two women who provided many interviews over a two-year period: Karen Rain and Tracy Hodgeman. Two things stand out in their narratives: the richness of their reporting on the assaults, and their highly attuned analysis of the dynamics in which they were caught. Karen's story also shows how someone can be central to a culture, and then, decades later, become central to its reform. My hope is that honoring the depth of such accounts, and the precarious ways in which they emerged, will help to sensitize readers to what it really means to listen to stories that no one wants to hear.

So here are the people you'll be hearing about and from, and a little bit about each, presented roughly in the order in which I came into contact with them. The text will also point you to each interviewee's fuller story, presented in **Appendix 2.** The fuller narratives establish beyond doubt both the chronic nature of the abuse perpetrated by Jois, and how many of the themes presented in **Parts Three, Four** and **Five** are detectable in each story of abuse.

Diane Bruni ran one of the first Ashtanga yoga programs in my home city of Toronto, beginning in the late 1990s. She was the first person to tell me directly the truth about Pattabhi Jois's treatment of some of his women students. Diane has now fully left the Ashtanga practice and community and has become an advocate for "functional movement". She reports having fully recovered from both her Ashtanga experience, as well as stage 3 breast cancer. In 2016, she founded a Facebook group dedicated to critical thinking in yoga and mindful movement practices. Her plan is to have it evolve into an online educational platform called "Movement Research Community."[26]

Anneke Lucas was the first Jois assault victim to publicly disclose. She wrote a blog in 2010 about the yoga master groping her in a group class in Manhattan in 2001, hosted by Ashtanga Yoga New York. In it, she described chastising Jois after the class, and extracting from him at least some slight recognition. Only a few people saw her article when it was first posted, and the site is now offline. She reposted it in 2016.[27] Her insight into the intersection between yoga practice and trauma recovery is invaluable, including to this book, and to the justice-involved men she teaches as the director of Liberation Prison Yoga. She has also pioneered a healing modality called "The Unconditional Model", which uses mindfulness, yoga, and psychology to heal what she describes as the internal landscape of power dynamics correlated to unresolved trauma. "The point is to render outer power structures futile," she says (story on p. 314).

Anneke connected me with her fellow New Yorker **Marisa Sullivan**, who traveled to Mysore in 1997. From observing the first class there, she'd seen clearly how Jois was groping and fondling the women in the room while "adjusting" them. On her mat, she adopted a closed-off stance towards him. She timed her poses to avoid adjustments. She remembers barely breathing and being on high alert when he did adjust her. Then, she reports, she decided to set her fears of molestation aside. For several weeks, Sullivan received lots of attention from Jois, and she felt her practice blossom. Until, one day, Jois assaulted her. Years later, Sullivan helped metabolize her experience by producing a funny and poignant off-off-Broadway one-woman show called "Kundalini Rising", in which the heroine moves from gendered humiliation into feminist strength (story on p. 308).

After leaving Jois's shala, Sullivan traded stories about Jois with **Maya Hammer**. Maya, 22 at the time, had actually been Diane Bruni's student back in Toronto. Jois assaulted her on her very first day in Mysore. After the third day, she phoned her father for support, and he helped her to build the confidence it took to confront Jois and ask for her money back. Out of all of stories I heard, Hammer's was the only one that featured the real-time help of a close bond with someone who was outside of the group. Hammer has gone on to be registered as a psychologist (story on p. 310).

Michaelle Edwards currently advocates for higher safety standards in yoga through her physiotherapy-inspired method, which she calls "YogAlign". But in 1991 she was assaulted by Jois in Hawaii. This has influenced the deeper message in Edwards' method and teaching: preventing physical injury is inseparable from preventing psychological and moral injury. (story on p. 307).

Another figure in the Hawaii Ashtanga scene is **Micki Evslin**. She reports that Jois forcefully pushed his finger or fingers into her vagina at an event in 2002. This is now widely regarded as a form of rape. Evslin said that she commiserated with two other women at the event, both since deceased, who described identical incidents. Shortly after the event, Evslin wrote to at least one mainstream yoga magazine, asking to be interviewed about Jois, but received no response. She also wrote to another prominent Ashtanga teacher on the island about the incident, asking that he teach Ashtanga without idealizing Jois, but never received a reply. Now 71, Evslin still practices a personalized version of Ashtanga at home, and still values it, but only attends the occasional class (story on p. 320).

Karen Rain offers a blistering and self-reflective account of Jois abusing her as one of his elite students—and a celebrity in his inner circle—from 1994 to 1998. I've had over a hundred conversations with Rain about memory, trauma recovery, and the costs of speaking out. Following upon the groundbreaking disclosure of Anneke Lucas, her activism has been central to the current discussion of abuse and enablement in Jois's sphere. It was after her disclosures on social media and her blog that many of the following women came forward (story on p. 60).

Michelle Bouvier was assaulted by Jois in Encinitas in 2002. Bouvier was disillusioned at the time. This did not drive her out of the yoga world, but towards its margins, where her teaching is inspired by student-centered and feminist values (story on p. 325).

Also in 2002, Jois assaulted **Charlotte Clews** in Boulder. Like Bouvier, Clews still teaches the art form that served her "tremendously", and "held me in the world." She says she now teaches a very different kind of yoga and uses it primarily as a means of facilitating body-awareness and self-ease. She no longer touches her students (story on p. 312).

Katchie Ananda described being both physically and sexually assaulted by Jois over the span of several days in Boulder, also in 2002. She has maintained her yoga practice and teaching despite suffering from back pain ever since. She's also become an outspoken critic of patriarchal abuse and internalized misogyny in the broader yoga world (story on p. 314).

T.M. is an old colleague of Karen Rain. She has asked to remain anonymous. She was a student at Jois's shala for an extended amount of time in the 1990s. While she wasn't there for as long as Karen, she was there for longer than any of the other victims who have offered their voices to this book. A lightly edited transcript of her statement appears in **Appendix 1** for readers who want to feel what it is like to sit for an hour in the altered state of listening to a history opposite to the one commonly told.

Tracy Hodgeman discloses that Jois sexually assaulted her repeatedly over several months in Mysore in 1999–2000. She shared her story over two years of interviews. She has overcome injury and community disillusionment to become a beloved senior teacher in the Seattle yoga scene (story on p. 79).

Kathy Elder, 72, was at the same event as Micki Evslin in Hawaii in 2002 and was also been digitally raped by Jois. After the assault, Elder stayed the course, refusing to cede the ground of yoga to an abuser (story on p. 321).

Nicola Tiburzi describes Jois digitally raping her at a day-long workshop in Seattle in 2002. She was in her early twenties. Subsequently, she began studying with a group of women who taught Iyengar yoga, eventually becoming certified in the method. She credits Iyengar practice with healing her ovarian cysts. As we spoke by phone, I could hear her two-year-old babbling happily in the background (story on p. 323).

After much internal debate, **Kiran Bocquet** disclosed that she too had been assaulted by Jois in Mysore in 1983, which makes her testimony the oldest in historical terms. She continues to teach Ashtanga and offer massage at her studio in rural Australia (story on p. 303).

Nicky Knoff, who lives in Australia, describes the "erotic adjustments" of Pattabhi Jois she experienced in 1989 in Mysore. Now 80 years old, Knoff remains a prominent yoga teacher for anyone from therapy students to super athletes. "I dealt with him at the time," she says, "It is up to us, we can let negative experiences spoil the rest of our lives, or leave them behind, forget it and start again, move on and be happy" (story on p. 304).

Kim Haegele Labidi teaches yoga in Los Angeles, where she also practices massage therapy. In 1991, she went to Mysore at the age of 30. On the first day, Jois lay on top her in the same way described by Karen Rain and T.M. (and potentially experienced by many other women), while she was in supine hand-to-foot pose (*Supta Padangusthasana*: *see* Figure 1, above). A ligament in her hip ruptured. She describes it sounding like a gunshot. To this day, she suffers with chronic pain. She can't sit through a movie, and on some days can't walk her dog. "I don't think it was worth it," she says. "But it has made me a better teacher" (story on p. 197).

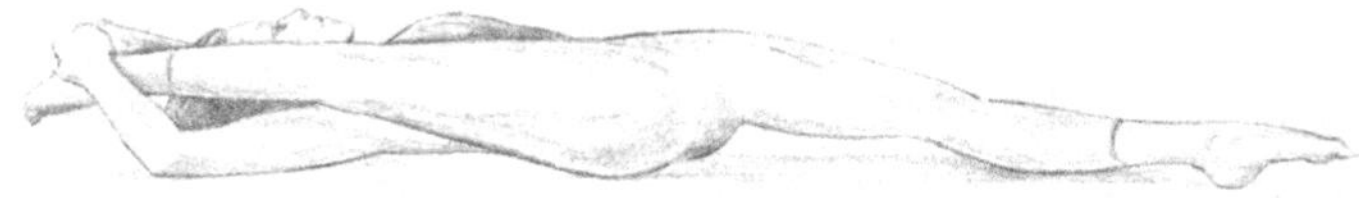

Figure 1: Trivikramasana (referred to by some interviewees in this book as "Supta Padangusthasana")

Two other on-record interviewees did not have traumatic experiences with Jois, but studied with his senior students. They provide a rich insight into the ways in which Jois's behavior has had an intergenerational impact. **Eija Tervonen** offers a personal story from the Finnish Ashtanga scene, which she has since left for gentler forms of practice (story on p. 138). **Michael Kazamias** studied with a certified Jois teacher in London. Michael still teaches yoga but in a gentler mode (story on p. 131).

In July 2018, **Jubilee Cooke** published a robust first-person account of being assaulted by Jois for months on end in 1997. It can be read in full at the independent website *Decolonizing Yoga* under the title "Why Didn't Somebody Warn Me?"[28] (story on p. 95).

Jubilee also did the appalling math on the number of victimizing experiences that this book may not be covering. When I asked her about the mixed responses to her testimony from the wider Ashtanga community, she wrote back the following. Her statement gives voice to what I've come to suspect over several years of research.

> What has frustrated me is how some in the Ashtanga yoga community have mischaracterized and minimized the nature and extent of Pattabhi Jois's sexual assaults. The public still does not understand the number of victims. I know of five women who lived in Seattle, including myself and Catherine Tisseront [*see* p. 79], who were assaulted by Pattabhi Jois either in Mysore or during his Seattle stop on his 2002 World Tour. I suspect there are more. Assuming at least five victims lived in each of the twelve cities he visited on this 2002 tour, we quickly arrive at 60 victims, a conservative estimate, which does not take into account those from out of town who traveled to his workshops. If we also factor in Pattabhi Jois's other world tours and other cities where he taught and consider his brazen assaults of multiple women daily in Mysore over the years, I believe that his victims number over 1,000.
>
> Aside from the times when Sharath adjusted me, Pattabhi Jois assaulted me daily in three different ways during practice in Mysore—that's three sexual assaults in one day to just one person. Even if Pattabhi Jois committed only three or four sexual assaults per day, six days per week, the number easily amounts to 1,000 sexual assaults in one year. Consider that Pattabhi Jois taught Westerners for over three decades and that reports of abuse and visual evidence date back to the early 1980s. We can then calculate a conservative estimate based on these figures and conclude that Pattabhi Jois likely committed over 30,000 sexual assaults.[29]

If this book feels at all long or overly analytical, it is in proportion to the magnitude of the tragedy—and still is reflective of only a small amount of the recovery and renewal it might take for it never to happen again.

SELF-CARE WHILE READING THIS BOOK

As you might guess from the transcript excerpt from T.M., and the preceding montage of victim stories, reading this book might be very challenging. Here I'll offer a few ideas about how to take care of yourself as you go.

Please bear in mind that I am not a psychologist, therapist, or counselor. I'm an independent researcher, with my share of biases and blind spots. As a yoga practitioner; a former teacher of active yoga classes; and a current instructor in yoga history, culture, and philosophy, I'm also invested in the long-term sustainability of yoga practice culture as it grapples with its shadows. My role in this book is that of an investigator and cultural critic. That's hard to square with my other job, in which I try to train aspiring teachers, with hope and cheer, in the yoga humanities. So the need for self-care in my case is heightened by the tension of having to keep my eyes wide open to not only the bad, but also the possible good.

No list of tips can address every need. The following come from sitting with interview subjects and ongoing conversations with friends and colleagues. They also come from my personal experience of having extracted myself from two high-demand groups.

1. Gather other resources. It might be difficult to read this book in isolation, or all in one go. Whatever or whoever you tend to rely on for support, make sure it or they are available if possible. Friends or family who can hold space for you without intrusion and can validate your feelings are golden.

2. Go slowly. When you open **Part Two**, you will enter the whirlwind of victim testimony. If you followed how the Jois story has unfolded on social media, you might have noticed the speed with which points and counterpoints were made, and how quickly discussions became highly charged and polarized. Nobody wins when speed reigns, least of all victims who in many cases have taken decades to prepare to speak.

Speed itself is often the medium of trauma, in the sense of "Before I knew what was happening, I was…." From a readerly perspective, speed may be a defense strategy that allows us to assess rather than digest, and fix rather than feel: *How bad is it? Well, can't we just get over it?* But this is not how victims are really heard. Luckily, printed books are not social media comment threads, and turning pages is not like scrolling. You can go as slowly as you want. You won't miss anything, and your nervous system will thank you for taking breaks.

3. Watch for being triggered. You might identify with a story or detail. It might unlock memories or reframe past events in startling ways. Anger, shame, and guilt are among the many possible emotions. Item #1 may help here, as well as #4. Defensiveness is also a clue. If you feel tight and armored while reading, there might be really good reasons for it. If you are a victim, you might be protecting yourself. If you've committed harm, you might be protecting yourself in a different way. Dissociation is another powerful clue. If you feel spacey, in a fog, or as if you are floating while engaging this material, it might be a sign to pause and turn to self-care.

Yoga scholar Theodora Wildcroft points out that the victim testimony in this book might be triggering to not only yoga practitioners who have suffered from abuse in yoga contexts, but also to those whose abuse stories come from outside the yoga world.[30] For this latter group, many of whom came to yoga to heal from abuse, this might be a particularly difficult book to navigate as they learn that a culture they trusted has betrayed others. There is no particular answer to this stress, beyond more and more time for self-care, reaching out for allies, and for the reader to try to remember in some way that no one and no story can really take away one's experience of having been empowered by a practice.

4. If you have been a practitioner of Ashtanga yoga (or belonged to a high-demand group) and this book brings up intense emotions that are difficult to understand or feel destabilizing, you might feel you need more help than items #1 and #2 give you. Friends and family will have limits in terms of how much they can hold and understand. Oddly, so can therapists. Many ex-members of various high-demand groups report meetings with therapists who couldn't really grasp their stories as being stories about structural power and abuse. If your therapist is unfamiliar with cultic dynamics, they may focus on your internal vulnerabilities as being essential to understanding why you found yourself in a toxic situation. This can actually delay recovery. The sources for this book contain practical resources that might help. Books and essays are often connected to communities of care where more appropriate personal therapy might be easier to find.

Cult survivor, theorist, and counselor Alexandra Stein says that there are two important types of support groups that ex-members of high-demand groups can benefit from.

1. If they can find other ex-members of the same group, they will often experience a deep sense of validation.

2. If they are able to communicate with the ex-members of other cultic groups, they are sometimes able to gradually grasp the underlying principles by which psychosocial control occurs in diverse circumstances.

Stein's advice expands upon the premise that because the high-demand group runs on insecure-to-disorganized relationships, part of the antidote involves finding a true safe haven of sober and secure relationships for reality-checking and relief. Some ex-members find this support by reconnecting with the family they were encouraged to avoid or even disown.[31]

One thing to avoid may be too much discussion with people who are still in the group that you're edging away from. This can get tangled up in what psychologist Jennifer Freyd calls "institutional betrayal".[32] Freyd shows how it can be retraumatizing for the victim of institutional abuse to reach out to or rely on current community members for support. In some cases, she explains, this can be like asking one's betrayer for care. In **Part Six**, we'll preview Freyd's initial findings on "institutional courage."

5. Expect changes in your practice. I've seen many people who encounter this material feel so disillusioned with Ashtanga yoga, or yoga in general, that they stop practicing. Some consider ending their teaching careers. But …

6. You may also find sources of continuity. Amidst the disillusionment, some people find themselves reconnecting to aspects of practice or community that were always nourishing to them, and remain so. Or, new communities of the disillusioned can form, and practice is re-enchanted for them, because they've found each other. Many report being able to excavate some core aspect of practice. They unearth it, brush off the dirt, and it's just as beautiful and vibrant as ever—perhaps more so, because it was fragile, and has been rescued.

7. History is not always destiny. In the darkest times of writing this book, I would turn my mind to the present-day lives of my interview subjects. All of them have recovered to some extent. The effects of their experience with Jois range from moderate (if it was brief and they were otherwise well-resourced) to severe and chronic. But even Karen Rain, whom Pattabhi Jois abused for years which left her with PTSD (post-traumatic stress disorder) symptoms almost 20 years later, has found a certain amount of relief. Her chronic pain from yoga injuries is gone, and her ability to relax and enjoy life has increased. I also reflect on the fact that those who stayed in the yoga world have been slowly and silently renovating it from the inside out. At the same time, I remain aware of how the power of redemptive narratives may not reflect the actual or eventual data. Many people love a resurrection story, perhaps because it's unlikely.

The selection bias built into the process of reporting these testimonies should be noted. Except for Karen's story, they come from women who for many reasons were both still active within yoga culture, and able and ready to speak out. I was able to find them through an emerging "network of empowerment" (p. 241). But there's no telling how many women had similar experiences with Jois (as noted by Cooke above) and who simply disappeared from the social network of yoga altogether. We don't know how they digested their experiences, and whether they have recovered enough to offer an uplifting public message. Their stories may be lost, and this should serve as a powerful reminder that efforts to protect yoga students from abuse are not just a cultural imperative but a public service offered to people whose names we may never know.

8. History is never over. This book will close by highlighting positive initiatives and offering workbook-style essay questions to explore new possibilities for improved ethics and critical thinking in communities. The problems presented in this book will never fully end, but incremental change through personal and public education is possible.

RECLAIMING "VICTIM": SOLIDARITY AND SPIRITUALITY

I'll be using the word *victim* in this book because of what I've learned from Karen Rain and other interviewees. Their use of the word to describe the state of having been assaulted by Jois aligns with a feminist politics that seeks to reclaim it from a common misunderstanding. "Victim," Rain argues, should be destigmatized, because it is first of all a legal term. A victim is someone against whom a crime has been committed.

"The culture wants to scare us into not using the word," Rain says. "But if we use it in a legal sense, and we are heard, the culture will have to address the crime."

The pop-psychology of our day, strongly amplified by the self-help industry, tends to ignore this legal definition. It typically presents "victimhood" as a disempowering *attitude* that no one who really wants to heal should adopt. To say that a person has a "victim mentality" has become a pious insult, disguised as care. The insult suggests that the after-effects of a crime are in the victim's perceptions only, and therefore theirs alone to repair. This is unjust and untrue. Using the legal sense of the word can be empowering, because it properly assigns responsibility to the crime. It clearly shows that the difference between criminal and victim is a difference in power and actions, and not attitudes and perceptions.

If you listen closely, the physical and material weight carried by the word *victim* can also allude to how a crime can be hardwired into the nervous system of the person against whom it was committed. Crime is traumatizing, and trauma is not a "mentality". It is a fact that calls out for collective repair, through listening, learning, nurturing, and structural change. Telling a victim that they have a "victim mentality" perpetuates the effects of the crime.

A SPIRITUALITY OF LISTENING

Speaking with Rain and others, and listening to feminist activism, shows that when we focus on and amplify the voices of victims, three things become possible.

1. As each individual story rings out, it carves space for the wound of collective silence to begin to be healed.

2. As previously silenced voices expand into that space, the voices that have insisted that everything is orderly, reasonable, and alright—voices that are often misogynistic, presumptuous, and victim-blaming—retreat, reluctantly, to the margins.

3. As victims' voices combine into a chorus, they validate each other in harmony and survivorship. Entire structures of denial begin to vibrate, and crumble.

These three levels of revelation illuminate and evolve a core teaching found in many South Asian wisdom traditions. Almost every form of yoga and Buddhism contains a core premise: that we cannot understand who we are nor begin to find peace until we listen to the voices of suffering within ourselves, in others, and in the world. Listening is not a posture of pity or charity. It doesn't silence with premature solutions. It begins by offering presence and solidarity.

Entering any yogic path seems to demand that we acknowledge and own vulnerability and pain. With luck, and the right tools, we can then examine the ways in which we defend against and repress it: through dissociation, reactivity, othering, and aggression. We can listen to the voice that is hurting, find out how and why it has been marginalized, and ask what it needs.

Maturity seems to be marked by a growing awareness that our experience and even identity is inseparable from our suffering, and the suffering of others. We come to know that we are interdependent. We feel how we are bound by internal and external hierarchies of ignorance and injustice, which, seen more clearly, and worked with patiently, over a long time, might transform into networks of knowledge and care.

The second yogic project that this book seeks to further is the examination and deconstruction of social conditioning. Practitioners of diverse eras have always sought to peer beneath what the power structures of the world have told them they are, to see if they can catch a glimpse of what they *could* be. The voices in this book are cradled within a larger story of modern yoga that follows this old tradition in a new way. It is being told by a practice population that is 80% female. This statistic alone turns the average yoga community into a site in which the meanings of gender and power are implicitly explored, and their limitations challenged. Today, the answer on the back of the t-shirt that asks the question "What Would Patanjali Do?" is "Study feminism."

By centering the voices of victims, and setting them against the wider backdrop of social change that has allowed them to be heard, this book will hopefully stand not only as a contribution to justice and safety in the yoga world, but also as a work of inquiry, hope, and healing that stretches beyond that community.

A LISTENING KEY

Neither the aspiration nor the meaning of listening came naturally to me. I'm indebted to women like Anneke Lucas, whom I began interviewing in 2016. At one point, I asked her why she thought that virtually no one had listened to her story about Jois at first. She talked about the shaming and silencing of rape culture, and the high stakes involved when a community realizes that its spiritual marketing might be disguising abuse. Then she took it to another level.

"We only really listen to trauma survivors," she said, "to the extent we recognize that we ourselves have been traumatized."

That sentence sank in deep. It wrapped itself around another idea I'd been trying to metabolize. bell hooks writes extensively about how people of all genders suffer under patriarchy. She shows how systems of dominance and control dehumanize victims, enablers, and aggressors alike in a feedback loop of vulnerable bodies and hardened hearts.[33]

I returned to this braid of wisdom almost daily over the years since reading it, like a compass. It helped me to see where social activism and self-inquiry meet, where the personal intersects with the structural, where psychology intersects with privilege. It helped me to see that the unraveling of social mechanisms of abuse depends upon examining complicity and responsibility. For me, this began with owning the fact that for the whole year I resisted writing this book, I was complicit in silencing the women to whom it is dedicated.

PART ONE

Learning to Listen

I first became aware of the abuse pretty soon after I met Jois in 2001, so maybe like six months after that because I was, when I was in Singapore I was doing research on him because I wanted to know more about the practice and I did come across some images and movies on the internet. And I heard people kind of making some, some really quiet comments about his "Roman hands" and his "Russian fingers". Um, and I mean I got to admit: my first response was 'I don't believe that.' Um, I thought the photos were doctored, you know, especially the one that I would see of Pattabhi Jois giving that mulabandha assist in Pindasana.... And I guess I guess I just didn't want to believe it. You know, I really didn't. And it also felt distant to me and I, and then like over the course of those years until Mary Taylor's blog came out, like I did come to believe it, you know, but, but it did feel like it wasn't close to me because it wasn't my experience and I just thought, 'Well, I don't know what that is.' Um, and I had had nothing but great respectful relationships with all my teachers and my love of the practice was undaunted, I have to say. So yeah, I know that what I just said is not going to be a popular thing to hear, but you know, that that is the truth of when I first heard about it.

—Genny Wilkson Priest, authorized Ashtanga teacher, in an interview[34]

But you know it's all true.

—Diane Bruni, personal conversation, 5/29/2014

THAT TIME I SILENCED MY FRIEND

This book started when Diane Bruni didn't keep quiet, and follow my plan. Some alchemy of age, dignity, outrage, and fatigue provoked her to finally speak out.

Diane had never studied directly with Pattabhi Jois, but she'd wound up teaching one of Toronto's first regular classes in his Ashtanga method in the late 1990s. She first studied it by practicing along to a 1993 video in which Karen Rain was a lead demonstrator.[35]

I first walked into Diane's now-famous studio in around 2003. I had seen her name outside, on a rain-soaked poster, next to a time slot for "Ashtanga Level 2". I unrolled a borrowed mat in a packed and muggy room.

Diane started counting. It was hypnotic. Two hours vanished in a blur of humidity and intensity. Pain broke open my initial shyness, and then, strangely, turned into ecstasy. As I've worked with the stories of abuse in the Ashtanga community, I've tried to remember this peak experience, to feel it echo through my tissues, to cherish what it told me about my body, its fears and possibilities. Thousands of practitioners who have found love and freedom through Ashtanga yoga have felt this. For some, that value was so rich, and so wrapped up in their love for Jois, that it became very difficult for them to acknowledge that he threw a shadow as long as the stretches were deep.

Quivering in a pool of bliss-shocked sweat in the dressing room afterwards, I turned to a guy covered in mantra tattoos. "So is this Ashtanga yoga?" I asked.

Tattoo Man snapped out his damp towel, folded it neatly, and smiled.

"Well…. It's also Diane," he said.

"Do you come every day?"

"Yeah." He grinned. "We're all addicts here."

Diane gave me my first lecturing job in the yoga world, hiring me to present seminars to her training programs. Over time, I would meet dozens of her students. Many were young and between jobs, or wondering whether to go to grad school, or return to grad school. Acting, waiting on tables, playing music, dancing. Many persisted in practice despite injuries and creeping pain. They practiced as though sacrificing themselves to the postures would buy them easier passage through life transitions and a tanking jobs market. Their balancing postures predicted the term "precariat".

Years passed, jobs changed, and I lost touch with Diane. I heard through the grapevine that she'd had a yoga-related hip injury, and then a battle with breast cancer. Then word came that she was coming out as some kind of yoga rebel. After a successful career as one of Toronto's leading teachers and the co-founder of the one of the country's best-known studios, she'd split off from her business partner and opened a neighborhood studio in her home. She'd stopped teaching Jois's method. Her home studio now offered a 1970s-feeling array of funky classes: Bed of Balls Restorative Therapy, pay-what-you-can Self-Healing Relaxation, Shaolin Exercise, Tai Chi, Movement Meditation, Contact Improv, Axis Syllabus. She'd named the place after its address: 80 Gladstone. This seemed to suggest that yoga for her was no longer about postures or techniques or devotions, but rather about the place you find yourself in.

"CAN WE USE THE WORD 'CULT' HERE?"

In January 2014, I put out a call on social media inviting people to contact me with stories of injuries they'd suffered while practicing yoga. By this point, I'd been practicing and teaching for over 10 years, and I was increasingly disturbed by reports from friends and colleagues about how the practice they had turned to for physical therapy and spiritual well-being had left them injured or in chronic pain. I was in chronic pain myself from hamstring tears and spinal stress. My idea at the time was to collect as many stories as I could, and look for common themes. When Diane came across a few of the blogs I had published emerging from my call-out, she got in touch and said she wanted to tell her story.

I interviewed her in the lobby of 80 Gladstone. It was powerful to see her again. She'd kept her hair short after her cancer went into remission. She was more muscular than I remembered. And more relaxed, but this had the aura of someone who'd come home from a war. Her studio was visible from the lobby through big sliding doors. Sunlight poured through the full-length windows and over a well-loved grand piano at the far end.

Our wide-ranging interview touched on how the intense sensations of yoga practice could be addictive to many people, how they could provoke a pain–pleasure feedback loop, how the focus on extreme stretching to the exclusion of strength and stability was causing a lot of repetitive stress injuries, and how at the highest level of training and teaching, people were being taught to tolerate and even spiritualize the pain of the postures.

"The postures were painful," she said. "We all knew it. We became experts in surrendering to pain."

One day, Diane's hip joint imploded while she entered a simple forward folding posture. Her mentors, who numbered among Jois's top students, had no advice or care to offer her. Some offered a "traditional" idea: that her injuries were signs of spiritual growth. But her sports medicine doctor related the injury to the incessant hip-stretching demanded by the Ashtanga postures. When Diane brought this news to her colleagues and suggested that they reconsider the technique they were teaching to hundreds of students, they weren't interested.

"Can we use the word 'cult' here?" Diane looked at my phone on the coffee table, recording. "Can we use that word?"

A few months after that first interview, Diane invited me to present initial findings from my early research at a community event at 80 Gladstone. I suggested that she speak first about her injury experience and the questions it raised about practice for her and maybe others. Then we'd have a sports medicine doctor give stats on clients who had come to his clinic with yoga-related injuries. I'd conclude by talking about some of the psycho-social contexts for injury that were starting to emerge from my interviews. I'd talk about metaphysical attitudes towards the body and pain, how physical flexibility in yoga was correlated with spiritual advancement (which I'd started to call the "openness bias"), how pain and pleasure seem to be so easily confused, and how strange power dynamics between teachers and students could lead into dangerous territory. We'd film it properly and publish it, to get a broader conversation going about safety and embodied kindness.

Diane didn't stick to my plan. When it came time for her to speak, she skipped over the story of her hip altogether—what was meant to be the centerpiece of the evening. She began in a much darker place. In a room packed with 60 Toronto yoga people, many of whom were her current or former students, she told the story about Pattabhi Jois she'd kept hidden for almost 20 years.

A BURIED TRAUMA

In 1996, Diane traveled with her yoga business partner to study Ashtanga yoga privately with one of Jois's most senior American students. This teacher was living in semi-seclusion.

They arrived at the teacher's house at the appointed time. He greeted them, and brought them to his practice space. He started leading them through the first Ashtanga sequence. But after a few sun salutations, he stopped abruptly and asked them to sit down. He said he needed to confess something before they went on.

The teacher told them that he'd split away from Jois for many reasons. He'd seen too many people injured by Jois. Also, he could no longer tolerate Jois's treatment of his women students, which he had witnessed since the

1970s. He said that Jois constantly touched women in a sexual manner while adjusting them in postures. He would squeeze and fondle the women's breasts, press his pelvis into their buttocks, and rub his hand over their vaginas. The teacher said all of this was common knowledge throughout the community, but few spoke openly about it, and no one had confronted Jois directly about it. He himself had remained silent about it, for years.

Diane described her shock. "I just lay down on the floor and started crying," she said.

> I didn't know what to do. I wanted to turn around and fly thousands of miles home. How could I participate in a culture that allowed its main teacher to abuse women? How could I encourage my students, who were mostly young women, to practice and explore their bodies according to this man's directions? From that moment on, I faced the task of disentangling myself from the method to which I'd given my whole life.

I gripped the edges of my meditation cushion while Diane spoke. This was not how I had wanted this event to go down. I felt scared, embarrassed, hypervigilant.

It wasn't that the story was news to me. The year before, another colleague had sent me a now-famous video montage of Jois mauling women and some men in ostensible "adjustments". I'd watched it with fascinated horror.[36] But between the graininess of the video, the anonymity of the uploader, and the fact that none of the students' faces were visible, it felt somehow distant. I understand now that when I first watched it, I went into a dissociative state. I couldn't feel into what I was seeing.

There was something overwhelming about that video, and what it implied. Jois wasn't some cartoonish mobster, like the hot yoga huckster Bikram Choudhury. He was a jovial, workaday, yoga-gym-teacher-grandpa-priest who stood firmly in the respectable mainstream of a now-global industry. His postures, the breath-driven rhythm of the movements between them, and his general attitude towards physical touch had influenced thousands of students directly, and millions were practicing derivatives of his method under the tags of "flow", "vinyasa flow", and "power".

Entertaining the possibility that Jois was a blatant and constant sexual predator felt like a dangerous idea. As Diane told the story, it seemed that an entire culture was trembling. Was it true? How long had it gone on for? Was it really that public? How many people knew? How much money had people made by keeping it a secret? How many of Jois's students had devoted themselves to him, deceived about what he was actually up to?

These questions battled upstream against a current of idealization. I thought of how Jois's smiling portrait graced the personal altars of thousands of middle-class, educated students around the world—the majority of them women. Many viewed his yoga as a means of self-empowerment. Some had even edited books about how Jois's teaching was *specifically liberating for women*—even great for pregnancy and post-partum.[37] This was despite the fact that one of his earliest non-Indian women students in the 1980s recalled being the first pregnant woman he had ever taught. He was so inept he manhandled her into a twist during her fifth month and broke her rib.[38] She still spoke of him in adoring terms. A true devotee can turn every story of harm or even cruelty into a necessary spiritual challenge.

So many people loved Jois. They still do. I was afraid they would be outraged by Diane's story. They might attack her, and me.

QUARANTINING THE TRAUMA STORY

Theodora Wildcroft is a queer yoga teacher and scholar, a trauma survivor and social justice advocate who lives in the United Kingdom. She explains that the stories of abuse and trauma are often felt to be contagious. Intuitively, we know that if we really listen to them, we might succumb to a kind of sickness marked by feelings of doubt, shame, and guilt. We know we'll have to start asking questions about how the big picture is organized. We'll have to bear out the possibility that everything we value is infected by everything we fear. So what we do to trauma survivors—even, sometimes, if we are survivors ourselves—is that we shut those voices down and quarantine them in an attempt to keep ourselves sterile and safe.

That's exactly what I did to Diane. After the event, I approached her calmly, the "rational" one. I started to mansplain. I told her I was concerned that releasing the video of her story about the story about Jois felt unwise. It was second-hand information, I noted, and impossible to corroborate. She hadn't disclosed the source of the story. There might be libel issues involved. We didn't want the uproar to distract people from the more pressing and definable issue of yoga injuries, did we? Did we really need an unsubstantiated rumor to damage her credibility, or my own, by association? I explained that neither of us were investigative journalists, qualified to responsibly report on the allegations. It should be left to others. I said that her story belonged to its own category of research. It wasn't a story about yoga so much as about the cultic abuse that could occur in any subculture. I didn't want outright smut diverting attention from our cleaner, clearer work.

"But you know it's all true," she said. "You've seen that video [the montage referred to above]." She glared at me but her eyes looked tired.

I held my ground. I told her I didn't doubt that the video was true. But—surely she could see there were problems with presenting it as factual. Who were the women? How do we know what they felt? How would we get in touch with them to ask? Did the uploader violate their privacy? Were there copyright issues? What would it mean if the women objected to the labeling of their experience as sexual abuse?

Wielding all of my excellent reasons, not to mention my ignorance of sexual assault, I lawyered Diane into editing her story out of the video we had planned to release. With my seemingly respectable rape-culture argument, I became party to a decades-long cover-up.

But as the views on her butchered video approached 10,000, what I'd done began to dawn on me. I felt sick. It was important enough to her that she started her talk with that story. Who was I to clip it out? Why was I worried about my own skin? For Diane, the sexual violence of her former lineage master was more important than the physical violence of the postures, and the emotional violence of mentors who had encouraged her to cope with her pain. These things were all related, and Diane had been clear about her priorities.

PATTERNS OF SILENCE

A few months after the talk, I confirmed Diane's story with the teacher she had heard it from. He declined to go on record at that point and at every turn as I continued to reach out to him over two years to confirm stories of Jois's behavior, which he did. I started to call him Ashtanga Deep Throat in my notes. His desire to speak seemed as strong as his desire to remain anonymous.

Conversations with other senior Jois students who admitted to seeing what he has was up to—many claimed they didn't—yielded dozens of excuses. They generally fell into the two categories of: "It wasn't really like that", or "He didn't really mean it that way." The first denies women's experience. The second bypasses that experience to continue to focus on the teacher, as if his inner life were more important than how he treated people.

Both categories enhance the silencing effect of spiritual mystification.

Like God, the teacher moves in mysterious ways. He cannot be understood. He's never doing what you think he's doing. There's always a bigger story going on, and you're not enlightened enough to see it. But if you mind your own business, and focus on your own practice, all will become clear. *Practice, and all is coming.*

After many interviews with Jois's dedicated students, I began to wonder whether the incredible focus for which they are known, their dedication, their ability to tolerate pain—all of the values still held by many younger Jois enthusiasts today—were tangled up with what they had to do to manage this shame, consciously or not. I wondered whether their ardor held back the dark of a shared secret. I was reminded of those Catholics I grew up with who became ever more devout with every revelation of systemic abuse in the Church. For them, real disillusionment would mean losing community, ritual, and even a sense of self. Perhaps it is natural to work harder to make it all okay. As if on some level, their own prayers and dutifulness and volunteer service could atone for the priests they needed to keep elevating for their world to remain in order.

In one of my last interviews with Karen Rain, I saw that the repressions of the culture's work ethic might be a veneer on top of something far more chilling. When I asked her how she thought she'd been able to perform such extraordinary postures under the stress of Jois assaulting her daily, her answer was unequivocal.

"I think it was the stress that helped me accomplish all that," Karen said. "My body was so charged with adrenaline and cortisol, it was like I could lift up a car. I was able to perform at a certain level because of the fear I felt."

As for the men who studied with Jois, I began to wonder whether their rationalizations were blended with the silent fatalism of misogyny. This is the never-spoken feeling—inherited from fathers, uncles, older brothers, and older boys—that it is natural for a man to objectify and dominate women's bodies. That, given half the chance and a whiff of consent, why wouldn't Jois take advantage of young women presenting their bodies to him for healing and transformation? It's the way of the world, an innocent sin, a biological imperative. What really needs to be said about it?

Nothing needs to be said, so long as you don't look those women in the eyes. Part of my argument to Diane about editing her story had been that none of the women had come forward. Who were they, anyway? How would we find them? Why hadn't they spoken out? I remember Diane staring at me as if across a chasm. Of course she knew why they weren't speaking out. In that very moment, I was demonstrating what happens when women begin to speak. And of course she knew how to find them. What was obvious to her from years spent in her whisper network was entirely abstract to me.

All I really had to do was start Googling. Once I did, my seemingly rational but misogynistic defenses against the stories themselves—against the work it took to listen to them and center those who tell them—began to erode.

RECOGNITION AND DENIAL, OUTSIDE AND INSIDE

The way in which the infamous video of Jois adjusting his students was anonymously produced, shared virally, suppressed, reposted, and viciously debated represents in a microcosm the battle between recognition and denial that so many of his victims had to fight as they found their voice. On one hand, the video exposed what many objective observers—yet outsiders to the highly committed Ashtanga world—would immediately name as assault and abuse. But for insiders, who perhaps felt the need to protect their devotion to Jois and his method, the video was a testimony to their teacher's intimate, inscrutable power. Their response carried the weight of love and idealization, as well as the spiritual premise that things in this world are not really what they seem, and that the genius of a yoga master can never be reduced to video. The seeming facts communicated by the images could not, they argued, be telling the full story. Their argument was strong enough to do two things: (1) augment the already-daunting barriers to victims reporting, and (2) transfer over into real-life interactions, so that when victims like Karen Rain were finally able to name their experiences clearly, they were met with doubt or outright disbelief.

The montage was put together by an anonymous YouTube user. Between 2013 and 2015, an unknown number of complainants had it deleted from YouTube at least twice and from Vimeo once. Certified Ashtanga teacher Eddie Stern wrote by email that he submitted one of the complaints, citing "inappropriate content". As of this writing, it is now visible on the *Decolonizing Yoga* website.[*39]

* The power of amateur/activist journalism showing up on independent websites—which is where this project started—cannot be overstated. *Decolonizing Yoga,* run by trans and anti-cult activist Be Scofield, not only protected the video from deletion, but also published key articles by Karen Rain and Jubilee Cooke that went viral and ultimately accelerated the process of disillusionment and reform. Forums like *Decolonizing Yoga* are taking on issues that no mainstream yoga publications seem willing to grapple with.

JOIS "ADJUSTMENTS" VIDEO: A DESCRIPTION

The video opens with a brief glimpse of Pattabhi Jois sitting in his conference room in the original Ashtanga Yoga Research Institute in Lakshmipuram, Mysore. He's lecturing on yoga. The quality is grainy and overexposed. He appears to be in his late 60s. After a moment, the shot fades to the small yoga practice room downstairs. Jois presses his crotch into the upraised buttocks of a woman in *Karnapidasana*. The pose is a shoulder stand with the legs hinged downward into a tightened plow position. It's like she's paused halfway through a backwards somersault. Her shins are flat on the floor and her inner knees are pressing into the sides of her head, covering her ears.

With his groin planted on top of her buttocks, he leans his full body weight onto her. He maintains his balance by reaching down to pin her ankles to the floor, as if he were in a pushup position. The back of the woman's neck, which appears flexed beyond 90 degrees, is carrying the weight of her trunk, plus the full weight of Jois's frame. When he disengages from the adjustment, the woman's spine springs upward with the release of downward compression.

"Without mind control," Jois says in the voiceover from the conference room, "sense organs will not come in your control.

"*Yoga chitta vritti nirodha.* Chitta is mind. Mind, you take control. Then sense organs you automatically control."

Jois is quoting the opening of the *Yoga Sutra*. He quoted it constantly. Why he quoted it, however, is a matter of confusion. The 2000-year-old scripture has little if anything to do with the rigors of the poses his devotees spent years struggling to perfect. The old book is about achieving mind-stoppage through deep meditation. Jois and his Indian contemporaries wrestled this text into a shape that would serve the modern yoga agenda with as much muscle as he wrestled his students into postures.

Jois's signature application of that agenda was to get his students to stop thinking. The students felt this viscerally: the intense sensations of the postures and adjustments could arrest all thoughts, in moments that were remembered as transcendent. When speaking of working through the "good pain" administered at the hands of Jois, Nancy Gilgoff, one of Jois's first women American students, told an interviewer: "*There's a moment when the mind is not present and he will take you through that time.*"[40]

The video cuts to the teacher applying adjustments to two women in *Yoga Nidrasana* (*see* Figure 2, p. 47). The practitioners are on their backs with both legs lifted up so that their legs are pinned behind their shoulders, and their feet crossed behind their heads. Jois lays on each of them in turn, pubis

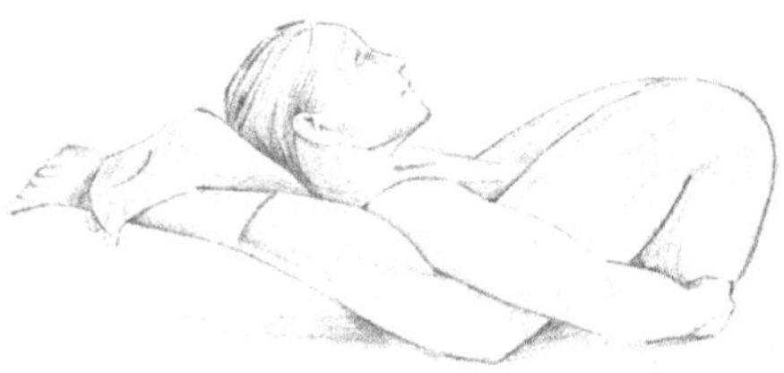

Figure 2: Yoga Nidrasana

to pubis, as if in missionary position, pinning them down while reaching up to wrench their ankles into a deeper cross-pattern behind their heads. With each press of his body weight, you can see the students' skeletons squeezed into ever more extreme compressions, with terrible pressure exerted upon their rounded spines. They are compliant in bound forms from which they cannot escape.

Then come several clips in which he is pulling the hips and buttocks of female students into his groin from behind while they're in downward dog (*Adho Mukha Svanasana*: (*see* Figure 3, below), ostensibly to help with spine-lengthening. Next he is quite obviously humping women while they're bent over in the crab-walk version of *Tittibhasana*—an extremely deep forward fold in which the practitioner's torso has actually passed through their thighs.

There are no clear shots of the student's facial responses until about

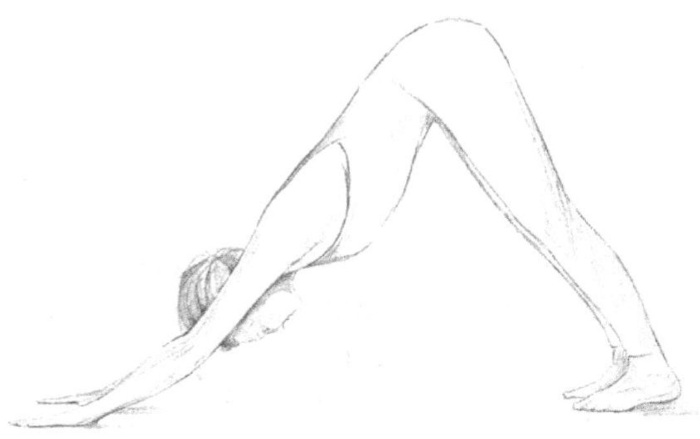

Figure 3: Adho Mukha Svanasana:

two-thirds of the way through. Then we see a lanky man in his thirties in *Upavistha Konasana*—a seated posture with straightened legs spread wide. I resonate with his body-type, which makes what follows especially painful for me to watch. As he reaches forward to wrap his fingers around his toes, he compensates for his rigid lower back by more deeply rounding his long upper back. Even with this curling forward, his forehead looks to be more than 18 inches from the floor. Jois approaches him from behind, places both hands firmly on his shoulder-blades, steps his right foot onto the student's upper right thigh (the student pushes Jois's foot slightly back from the knee), then stands his full body weight up and leans forward, pressing his left knee into the student's middle back and then on the outside left of the student towards their left thigh. Jois then moves his left hand to the back of the student's neck and leans his body weight over even further, his left knee again on the student's back, to push the man's head down. Jois is counting out the breaths. The man's spine curls forward slowly with the tension of a steel ruler until his forehead touches the floor. Jois repeats the numbers 6 and 7, and then looks up, beaming a grin to the rest of the room. It's unclear whether he extended the count as a joke or because he was distracted by the effort of wrestling the student into position. Eventually he releases the student, who springs back up with a look of giddy elation and relief.

The video ends with Jois leaning his bodyweight onto two men, one after another, as they lie back with one leg wrapped behind the shoulder and the other extended. One of the men is Chuck Miller, who also appeared in the 1993 video with Karen Rain. Jois seems clumsy and off-balance. Also bored, as if he were wrestling meat in a packing plant. At the end of the montage, the editor slows the film down so you can almost hear the ligaments groan. There's an overlay of brisk Carnatic music. The cascading tabla rhythms seem to say, sardonically, "And on it goes."

REACTIONS TO THE VIDEO

For years, the video was both a social media flashpoint for pent-up suspicions about Jois, and a litmus test for the faith of true believers. Whenever it was posted, opinion was sharply divided, and tempers ran high.

Debate usually opened with visceral disgust. Detractors called out the depicted contact as assault. This was followed closely by equally passionate rebuttals from those who were disgusted at the disgust, calling out the "projections" of the first group, who, they claimed, were obviously watching the images through a corrupted "Western" lens of sex obsession.

The high road to defending the video was to profess a benign ignorance, or offer the benefit of the doubt.

The relationship between teacher and student is sacred in India, high-roaders would say. *We simply can't know what's going on in this video. These are, after all, advanced practitioners.*

Jois assaulted some of the subjects in this book—like Maya Hammer—on their first day in his presence. So the "advanced practitioner" argument is incorrect. But what's more important to note here is the rationale that if the students were in the room, they must have been fully consenting to whatever happened, and benefiting from the intimate and personal attention.

Speaking with senior students gave some insight into where this attitude might be coming from. One of them described being in her fifties and attending an intensive led by Jois in Encinitas in the early 2000s. (She did not recall the exact year, but it might have been the event at which Jois assaulted Michelle Bouvier.) She had studied with him in Mysore for years, and was deeply embedded as a teacher in her local Ashtanga community. She rolled out her mat beside a woman in her twenties. When Jois circled the room before class to receive the welcome of each student, the younger woman said directly to him:

"Guruji, I am injured and would prefer not to be touched today."

Reportedly, he nodded, and moved on.

The older student was outraged.

"Who did she think she was?" she wondered. "You enter the guru's class, and he's in charge. You don't get to say that he's not going to touch you."

Another faction of defenders acknowledged that Jois may have been sexually intrusive, but that it was all for the women's benefit. Some went further, and said that he was helping them heal from sexual trauma. Ashtanga Deep Throat took it further still, saying outright that Jois and his female students were engaging in consensual exhibitionist sexual activity, that the women wanted and benefited from it, and some described having the best orgasms of their lives when he touched them. Because they kept coming back for more, it was obvious, to this source anyway, that it was consensual.

These responses share several features. First, they display profound ignorance of how power differentials, internalized misogyny, and trauma responses that range from freezing to tend-and-befriend make consent in such situations highly problematic, if not impossible. The second thing they share is a complete unwillingness to actually seek out the women and listen to what they have to say. Basic ignorance of rape culture plus a lack of human contact with actual victims intersects with other rationalizations to create an efficient and adaptable barrier to reporting.

Third, speculative tangents that focus on what Jois *intended* when he groped or digitally penetrated his student ride on an all-too-common misunderstanding of sexual assault. Sexual assault is not defined by the assaulter's *intentions*, nor even by the *interpretation* of the victim. This latter point is crucial for protecting children, or those who live in such sexually violent environments, or who have been so deeply influenced by rape culture and misogyny that they may not be able to articulate that they've been sexually assaulted. Sexual assault is defined by *what actually occurs between two people*: non-consensual sexual contact with or penetration of a victim's body. Many experts emphasize that the power differential between the two people is a key factor in assault.

Some people on social media continue to equivocate about what they're seeing in that video, framing it as consensual and harmless. They may be trying to resolve cognitive dissonance by denying what they see. For the dedicated disciple, Jois literally *cannot* be doing what he appears to be doing. If he is, the entire culture is thrown into question.

It is tragic that what the member of the high-demand group must do in order to maintain the integrity of the group's narrative (i.e., "Jois was a spiritual master") harmonizes, toxically, with what abuse victims are encouraged by the group to do to suppress their truth. ("It wasn't really like that." "He was giving you blessings and attention.") The suppression might feel welcome for a while, if it seems to protect the victim's dignity from the terrible knowledge that they have been abused. One part of the abuse victim may be acutely aware of what has happened. It's as obvious as video evidence. But another part, conditioned by dissociation, shame, and group pressure, may begin to deny, suppress, or minimize it.

The public denial of what that YouTube video clearly shows is a powerful example of rape culture and gaslighting en masse. But it also reveals the high-demand group members' inner split. They are forced to say that they don't see what they see.

The difference between a high-demand group member who defends the teacher and organization and the ex-member coming to terms with an abuse memory is that the latter has felt, started to address—and perhaps heal—this internal split. If they eventually become a whistleblower, they will become a traitor to the group, but a truth-teller to the outside world.

The ex-member's clarity in relation to their experience threatens the group narrative. Both the group and the individual are coping with internal splitting. But the group, stronger in numbers and social capital, further abuses the individual by ramping up the very splitting that the individual has started to heal.

For some group members, the blatancy of the video evidence seems to *increase* the drive to rationalize it as harmless. The more they see what's happening, the harder they have to work to reframe it. In the most severe cases, this leads to statements that sound internally split to the point of schizophrenia.

One source who wished to remain anonymous described a conversation he had with his teacher, who was certified by Jois. He had advanced to the point at which she asked to interview him about a possible job at her studio. The student was not a Jois disciple, but was aware of the rumors surrounding his behavior, as he had spent years in Mysore himself, studying at a different school.* His potential boss asked him: "How would you describe your personal attitude towards Pattabhi Jois?"

The prospective hire had heard all the stories. He didn't mince words.

"I have two problems with Pattabhi Jois," he reports telling her. "One is the trail of physical trauma he has left behind him through injurious adjustments. The other is the trail of sexual trauma he has left behind through assaulting women."

The boss turned stone cold.

"That didn't happen," she said, referring to the sexual assaults. "But when it did, he was doing it on purpose."

DENIAL AND RECOGNITION: MICROMOMENTS

That didn't happen. But when it did, he was doing it on purpose.

These two sentences together make the opposite of sense. There may be a reason for this. The speaker may be describing a nonsensical condition.

Alexandra Stein has pioneered a tool called the "Group Attachment Interview" to assess how people remember and recover from their experiences within high-demand groups. As she used the tool to compile data, she began to notice contradictions, logic lapses, and non sequiturs in the transcripts of her interviews with ex-members.

She theorizes that these verbal/cognitive knots indicate a

* That of BNS Iyengar (1927–), also a student of Krishnamacharya, and not to be confused with B.K.S. Iyengar. BNS also teaches a method reminiscent of his childhood physical education studies. Like Jois, he calls it "Ashtanga", but his influence beyond Mysore is limited.

failure—sometimes traumatic—to process the pressures and contradictions of the group. As the person begins to approach the wound in their narrative, they might trail off, fall silent, or stammer. They'll struggle to remember dates and places. They'll forget the question, change the subject, become disoriented, or use odd euphemisms to describe the abuse. These can be signs that the subject is implicitly aware of the harm to which they have been exposed, or in which they have been complicit (or both). They have split themselves internally in order to keep that truth safe from conscious contemplation. The echo of that split is registered in the instability of their speech.[41]

Many interviewees described a protracted battle between the internal forces of recognition and denial that contributed to confusion in the midst of their experiences with Jois, and then later, to their difficulties in disclosing. The battle took many forms, large and small.

Tracy Hodgeman described pushing down the thought that Jois's hands were intrusive.

"My brain was confused by the way he adjusted us," she said. "Hand to pelvic bone/floor, groin to groin, face to groin. But my heart was not. It's difficult to explain."

T.M. could feel that something was wrong, but she was vulnerable to the group reasoning that it *couldn't* be wrong. She describes eight months of internal conflict between knowing she was being assaulted and telling herself what she had been taught to think: that Jois was healing her.

Marisa Sullivan went from recognition to denial and back again. She watched the assaults unfold over two months before she overrode her hypervigilance and let down her defenses.

Nicola Tiburzi describes recognition winning out over denial as she processed being digitally raped in real time.

"I remember being in downward facing dog (*Adho Mukha Svanasana; see* Figure 3, p. 47) and seeing his feet behind me," she said.

> ...and then having his hand come right into my groin and almost a feeling he's gonna lift me up a bit. Quite a strong touch. It wasn't a light brush. It was like, "Oh! Okay." And it was a confident touch.
>
> I'm a very intuitive person and I haven't had any big trauma that way, I just knew in my body it was not a healthy feeling. But, even though it wasn't a good feeling, it wasn't healthy, it also wasn't making sure the tone of my pelvic floor was in good

> standing for the sake of my spine or anything.... I just knew that it wasn't right. I did some self-reflection, like "was there a need, was my pelvic floor really misaligned?" But, I just felt like, "Oh, I need to get out of here," it just didn't feel right at all.

For Karen Rain, being able to name that she had been sexually abused by Pattabhi Jois took years in therapy. Crossing the bridge from denial to recognition in a public setting, however, took an even longer time. In 1995, she was nowhere close to making that step.

That was the year that journalist Larry Gallagher attended class at Jois's Mysore shala for a month. He was there to work on a yoga-travelogue feature that eventually ran in the September issue of *Details* that same year. The resulting piece is breezy and sharp. There's skepticism, but no real hint that anything is amiss. In the following passage, he even quotes Karen.

> "Ashtanga is a lot like slam dancing," she says, "only slam dancing isn't as painful." But she found the discomfort of tweaked hamstrings and a strained back preferable to the general psychological angst that no amount of talk therapy seemed to quell.... Daily handstands have left Karen with triceps that any Detroit Red Wing would kill for, and she's got a callus on her chin from scraping it on the mat while executing wicked, scorpionlike maneuvers.
>
> "Yoga is transformative," she says. "I've watched people change in ways I've never seen before: their energy, their attitudes, their voice, even. As a matter of fact, I haven't seen anybody come here, stay for four months, and *not* be changed." She winces at the conspicuously unpunk overtones of what she feels compelled to add: "I believe there's magic in it."[42]

"I gave him a bunch of brainwashed answers," Karen said. "He even asked me about the adjustments. He knew something was wrong. I deflected. I told him they were healing."

"It was in the air," Gallagher confirmed when asked about whether he knew about the assaults. "Pretty much anyone who was there for any length of time knew about it."

Gallagher's Australian girlfriend at the time was one of Jois's targets. She told him to stop, and he moved on to other women.

"He knew what he was doing. It was irritating and galling to see it."

The couple tried to minimize the assaults with humor. They called Jois "Uncle Wiggly".

When asked why he hadn't written about what had been so obvious, Gallagher explained that it wasn't what he'd been contracted for. He also said that he'd made friends with Eddie Stern over the course of their interviews, and it would have been uncomfortable to bring it up.

"Here's my statement of complicity," says Gallagher. "I made a choice to not include that stuff, because it was a can of worms. I hadn't been sent on an assignment to out a sexual predator."

PRE-EMPTING DENIAL, NURTURING RECOGNITION

The first step of the **PRISM** model is to "**P**ause to reflect on the idea that each yoga/spiritual method and community carries both value, but also, potentially, a history of abuse." Any Google search of "yoga scandal" or "yoga abuse" will instantly validate the pragmatism of this advice. The deeper truth that Google won't reveal—at least not instantly, because Google is an advertising platform as much as a search engine—is that *the reported value of a given yoga or spiritual community can easily be used to cover over its abuse problems.*

The benefits of Jois's Ashtanga yoga are lauded in countless books, blogs, podcasts, and videos. The method has been said to cure all manner of diseases, from the physical to the spiritual. Such idealization is a red flag. If anyone speaks of their teacher, method, or community in all-good terms, it's an invitation to look a little deeper. People and systems are complex, and there's generally a painful distance between how we want things to be, and how they actually are. That distance is even more painful for those who assumed the yoga or spirituality community they found would provide an antidote to their trauma load.

All-good stories are often not just the products of sentimentality. They can also be features of any system that seeks to grow its influence. If a community presents its method or leadership in unqualified positive terms, they're not just expressing devotion. They are inviting you to get closer, to join up, to buy something. If you are already in the group, they might be trying to get you to stay. The end result isn't necessarily harmful—not everyone will fly into the fire—but all students are made safer by a fuller, more transparent picture.

Beneath many all-good stories, there is a struggle between recognition and denial, playing out in many forms, from battles over what constitutes evidence—as we see with the Jois adjustment video—to the more mundane conflicts faced by reporters like Gallagher, where the cards were stacked against his being able to write about what he actually saw. The internet has proven to be an amazing tool for recording this struggle; previous generations had to rely on whisper networks alone.

Sometimes, denial can be overpowered by recognition—via the magic of empathy. We can see this in the story of Kiran Bocquet, who got clear on what Jois was doing to her when she saw him doing it to a friend.

"I remember him coming at the back of me in *Baddha Konasana*," Kiran said. She's describing the "butterfly" posture (*see* Figure 4, below), in which the practitioner sits upright with her legs folded outwards and the soles of her feet touching. Jois sat down behind her, wrapped his legs around her and over her thighs to press them down, and then reached around to hold her breasts.

"As he was counting he was pumping my breasts. It was very confusing.

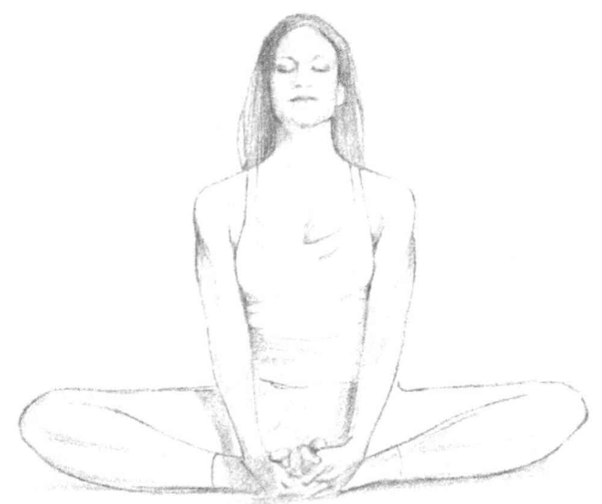

Figure 4: Baddha Konasana

I wasn't expecting it. I was thinking, 'Is this one of the adjustments?'"

She feels that she remembers the assaults continuing for a week. "There was a sense I had to endure it," she says.

Then, a friend arrived from Singapore. She confided in Kiran that she had recently been the victim of a drugged date rape.

"She was dealing with a lot," Kiran said.

"Her mat was behind me. For some reason I turned around and saw Guruji behind her in *Baddha Konasana,* and he was also pumping her breasts.

The tears were running down her face. That was the moment I decided 'I'm not tolerating this. This is wrong.'

"So the next time he went to adjust me in *Baddha Konasana*, I pulled his hand away and pointed my finger and just yelled 'No!'

Pausing to consider whether the yoga method or spiritual community that you love also carries a history of abuse is not scare-mongering. It's a lucid and mature way of beginning to sort out the difference between yoga beliefs, yoga marketing, and yoga data. We'll explore this more fully as played out in the Ashtanga world in **Part Three**.

But this pausing also does something else. By encouraging the practitioner to look for the shadows in what is otherwise idealized, it can help them to understand—as it helped Kiran in that flash of recognition—where they themselves might be caught in a dynamic they cannot fully see or articulate. This empathetic reflex, which can protect the self as much as it protects others, is naturally strengthened by step 2 of PRISM: "**R**esearch the hidden literature on the method to find that history." **Part Two** is offered as literature that is just now coming out of hiding regarding the Jois Asthanga event.

PART TWO

Two Survivor's Stories

The Ashtanga yoga I knew was sanctioned physical and sexual abuse.

— Karen Rain, who studied with Jois in Mysore from 1994 to 1998

There's the belief that this person who's your teacher must know more than you, right? So maybe it's a good thing, right? Probably a great thing and then you realize, 'No, wait. There's a muscle ripped. Or no wait. My heart is broken.'

— Tracy Hodgeman, who studied with Jois in Mysore in 1997

ISOLATION AND THE PERSONAL SPHERE

The beginning stage of exiting a high-demand group dynamic can feel like waking up from a feverish dream. There might be vivid images, or only feelings might remain, vibrating. You might want to shower and shake it off and get on with things, or you might feel unable to move.

The one thing that is clear is that the dream was *yours*. It happened *within* you. You might tell it to a friend or bring it to therapy, but no words you use will capture it fully. You might find a dream interpretation that helps. You might not. It's really up to you to figure it out.

Whatever the dream leaves you with, and whatever you go on to do with it, the umbrella rule is that the dream was private, internal, and impossible to fully share. It was *isolating*. In this sense, it mirrors a core feature of the cultic dynamic.

In varying degrees, every testimonial in this book began in—and almost didn't escape—the thrall of isolation. T.M. told a few Ashtanga colleagues what happened to her after returning from Mysore, but then stopped when no one seemed to be listening. Anneke Lucas was assaulted in 2001. Nine years passed before she published her report online to an audience who for the most part ignored her. Karen Rain didn't fully name Jois's assaults for what they were for almost 20 years. After Jois assaulted Micki Evslin, she reports telling the host of the event, talking about it with two other women in her class, telling at least two of her best friends, and writing to a mainstream yoga magazine about it. She also told a renowned yoga teacher in Hawaii who had also heard many stories about Jois and who sent her a picture of him purportedly molesting a student in class. Evslin raised many alarms, and nothing happened.

The silencing mechanisms of rape culture are becoming better known in the post-#MeToo world, and isolation is widely understood to be a key tactic of intimate partner abuse. Before abuse victims even begin the harrowing process of reaching out for help, many must first navigate with the internal isolation mechanisms of guilt and shame. In high-demand groups, these isolating responses reinforce the isolating measures the group itself employed. Alexandra Stein says that isolation effects are threefold.

> Contrary to public perception, the key experience of membership in a totalist group is one of isolation, not community or comradeship. The follower is isolated from the outside world; he

> or she is isolated from an authentic relationship to others within the group—allowed only to communicate within the narrow confines of the groupspeak and rigid rules of behavior; and, due to the dissociation that is created, the follower is also isolated from his or her self, from his or her own ability to think clearly about the situation.[43]

It is the third type of isolation that seems most immediate, personal, and visceral to many former group members. This is what makes it feel like waking up from a dream. You may be hurt, but your primary focus is internal. You are alone. It may be some time before you start asking questions about external factors, like who gave you the narcotic? Who shut you in the room? Where is this house, anyway? Why won't anyone listen to you?

If we think about the dreamer as a member of the high-demand group, we must also consider what they are waking up *into*: a globalized capitalist society that thrives on the isolation of its consumers, who are told in every advert that they must be self-responsible, and self-interested in a world of vanishing common values and social contracts. In this way, learning about how high-demand group members wake up, not only from a nightmare, but from the isolation of the group itself, is salutary for everyone's relationship to a culture that all but enforces isolation. Members who wake up out of high-demand groups and begin to speak are like canaries in the coal mine.

A FOCUS ON TWO VOICES

This part of the book will focus on the very personal register of experiencing abuse: how subjects remember distinct images, tiny moments, and intimate interactions, often not all at once, and usually without the benefit of any bird's-eye view. For this purpose, we will hear from two voices primarily: those of Karen Rain and Tracy Hodgeman. Both describe a strange awakening process that began in isolation, but through courage, the help of allies, and luck, broke through into a world of fragile but strengthening solidarity.

These voices will add new depth to the tension between recognition and denial. We'll see how abuses fostered within and protected by a group involve key moments of betrayal and deception. The theme of "grooming" will emerge as we hear about how these women were prepared to interpret abuse as care or spiritual transmission. We'll also see why stereotyping these experiences is a misguided attempt to form a structural analysis of group behavior that often slides into victim-blaming.

What we'll see in the transition between this part of the book and **Part Three** is that a robust structural analysis of the group dynamic involves showing how these personal and isolated experiences scale up to a systemic level. At this point, we're no longer talking about private nightmares, but about the paradoxical loneliness of being in a group where recruitment depends in part on covering over secrets, and staying means putting limits on what you can talk about.

THE YOGI WHO DISAPPEARED

In May 2016, I got a lead for tracking down a former elite Ashtanga practitioner and Jois student named Karen Haberman,who had mysteriously disappeared from the yoga world. I was told she had a story to tell, but she'd changed her name. A search came up with a half-dozen possible phone numbers. The right Karen picked up after I left three rambling messages on other Karens' phones.

"Hi. My name is Matthew, and I'm phoning from Toronto. I'm looking for someone who used to go by the name of Karen Haberman."

There was a long pause.

"That would be me," the voice said, slowly.

"Oh! Well, can I ask: did you used to do an awful lot of yoga?"

"Unfortunately!" she said, bursting out in laughter.

I told Karen about my research and book plans, and asked her if she wanted to be interviewed about her experience with Jois. I suggested that my main focus would be on how and why she'd left the physical practice. I told her that my suspicion was that many top yoga practitioners had practiced themselves into chronic pain, and I was looking for subjects who could speak directly to that.

This was all true. But I left out the part about wanting to ask about Jois's sexual assaults. I didn't know how it would fly to bring that up in a first call. I felt that the injury story would be easier to talk about, but might lead into other territory. Karen intimated that it would, and suggested that, because it would, I really couldn't be interested.

"I don't think I can help you with your book. Yoga really isn't part of my life now. I don't think you want to hear what I have to say."

I tried to tell her that I really was interested, in fact.

"Nobody is interested in what I have to say." She was emphatic.

"Okay, well... um... how about I send you some notes about the project and the questions I imagine asking you? If you have time, you can read them over and get a sense of what I'm doing."

She sounded skeptical, but agreed. I sent the notes and questions. She replied warmly, and we set up a call.

Neither of us knew what the consequences of my finding her would be. I had little idea how horrible the story was, nor how much it would cost her to tell it.

"This is all your fault," she said in our last interview, two years later. We laughed, but it was also painful.

A ROAD TO MYSORE

"When I was in my late teens, I used to listen to a lot of punk music," said Karen on the first call. "I loved it. But now when I hear it, I think 'Oh my God, I can't believe I ever listened to this! It's so painful!'"

She laughed, hard.

"That's about how I feel about yoga these days. Like: I can't believe I put myself through that."

Nobody knew "Karen Rain" in the yoga world in 2016. After practicing Pattabhi Jois's method from 1990 to 2000, and studying directly with him for two years in Mysore between 1994 and 1998, Karen Haberman left the scene, ended or lost contact with most of her fellow students, and changed her name. In our first call, she described leaving with chronic pain and a fear of Jois's dangerous adjustments. She had felt done with what she describes as the absurd idea that he was a spiritual teacher.

"It's just a bunch of postures that aren't even good for the body," she says, laughing again. "Repetitive actions in a dangerous range of motion. What are the benefits?

"Sure—bringing awareness into my body was really beneficial for me, but I could have done that by doing anything. It just happened to be yoga."

Karen was at the very top of the Ashtanga pyramid for years. In 1993, Jois traveled to California for a series of intensives. While there, his hosts Chuck Miller and Maty Ezraty booked a TV studio to film him teaching his Primary Series. Jois asked for six demonstrators. Karen was one of them.

The set seems to float in infinite space, with no distinction to be seen between the white floor and white walls. The six models—Karen, Chuck, Maty, Tim Miller, Richard Freeman, and Eddie Stern—move with ballet-corps precision on symmetrically spaced mats. Jois calls out the postures and the breath count in a mixture of Sanskrit and fragmented English. His singsong tone is gentle and mesmerizing. He doesn't touch the students, but rather stands in the center of the set like a chamber music conductor. The yogis breathe with the slow and steady Darth-Vaderesque rasp called that Jois called "free breathing with sound",*[44] produced by drawing air steadily and fully in and out through the nose while narrowing the throat with the back of the tongue. This was one of many videos available on VHS via mail order at the time that had inspired Diane Bruni, and was therefore partly responsible for the spreading Ashtanga scene, in Toronto and around the world.

Karen's performance is wiry, dynamic, effortlessly flexible, and intensely focused. She'd started doing yoga in the late 1980s, while going to the University of Toronto, where she studied zoology. In her last semester, she went to a variety of yoga classes in the methods of Sivananda, Kundalini, and Iyengar. In general, she remembers that yoga postures elevated her mood, and made her feel capable and strong.

After graduating in 1989, Karen moved to the Bay Area for a job as a field biologist. She soon came across a small pocket of Ashtanga practitioners. She thought the sun salutations were beautiful, and they felt good as she learned how to do them.

"I was listening to my body at that time," she said. "I remember liking the way yoga made me feel about my body." She explained that the simple physical activity also helped elevate her mood.

She was a natural at the postures. As she became proficient, it became a more serious thing. "An attachment and an identity," she said.

Later, Rain described how at the height of her fascination with Ashtanga, she felt it was her ticket to spiritual liberation.

To hone her skills, she traveled to Calgary for an intensive with Jois's childhood colleague, B.K.S. Iyengar. She was shocked by his manners.

"He was brutal. He made people cry. He was so arrogant. Everybody was talking about how great he was and I'm like—am I the only person here who thinks this guy is abusive?" She watched him yell at one woman and hit her with a stick.

Karen made her way back south and reconnected with the seemingly gentler Ashtanga fold. In 1991, she started to study with Richard Freeman (her future video co-star) in Boulder, Colorado. Freeman has gone on to become the éminence grise of American yoga. Handsome and mysterious, Freeman cites Pattabhi Jois as the primary influence for his globally acclaimed teaching.

* The breathing technique has been called ujjayi by Jois's students. Ujjayi, however, is the name of an even more focused breathi ng technique (pranayama) that typically is performed in a seated position only.

Privately, he's been said to murmur about the "dark cloud" of Jois's legacy.[45] I booked an interview with him in person, but he cancelled at the last minute. Later, his wife Mary, also a senior student of Jois, wrote that they were against being interviewed by me about Jois's abuses because they feared my approach would be sensationalist.[46] (They later released a series of statements about Jois, which are covered briefly in **Part Five**.)

After months of study with Freeman, he gave Karen the okay to teach.

"All of the sudden, it seemed, I was famous for my skill. My life was set. I had this gift. People wanted to study with me. I didn't have to figure out what I was going to do with my life."

She pauses.

"But the yoga was all about what I could do, as opposed to what I felt or experienced in my body." She compared the training to that of a circus performer.

Karen first met Pattabhi Jois when Freeman invited him to teach in Boulder in 1993. I asked her about her first impressions of him. Her speech changed, became less fluent. She made false starts, and stammered a little.

"Yeah, I would say he was pleasant—[sardonically:] *yeah, pleasant!*—ah, he made jokes, he laughed... um... [long pause]

"I'd heard the rumors about him groping women... and stuff. Um, I didn't experience that at that time... Yeah, sometimes he was... the way he would give instructions was very, like... he was like a drill sergeant. But at the same time it felt to me like there was an element of lightness about it, compared to Iyengar. In fact, I think Iyengar was so outright brutal, he groomed me for Pattabhi Jois, who seemed like a sweet old man in comparison."

I asked whether the rumors of sexual harassment were true. Her speech re-centered and started to flow again.

"Oh yeah, that was one of the first things you heard about him, you heard about it a lot. But it was always told in a light-hearted way, as if it were cute or endearing."

Karen paused.

"And just so you don't have to feel burdened with asking me all these questions. Yes, he groped me. No doubt about it. His adjustments on me were inappropriate."

She paused again, and then returned the focus outward.

"Once while I was in Mysore, I heard about a woman whom he was digitally penetrating, every day, over a month or two. I was told that Sharath would leave the room to get coffee while it was happening."

"Everyone was talking about it, including the advanced practitioners who were there. One of them—I won't say his name—would say things like 'Maybe this is what the practice is really about', meaning: accepting the guru. The idea was that devotion was paramount."

I asked her how that idea had sat with her at the time.

"I had sunken costs, and there was denial and there was justification, and there was 'Well, when he touches me that way, it doesn't feel sexual.' Now, when I think about it, I wonder how that argument ever made sense to me. Why *should* a sexual assault necessarily feel sexual to a victim? It might feel confusing. It might feel painful. It might feel like nothing."

"Everybody made justifications. When he touched women that way, people would say 'Oh, we don't know what he's doing for that woman. He's opening their chakras.' Or when he would rip people off for money, people would say 'Oh, that person has a problem with money, and he's helping them somehow, karmically.' The justifications were phenomenal."

Our conversation moved on to stories about Jois fudging bank exchange rates in his favor, demanding more cash from students than what had been agreed upon, or arbitrarily saying that people's pre-paid months had expired before they actually were so that he could demand more money. Karen deconstructed the ways in which she and her colleagues alike had projected some kind of holy status upon him. She said that she was a wreck when she finally left, and tried to do so quietly. "I didn't want to give up my status. Or have all of those conversations. I was afraid."

In conversation with me, Karen was direct, firm, ironic, and, at times, cutting. She sounded confident and in full possession of her story. That first interview gave the impression of someone who'd had a difficult experience in her late twenties that she had largely processed, and from which she had mostly recovered. She seemed able to speak about something dark and difficult from the distance of a hard-earned maturity, and it seemed that her credible but also dispassionate witnessing could help anchor a revised history of a global modern yoga brand.

What wasn't clear over the phone was the tension and fatigue with which she's had to hold that story. It became clear when we met in person, two years later. Then, it was plain to see that some amount of that confidence and infectious laughter was protective. By phone, it sounded like she was disclosing as much as was relevant and important to her. What was closer to the truth was that Karen hadn't felt ready, or as though she trusted me enough, to get into the hard details.

At that time, I was ignorant of the processes that trauma survivors must go through to retrieve and disclose memories. I didn't understand that being ready and feeling a sense of trust were prerequisites to being able to draw those details out of the past and into sharp relief. It took me a number of mistakes to realize that the type of space I was able (or not able) to provide in an interview could play a material role in how those memories might be allowed to emerge.

Like what Jois actually did to Karen's body. Like how, 20 years after ending her Ashtanga practice, she was still waking up every morning at 3:30am—the hour she would have risen to practice with Jois—with a hyper-vigilant feeling that something terrible was about to happen.

DEATH PIERCES THE FOG

In June 2017, a friend and colleague of mine died from fentanyl poisoning. Michael Stone had taught yoga and Buddhism all over the world while secretly struggling with mental illness. He was a complicated man, torn by internal conflicts that gave his work and presence an anxious radiance. In 2014, we had published an intimate book together about fatherhood and spirituality. The last project we worked on together was a talk he gave in Toronto as part of a series I curated. I'd asked him to speak on the subject of how he understood and managed his charisma.

The day after Michael died, I found myself staring at the first page of our book. Right there in black and white, he cites Pattabhi Jois as a positive influence in his life and teaching. He'd met Jois only once.

Jois's name had always seemed out of place on that page, yet at the same time, I knew how important it had been to Michael to keep it there. He had always considered himself as progressive and feminist. Yet like so many others, he had also been captivated by the charisma of a likely sexual predator. He knew the rumors about Jois, but it was more important for him to drop a famous name than it was to find a more appropriate reference.

The capacity to idealize leaders like Jois runs deep, whether enabled by deep psychological needs, or the banalities of laziness or self-interest. As in how I responded to Diane's story. Or how thoughtful people who work in an embodiment industry with an 80% female demographic hear about assault allegations against one of their leaders—someone whose name they don't even depend on socially or financially—and basically shrug. When we were editing our book, I told Michael that I didn't think referencing Jois on the first page of a book about family intimacy was appropriate. He stared at me, half blank, half quizzical. "He was many things to many people," he said. I didn't argue. There didn't seem to be anything solid to push back against.

Much of my communication with Jois's male students has been filled with that same kind of fog. Some were vague in response to direct questions like: "What did you see, and what did you do about it?" Others provided meticulous detail in their answers, which almost hid the fact that they were changing the subject. With this second group, there was usually a brief acknowledgment of a "problem", but then we'd suddenly be talking at length about yoga philosophy, or the layered and ultimately inscrutable differences between Indian and non-Indian cultures.

This wasn't just happening to me. In January 2018, Diane Bruni's daughter Kathryn Bruni-Young (once an Ashtanga adept, now a functional movement explorer) published a podcast featuring Richard Freeman.[47] Two months before, Karen Rain had posted her succinct #MeToo statement to Facebook, sending the online Ashtanga world into confused shock. Kathryn asked Freeman how he felt about stories like Karen's.

Freeman spoke slowly. His voice was contemplative to the point of hypnotic. There was a glimmer that he was perhaps struggling, but his signature calm and authoritative tone mostly covered this over.

> Yeah, well, it's very sad, and it's a very unique kind of problem that he manifested, but it definitely was a problem. Very complex, very confusing to... you know, I wasn't aware, in his later years I wasn't around the community very much. But I was aware that some of that was going on. It was like: "Oh my God, why?" Because it wasn't assault in any sense that he was... He never slept with the students, he never raped the students. But he was obsessed, I know, with *mulabandha*. With the pelvic floor. And somehow, through some kind of self-delusion he had, or through some cultural gap between the liberal Western world and the medieval provincial orthodox world, he started doing this occasionally. And he would do it, and people would complain, and he would stop. But somehow he would start again. It's very mysterious.The statement reflects how deep the divide can be within a community between those who, like Rain, suffered trauma directly and those who were merely aware of it. How time and avoidance and mystification can make a memory abstract to the latter even as it becomes more acute to the former.

Karen was one of Freeman's early students. They shared that studio stage with each other in 1993. Rather than admitting that Jois sexually assaulted students like Karen, Freeman described it as a "unique problem" related to a "cultural gap" that was "very mysterious". This was a large part of what made Karen's memories so difficult to directly disclose. She would have to cut through the fog that continued to surround her attacker.

***

Karen emailed out of the blue in August 2017. I was out west attending Michael's funeral. She told me her mother had died in March of that year.

"I've never experienced grief like this before," she wrote. "I started taking *qi gong* to have a practice to help me. I like it and think it has helped me with distress tolerance."

I showed her the chapter I'd produced with the help of her interview data from the year before. She wrote back in September.

"I just wanted to let you know that if you'd like/it would be helpful for your book, I'd be happy to explain more specifically/graphically how Pattabhi Jois was sexually abusive in his adjustments with me and what I saw with other women."

We scheduled a time for October. We started out talking about her mother, and Michael. She told me about a podcast called "Terrible, Thanks for Asking!" in which the host, Nora McInerny, tells stories about how people find resilience and even humor when terrible things happen.[48] Karen and I had still never met in person, but it felt more relaxed and familiar to talk than it had before.

When I changed tack to ask her about the details she wanted to share, it was clear that she had a well-ordered list. She later published the full details on her blog, and then photographs of the assaults.[49]

> Pattabhi Jois got on top of me in supine postures, placed his penis against my genitals and would grind rhythmically, almost daily. In a couple of standing postures he stood behind me and placed his penis against my buttocks and pressed back and forth. Similarly, he would press his penis against my genitals in the final backbend, while I was standing on my feet and reaching my arms backward to hold my legs. He grabbed and pulled my genitals when I was in *[M]ulabandhasana* (*see* Figure 5, p. 68). When I

> would say goodbye after practice, he would kiss me on the mouth and massage my buttocks. He groped one of my breasts once. I saw him do all these things to other women. He put his hands on women's breasts, in various postures, mainly twists and forward bends. I saw him, in forward bends lying on top of the women and reaching from behind to play with their breasts. I saw him playing with one women's nipples.[50]

On the phone, I asked Rain whether the humping action threw the women off-balance when he was standing behind them.

"Totally," she said. "It was part of the game to try to keep your balance. And people would use *that* as an excuse for what he was doing. He was 'challenging' you, they'd say. It wasn't a sexual thing, they'd say. He was helping you get better at the posture."

The posture called *Mulabandhasana* (*see* Figure 5, below) in Rain's description is highly contortionistic. Imagine sitting upright and cross-legged with the soles of your feet together and your thighs in butterfly position. So far, so good. But then: bring your heels to your groin, and then, with your hands, lift your heels up and over so that your toes point back towards your buttocks. Then lift your pelvis so that you're sitting on the outside edges of your turned-back feet.

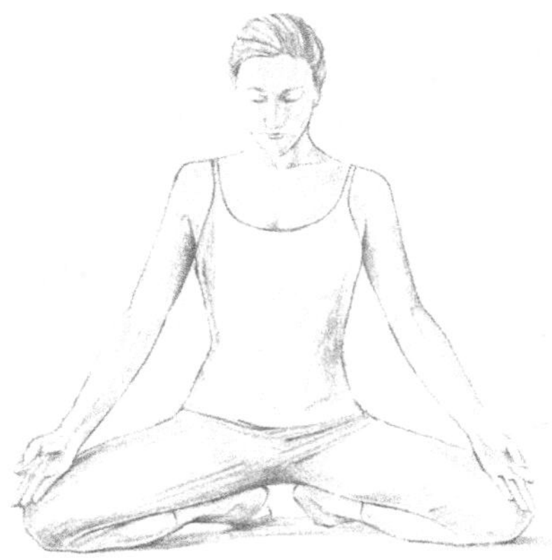

Figure 5: Mulabandhasana

On our call, Rain said that she'd heard that Jois had added one of the supine postures he assaulted her in into the First Series (now known as the Primary Series). Was she suggesting that this posture, which made women practitioners particularly vulnerable, was added in so that Jois would have access to more women's bodies?

"I would say that," Karen said. "Other people wouldn't."

It's important to note that the exact sequence of postures in each of Jois's series is regarded as a sacred liturgy to his most devout followers. Keeping the precise order, they believe, is essential to the almost-magical healing powers of Jois's yoga.

But it's also well known that the series went through many changes between 1964, when the first non-Indian students began showing up in Mysore, and 2003, when the operation shifted from his 12-person shala in Lakshmipuram to the richly appointed 60-person shala Jois built across from his new residence, in the upscale neighborhood of Gokulam. Since his grandson, Sharath Rangaswamy, assumed control, there have been other changes. Many older students have remarked that the changes made over the years seem to have been about managing an increasing student load over time. Practice sessions got shorter and more regimented as Jois attempted to funnel more students through each time slot.

But Karen's speculation is stunning: that Jois might have also changed his sequences to give him more sexual access to more women.

"Someone who didn't want to say he was a sexual predator would say he was changing the sequence because of the science of yoga. I wouldn't personally. I'm guessing he threw that one into the First [now Primary] Series because it was a good opportunity for him."

As they process reports that he was a daily sexual predator, many Jois disciples theorize ways in which his method can be separated from his behavior. For them, it might feel catastrophic to even begin to suspect that the method itself was inextricable from his actions. It might be intolerable to consider that the ritual they perform every morning with such effort and devotion was structured in part by Jois's craving for nonconsensual sexual contact. It would make sense that the lengths to which some would go to deny it and blame whistleblowers would directly reflect the passion built up in the practice itself, over thousands of candlelit mornings.

AGAINST STEREOTYPING

How did Karen Rain and so many others get drawn into such an abusive situation? What baggage did they bring with them to Mysore? And if there are others like them, what's wrong with yoga people?

This brings up the victim-blaming nature of stereotyping.

The very sound of the word "Ashtanga" can communicate something austere, painful, blissful, raw. I personally register it as some ultimate alchemy of absolute discipline, bounded by precise choreography, enforced by intimate physical contact with teachers, and overflowing with rich and sometimes chaotic sensation. And while this description might be resonant to many readers, it remains a stereotype as much influenced by marketing and gossip as it is by reality. It's also a vision to which I'm allergic, which means that I have tended to other the Ashtanga experience as unpleasant or unnecessary. For years, I carried the semi-conscious judgment that the method was sado-masochistic and somehow attracted people who had some wounded need to explore both bodily and interpersonal intrusion.

This is a stereotype. In fact, Ashtanga practitioners report a broad range of bodily experiences, largely dependent on the uniqueness of their bodies and the diversity of the experience they brought to the practice to begin with. Some came with bodies that were congenitally hypermobile, which meant that going into extreme ranges of motion was necessary for them to feel anything in asanas that would have others crying out in pain. Or they came as athletes entrained to accept high pain thresholds, or with relational histories to parents or sporting coaches that made Jois's physical demands seem tolerable or even loving. Some came with chronic pain to start with and the opiate-endorphin rush of practice gave them more relief, albeit temporary, than any medication had yet afforded.

Some Ashtanga practitioners self-identify on the autism spectrum, and they report that the close, body-draping, hugging adjustments that some teachers apply to them in some postures give an exquisite sense of containment to bodies that often struggle to feel at home in a single part of the world. One practitioner related that the full-body embrace that one female teacher applied to get him further into a twist filled him with deep relief, because it reminded him of how his mother used to restrain him when he had uncontrollable tantrums as a little boy. His story highlights the invisibility of what happens in other people's bodies. Sensations and interactions that in some would provoke violent responses can be deeply craved by others. If we paint the Ashtanga experience in broad strokes, we miss the infinite and unnamable inner colors.

Realizing this experiential diversity begins to unknot another stereotype: that there was a "type" of person drawn to this practice. The reader might nod when T.M. (see the full transcript: Appendix 1) described herself as someone with an "extreme personality", or when Tracy Hodgeman describes below coming to Mysore from an environment in which sexual boundaries were frequently violated. Or when Tattoo Man said, "We're all addicts here," in the locker room after that class with Diane Bruni.

Group identifications may feel reasonable, but they can also reinforce ways in which certain personality traits amongst practitioners get emphasized to the exclusion of others, not only because they are shared but also because they aid in the formation of a group identity through which they find belonging. This group identity can also be framed positively by the insider voices of Ashtanga bloggers who write about community members in a universal plural.[51]

Digging deeper, however, reveals something both simpler and more complex. There really is no "type" drawn to this method, as opposed to any other. Ashtanga draws former gymnasts and dancers, but also non-athletes. It draws atheists, new-age seekers, alcoholics in recovery, vegans, paleo-eaters, acid-heads, pot-heads, dropouts, and accountants. There are single people, monogamists, polyamorists. Disciples are straight and gay. There are people with sexual trauma histories, and those without. People who credit the practice with helping them rise out of depression, and others who entered with no history of emotional disregulation. People with advanced college degrees and people who work in trades. People who plunge in deep, people who stay on the fringes. People who explore pain in practice, and people who use it to find relief from pain. Historically, the vast majority of Jois's non-Indian students have been white. In recent years that has started to change as the Mysore shala begins to draw students from other parts of Asia.

There is also a wide range of personal recovery narratives leading away from bad Ashtanga experiences. The very different post-Mysore paths cut by Karen and T.M. stand out. Both had similar experiences with Jois: long months of being assaulted daily, about the same number of years ago. Both amputated themselves from the Ashtanga community. But they wound up in very different positions in the world: with very different jobs, circles of friends, relationships to pain, and economic circumstances.

It seems obvious to say it: people are diverse when coming into Ashtanga practice, and they are diverse when leaving it. Their association with the Jois method really isn't predictive of any other similarity they might share. This is a crucial point, because if we understand it, we'll get out from under the semi-conscious rape-culture question of "So what's wrong with these women who gravitated towards this abusive place?

COGNITIVE DISSONANCE

When Karen Rain opened herself up to public scrutiny, she weathered many variations of that question. "Why didn't you leave?" "What made you stay?" "Why did you put up with that?"

Such questions show no insight into the dynamics of abuse. There are well-documented reasons for why victims stay in abusive relationships. They learn to freeze, fold, or tend-and-befriend as survival strategies. Their relationship patterns may become disorganized, which means that they feel compelled to run towards the apparent caregiver who also harms them. (This is covered at length in **Part Four**.) They may have become emotionally or financially dependent on a social structure marred by abuse. They may have lost relationships that could provide outside perspective. They might have felt isolated, as T.M. describes, within a network of "thin social ties".

"There was cognitive dissonance," Karen reflects.

> I loved Ashtanga so much, and was so ... dedicated to it, I thought I had found my ticket to freedom. And part of that narrative of Ashtanga being my ticket to freedom was that Pattabhi Jois was this guru, enlightened being, and so when I saw things, and when things happened to me, that didn't fit that narrative, I just couldn't accept it. There was disassociation, there was denial, there was ... Yeah, I mean. I just was trapped. I never would've chosen it though. That for me is really important. It wasn't like I designed it. Life would've been much better for me had that not happened.

Interpersonal toxicities, scaled up to a certain social density, begin to describe cultic dynamics.

The victim-blaming questions Karen and others fielded also show no insight into the fragility of individual human agency. They assume that we're all equally empowered at all times to make choices in our own individual best interests. This is ignorant not only of the power of group dynamics and gender imbalances, but also of the fact that abuse itself degrades the victim's capacity for agency. In fact, this could be a good general definition of abuse: that which takes away agency.

It can be difficult to understand this in psychosocial terms. But in physical terms, it's much easier. If you watched someone break another person's leg, you wouldn't ask the person with the broken leg why they didn't run away from their attacker. You would instantly understand that the attack has impacted the person's ability to run away. You don't have to be Karen Rain's therapist to understand that when Jois imposes physical and psychological control over her body after a period of grooming, and the group of students that surrounds her tells her that this is just the way it is, and they reward her for staying, the assaults become her reality. She learns to adjust—and be adjusted (which really means being assaulted) until something has to give: body, mind, or both.

This point is also crucial when we are talking about experiences within the yoga world more generally. Both philosophically and through its own marketing terms, the basic zeitgeist of the modern yoga landscape is highly individualistic. This has led some theorists to categorize yoga itself as a kind of privatized religion that features minimal social investment, as it's focused almost exclusively on the development of the self.[52] Some go further to describe yoga as the spirituality of the neoliberal era, in which the power of personal will is valued above all else and worked on obsessively through expensive self-improvement rituals that leave no time to be concerned about, let alone work on, issues of structural inequality.[53]

The bodily isolation and subjective diversity of some practice experiences can reinforce this theme. Most of us practice on 2' by 6' strips of rubber. If we are dedicated Jois students, we're practicing together, but we don't make eye contact. We focus inward, on our breath. For example, Charlotte Clews remembers practicing in Richard Freeman's yoga Workshop in Boulder, Colorado. (Jois assaulted her in 2002 in the gym Freeman had rented to host the master on tour.) She noted there was no waiting room to hang out in and thus very little socializing before or after class. Conversations with Richard were limited to the practicalities of practice and esoteric philosophy. As for Freeman's teacher Jois, his limited English kept conversations brief and aphoristic.

When interpersonal and institutional abuse occurs in the yoga world, we have to understand how the premise of "yoga as a personal journey of discovery" inhibits an examination of the structural supports of that abuse. It's a premise that can be torqued to force victims to answer for why they have been victimized. For decades, this ethos of hyper-individualism blended with the basic victim-isolation of rape culture to reinforce the loneliness felt by Jois's victims (and those of Choudhury, Yogi Bhajan,*[54] and others). For decades, questions like "Who are these people and why didn't they exercise their free will when they were being abused?" not only express rape culture in action but also play upon the spiritual idea that yoga is meant to invigorate a private empowerment, and that if it hasn't, you weren't really practicing hard enough. Those questions turn the focus away from the fact of the abuse itself, to ask why people were so stupid as to have had their legs broken, and not run away. They feed the illusion that everyone comes to yoga in freedom, when it is actually freedom that they're looking for. They feed the illusion that all yoga masters offer freedom, when they might be offering far less.

"IT WAS ALL PROJECTION"

There are physical qualities that are particular to the Ashtanga environment: it's intense and austere. Also certain personality traits seem correlated with the attraction to practice. But these are peripheral issues. Generalizations about how Ashtanga feels for everyone, or why people join, or why they persist in practice, depend on and are linked to the faulty stereotypes noted above.

What will be most useful for creating a safer yoga culture in general is to foreground the more observable structural mechanisms driving the failures of the Jois-devoted sector of the Ashtanga community to address abuse. These are mechanisms that allowed the somatic and psychological desires of its members to be weaponized against them. They allowed the desire for wordless, ecstatic experience to be mobilized against critical thinking. They allowed the desire for bodily intensity to exhaust members beyond the point of resistance. They allowed the desire for intimacy and touch to be mobilized into a form of grooming.

As mentioned briefly in **Parts One** and **Two,** the first and most pervasive of these mechanisms is *deception*. This is a chilling thought for those who pursue yoga as a form of truth-seeking. If there is a common denominator running through the testimonies in this book—and the stories of Karen and Tracy—it is not how the students felt about the practice, what they were like when they came to it, what they projected onto Jois, or how they recovered from their experience. The common denominator that made

* Yogi Bhajan (1929–2004), born Harbhajan Singh Khalsa, was the creator of the branded method known as "Kundalini yoga". The organization Bhajan founded, 3HO, settled two lawsuits against him, including one case of rape and confinement brought by a woman who entered his harem of "secretaries" at age eleven.

the assaults likely to happen, and allowed them to be rationalized once they did, was the fact that *the victims were deceived by people who were supposed to be caring for them*. They were drawn in towards the center of an organization through layers of deception.

On one hand, the Jois story is unremarkable. Most of the world groans under the weight of rape culture, which enables, normalizes, protects, and reframes sexual assault. But the yoga context adds to this basic landscape in ways that are important for all practitioners and teachers to understand, especially given how many people come to yoga practice expecting safety and healing. Looking closely at how rape culture works in the yoga world in particular is foundational to mitigating harm in all yoga communities. Abuse in yoga communities is enabled largely through mystification and idealization, and enforced through somatic domination framed as care. These deceptions can be disguised with a spiritual glow.

During one of our interviews, Karen suggested that Ashtanga yoga was taken to be spiritual by Jois's students to the extent that they maintained a fantasy about him.

"Do you think he was a good man?" I asked.

"No," she said. "I think he was sick, and he needed a lot of help. The last thing he needed was to be venerated. His students, myself included, attributed much more to him than was warranted. He had a limited English vocabulary, but people made it out like everything he said was so full of wisdom."

How far had Karen and her fellow students taken that idea?

"I would say he was an almost God-like figure. He was all-seeing, all-knowing, all-powerful, and all-loving."

What did she think Jois was getting out of it all?

> It was obvious. He was getting money and a power trip by doing whatever he wanted to his students. I might have more to say about what was going on for him if he'd had a personality to me, but he didn't. There wasn't a lot of give and take in the relationship.
>
> It was all projection. He could do what he was doing not because he was my father or uncle or doctor. It's because he had a mystique around him. Half of the grooming for sexual harassment is done by the time people come to him, desperate for whatever they're desperate for in Ashtanga yoga.
>
> Then there are all the people who are there and doing it and

accepting it, and are fine with it and when someone new comes in, they're shocked, but then the whole culture says "It's okay" with whatever justifications they have.

We were grooming each other.

DECEPTION AND GROOMING

The concept of grooming is well-known in the study of sexual violence. It shows how the physical and psychological boundaries of a potential victim can be gradually infringed upon, softened up, and broken down, up to and including the prosecutable moment of assault. It shows that sexual assault is often the endpoint in a creeping betrayal of trust.

"We were all grooming each other" expands an understanding of this process outwards into the social sphere. Jois's assaults against bodies were a private end-point. But the grooming prior to the assault and the justifications after it are parts of a social mechanism that not only enabled Jois but also spread and expanded his influence, even while his behavior was more and more widely known.

Jois's disciples spoke of him as representing a tradition, as being a spiritual master, as having healing hands. This is all well and good: people can believe what they want. But, as we'll explore, it's that framework that in part allows those same colleagues to tell Karen, after she's been assaulted, that she hasn't experienced an assault. Recall what T.M. says: "Immediately, I was told 'It was not sexual.'"

That lie told to T.M. did not come out of nowhere. It came, rather, at the end of a cumulative series of deceptions that made it predictable, if not inevitable. If Jois was a traditional teacher and spiritual master with healing hands—all premises that were established for T.M. and Karen long before they ever showed up in Mysore—*then he simply couldn't have been assaulting them.*

The cognitive dissonance of victims can scale up into systemic deception. Not only does Karen model a kind of submission to Jois's assaults for newer practitioners—as though that's what "advanced" practitioners simply do—she actually advertised for the group by telling Larry Gallagher that the adjustments were fine. She didn't sexually assault students herself but she does admit to replicating Jois's intrusive adjustment technique. She encouraged other students to go to Mysore as well, where they too might be assaulted. Those who are successfully deceived, and are rewarded for it, will often deceive others in turn. "The confirmation of manipulation," writes Cathleen Mann, "occurs when ordinary cult members are successful in activity to convert others."[55]

In a blog, Karen Rain addressed this directly. "Here is my own statement of responsibility," she wrote.

> I was intensely involved in Ashtanga yoga for several years. During that time I did my share of glorifying Pattabhi Jois and recommending studying in Mysore. If anyone went there on account of me and was hurt in any way, I am so sorry. I also offer my sincerest apologies to anyone I hurt with my adjustments while teaching. I know of at least six people and there are probably more. I was not very skillful or attuned. I wish I could go back and do things differently. Because I can't go back, I am speaking out now, to be a part of a movement toward a safer, more transparent and more just future.[56]

THE #METOO MOMENT

Karen Rain's public activism began in November 2017, when she posted this disclosure to her Facebook page.

> MeToo.
>
> After reading other women's posts, I am inspired by the importance of sharing experiences and naming names. Pattabhi Jois sexually assaulted me regularly in his yoga asana "adjustments." I also witnessed him sexually assault other women regularly in a similar manner. His actions were protected by a culture of denial and cryptic justifications.
>
> — Karen Haberman
>
> I studied Ashtanga yoga in Mysore for a total of 2 years between 1994 and 1998.[57]

The flood of public response was mixed. Many supported her. Many disbelieved her. The waves were both powerful and impossible to fully grasp. I'll document some of it in **Part Five.**

Karen was fairly new to social media. Looking back, she recounts how overwhelming it all was, how she needed to boundary herself from the onslaught. It was disturbing her life, and she hadn't bargained for it. She'd thought she'd left the yoga world behind. At one point, she started to use the term PTSD to describe her symptoms. She said that waking up at 3:30am had actually become more regular and more intense since disclosing her story publicly.

Social media also reconnected her with an entire world of former friends and colleagues. People reached out to her from across oceans and decades. They remembered learning yoga from her, her dedication to the practice, the mystery of her disappearance. The isolation began to break down. In February 2018, she received an email from Ross Smith, a friend with whom she had traveled to Mysore in 1994. He invited Rain to publish the letter to her blog. To that point, it constituted the only on-record corroboration of Rain's experience from among her colleagues.*[58]

Behind the scenes, other former colleagues reached out to Rain. As they did, her own memories continued to rise up in visible form, while layers of secrecy and shame continued to peel away.

It was as if her interview data was alive and growing in tandem with her internal process. She'd email me asking if I had time for a call. I'd phone, and she'd pick up from a sentence she'd uttered more than a year before.

"You know how I said that we were grooming each other?"

"I remember."

"Well I don't think that's totally accurate."

"How so?"

"Pattabhi Jois actually groomed me directly when I studied with him in Encinitas, shortly after making the video. I was waiting to use the bathroom. He was in the bathroom. The door opened and he came out. He saw me and smiled and laughed. Then he came right up to me and hugged me and kissed me fully on the lips. I felt confused, but also special. The kissing seemed to be innocuous. If it had stopped there, I wouldn't have PTSD. I had no idea

* " Dear Karen, I studied yoga with Pattabhi Jois in Mysore for three months in mid 1994, and five months in early 1997 (if you want exact dates, I can get them). During these visits, I saw Jois give adjustments that placed his genitals against yours, and other women's, over 100 times (mostly in assisted backbends, and *Supta Trivikramasana* [also known as *Supta Padangusthasana*]). I recall a few other students finding this inappropriate, but I don't recall anyone saying it was abuse or assault. My personal reaction was mild disgust, and even some jealousy. He clearly favored the female students, so the male students received very little help, mostly from Sharath, his grandson. It didn't seem at all yogic for Jois to fawn over the women so.

I recall you first told me about Jois shortly after you finally left Mysore. I recall your saying that Jois had inappropriately touched you and other women, it was wrong what he had done, and you were never going back. I don't recall if you called it "abuse" or "assault", but I remember you were very upset by it.

I remember feeling disgusted, and abused myself. I felt that not only had he abused you and other women, but he had abused everyone by destroying our trust, and severely damaged yoga's reputation in general. I lost all respect for him, and stopped telling people to visit Mysore…".

that I was being groomed for something worse. When the assaults escalated, I dissociated, and didn't feel special in any way."

"That's intense."

"Yeah. So I don't think it's right to say we were grooming each other."

"Wasn't it that both things were going on? He was directly grooming, and the idealizations and rationalizations were also in play?"

"That sounds right."

A further detail came not through the release of a memory, but because Karen received news of a friend's death.

"You remember the woman I told you about?" Karen messaged. "The one where Jois would lay on her back and play with her nipples?"

I remembered.

"She was a friend. Her name was Catherine Tisseront. She was from France. I saw Jois assault her more frequently and severely than any other woman. We never talked about it. I just found out she died of cancer at the age of 45."

A MUTUAL FRIEND, A SHARED STORY

Catherine Tisseront's name had come up in a series of interviews with a woman named Tracy Hodgeman two years before. Tisseront was one of Tracy's teachers in Seattle, and her friend.

The first interviews were about Tracy's shoulder injury. She recounted how, after thirteen years of practice, her right shoulder had collapsed in fall 2006 under the strain of the Third Series, a torturous parade of arm balancing postures. She had been practicing four to five days a week, two to three hours per session. Her shoulder had been sore for a while, but she ignored it, and progressed with happy determination. To manage the pain of practice, she was visiting a chiropractor two or three times per week.

In a 2007 blog post,[59] Tracy described the moment of the injury.

> "...it was somewhere near the end of my practice... When suddenly there was a loud *clunk!* that came from my right clavicle, and I felt it jump under my skin. My right shoulder started to feel warm and wobbly.... My arm was unsteady and my elbow swung way out to the right and there was nothing I could do about it.

"'Hmmmm' I thought to myself hopefully, 'maybe my body is shifting, getting stronger, realigning.' You see, in Ashtanga loud clunks and 'strong sensations' are commonplace, our guru Sri K. Pattabhi Jois calls them 'openings.'"

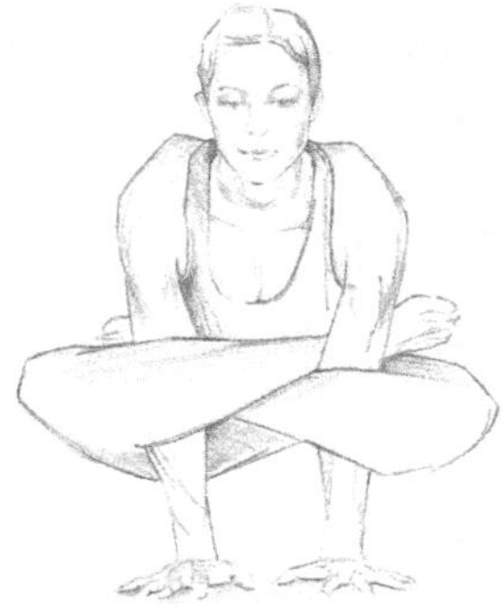

Figure 6: Kukkutasana

Tracy went on to describe how she kept coming to the studio to practice every morning, even though her shoulder was destabilized. She believed that the practice that had harmed her would also heal her. It took nine months and a gift of $2000 from a friend to cover the costs of an MRI before she got a diagnosis and a treatment plan. A key muscle attachment in her shoulder had been torn clean off the bone. It would have to be repaired with an expensive and painful surgery.

Tracy had practiced with Jois himself in Mysore years before, over the New Year's session in 1999–2000. She also studied with him for a week in New York City in early September 2001 and again when he came to Seattle the following year. In 2016, I met with her in a Seattle café and asked her what she remembered about his adjustments—if she'd ever felt strange about them.

"Not at the time," she said. "Except when he would give me the *Kukkutasana* assist. Then I would wonder: 'Is that okay?'"

The maneuver in *Kukkutasana* (*see* Figure 6, above) is ostensibly meant to help the practitioner leap back to a plank position from a hand-balance in which her legs are folded around her straightened arms in full lotus. Jois gave it to his women students by reaching underneath from behind, grabbing them by the groin and then pulling back.

"I did think it was odd that he was handling all of these young and beautiful women. It was like we were keeping him young."

A few months later, she sent an email that filled out the scene in Lakshmipuram with more detail, and suggested even more strongly that her story wasn't primarily about her shoulder injury.

I remember the weird uneven floor of shabby layered carpets in the big empty windowless room where we practiced. I remember a few faded portraits of deceased family members on the wall decorated with bright garlands of fresh carnations.

I remember the dark narrow steps leading up to the right of the entrance to the main practice room where we would sit quietly waiting for our turn to go in and put down our mat. I remember watching the yogis from all over the world contorting themselves into unlikely shapes below, with the sound of their *ujjayi* breath and the occasional short instruction by Guruji ("Why fearing???") drifting up to my ears.

I remember bowing to touch Guruji's soft feet as I left at the end of my practice. He would sit waiting on a stool just outside of the practice room at the foot of the stairs. I remember feeling great affection for this old man.

It didn't seem as though he was touching just to touch. His adjustments seemed to fit the function of whatever was physically required (move us from seated lotus to *chaturanga*, increase stretch in *hanumanasana*, etc),* although they were certainly more invasive/unconventional than I had ever experienced before or since.

I remember the coconut man outside on the corner waiting for us to pass by on our way home from practice. I tried not to watch as he chopped the coconuts open with his machete because I was worried that my fear of the knife would somehow cause him to slip and cut his hand.

IT'S NOT REALLY ABOUT A SHOULDER INJURY

Tracy described how her teacher, Catherine Tisseront, who was originally from France, had come to yoga from a strict Catholic background. Catherine would often talk about how people simply couldn't change without facing hardship. On hikes through the hills above Seattle, she would tell Tracy about the saints and martyrs who fascinated her. How Saint Agatha of Sicily had to suffer her breasts being cut off in order to receive the healing vision of St Peter and transcend her body and the world. It was through Catherine that Hodgeman came to believe that the pain of Ashtanga practice was a developmental necessity.

In reviewing my notes, I wondered if Tracy had seen Karen's #MeToo

* *Chaturanga* is a push-up position; *Hanumanasana* is a forward splits position.

post, and, if she had, what she'd made of it. She herself had made allusions to having been sexually assaulted by Jois, but hadn't used that language. Had anything changed? I reached out to ask if she'd like to pick up where we'd left off. We set a time.

I explained that my research project had taken a turn away from the physical injuries. I told her that I'd been documenting victim testimonies, and was about to publish a mainstream article on Jois's sexual assaults. Reading back to her the quotes about being adjusted she'd given in previous interviews, I asked her how she felt about it all now. She spoke as if she was letting out a long exhale after holding her breath.

TRANSCRIPT: "IT'S GOING TO TAKE ME A WHILE TO PROCESS THAT."

[Tracy Hodgeman] I'm so glad we get the chance to revisit this 'cause the #MeToo thing has come up and I've been doing a lot of thinking about my own sexuality and my own history of what you'd probably call abuse and how context effects everything. I was raised with hippie parents during the sexual revolution, so I saw all kinds of shit going down and I was touched in lots of different ways that I shouldn't have been. Now, I know, but back at the time, I just thought this is the way adults are. They're a little strange. Nobody's really hurting me and so, I just carried on.

So, it sort of feels like what you think is right or wrong will effect whether or not you feel abused. What you know affects how you interpret things, which affects how you emotionally respond. And my husband and I would have this conversation in Mysore. He would say, "Well ..." and I would say, "Wow—weird thing happened, you know. He does this adjustment. He's lying right across you and you're in the splits and his face is on your face and his groin is in your groin and it's like, wow, I would never do this to one of my students." Although Catherine did that adjustment just like that on me and she was, it was still really intense, but she was a woman.

I would say, intellectually, "This doesn't work. I know this is not correct." But in my body, I don't feel like this huge repulsion or fear or arousal. It didn't feel sexual. It felt intimate. It felt ... like maybe, wow, you're awfully close to me, you know.

But it didn't have a sexual flavor somehow 'cause he's an old man and I don't think of old men as sexual, whatever it is that's going on in my head. And I've had a lot of strange things happen to me in my life, so I think,

"Oh, this isn't as weird as some of the other things that have happened to me," so it kind of gets filed away in a "Not-a-Big-Deal Place."

[Matthew Remski] *You said that you had the conversation with your husband. Did he have a different impression or was he ...*

[TH] He didn't like what he was hearing. He was like, "That doesn't sound right to me." And I'd say, "Oh, I know, but you wouldn't understand because you're not there."

[MR] *Many of the women I've spoken to did feel assaulted by that behavior and ...*

[TH] I think a normal person probably would. For some reason, maybe I'm not, yeah...

[MR] *Well there's a whole range of responses and ways of tolerating and ways of, you know, resolving cognitive dissonance and ...*

[TH] Explaining it away, yeah.

[MR] *People also describe freezing, or dissociating, or not ... just putting themselves into another frame of mind or ...*

[TH] [Nodding] Yeah.

[MR] *So you're nodding, which makes me wonder whether any of that resonates with you at all.*

[TH] Well, one of my favorite responses to trauma is to dissociate and to freeze. I'm not much of a fighter, although I can fight for someone else.

But ... in that setting, I felt pretty safe because there were people around and everyone else seemed like they were okay with it so it felt okay. If it had been alone in a private lesson, that might have been a whole 'nother story. That might have freaked me right out. I don't know.

I have this memory that keeps popping into my head as we're speaking—of Catherine really wanting me to go to Mysore. She really pushed me to go. She was the reason I went 'cause she was like, "You have to go here. You have to study with him. It's so important." And when I finally said, "Okay, we're going," she said, "Oh, he is gonna *like* you," and she had this funny look on her face. And I was thinking, "What does she mean? He's really gonna *like* me?" It was just odd, so I don't know the answer to that.

I told Tracy how Karen had seen Jois intensively fondling and assaulting Catherine. She was astonished. She hadn't heard anything about it.

[MR] *When you think about Catherine wanting you to go to Mysore, what do you think is involved there? It seems like there was something secret about what she was involved in, but she wanted to share it with you in some way.*

[TH] It's fucked up. Yeah, she really wanted me to study with Guruji. She sent me to New York to see him when he was there. Paid for the airplane. I don't know right now. It's going to take me while to process that.

[MR] *I'm sorry for laying it all on you actually.*

[TH] No, it's okay. It's intriguing. Catherine was always ... very pro-Guruji. She was always like, "He's the master, he's the one." And if I ever had any doubts she would say, "Trust the practice. Trust the practice. You do. Don't ask, don't talk about it. Just do it and it'll heal you."

But in the end she said, "I think it's all a lie and I think it's all just to make your ego bigger and I think you can hurt yourself with yoga and I don't believe in any of it anymore."

[MR] *Wow. Was she saying that to you while she was in hospice?*

[TH] It was before that, when she still was hoping to live, I think. She was hoping to live up to the day before she died. She was amazing. Life force.

[MR] *Do you remember a little bit more about that conversation where she described having really lost her faith?*

[TH] I think she was talking about like what she wanted to do in the future. She kept telling me that she wanted to open up a little studio, like a place where people could come for healing and she learned massage in the last few years and she knew that I was into therapeutic yoga and after my injury, I got more interested in how to stay in one piece and she thought we could open this shop together and we would offer these healing modalities and that was when she was like, "I can't teach yoga anymore. I've lost faith in it and I don't believe in it."

She had a dream that Guruji came to her and he said, "You need to have more fun."

[MR] *Was her loss of faith in the practice reflected in any change in the way she spoke about Jois himself?*

[TH] I never heard her say anything negative about him. It always seemed like she was speaking of her favorite grandfather or something.

[MR] *So when my article comes out and this book is published, you'll hear the voices of other women who went through something similar to you. People like Karen Rain use different language than you do. They'll say: "I was assaulted." How does that strike you?*

[TH]Well, I totally ... honor and believe Karen's version for herself what it felt like that she was assaulted. And that doesn't really ... shift my perception of my own experience. The main thing I feel when I see this body of work is sad. I feel sad that ... that what could have been, maybe, a beautiful healing environment was actually so toxic and has created so much pain for so many people in so many ways.

I remember there was talk at the time when I was there like, "Oh, well, his wife has died. He's lonely. He's just getting affection through all of us." I had this image of us being like flowers and he was like this bee. This old man who was like getting life energy from us in small amounts. Well, what's the harm in that, you know? We can support this old man in his later years and, you know, but I didn't get quite the same treatment, but I mean, probably a lot of people would have been pretty mad to be adjusted the way I was.

I can't make sense of it really. I know that he was a man and I think that the Indian culture, maybe every culture on the planet, I don't know, is pretty messed up between men and women and I knew that there weren't any Indian women in the room and I knew that if there were, it would probably be a lot different. So I felt like he was an opportunist for sure. That he was working on these people that had different morals and because he was like the guru, he had all the power.

[MR] *Has this all given you sort of some further thoughts about what yoga culture might need in general to both recover from this and to make sure it's really less likely to happen?*

[TH] Of course, we have to heal ourselves. We're not coming to feed off our students, but we're there to hold a safe space and allow them to do their own work and you know, keep the roles very clean and clear and separate and yeah, that's ... that's one place where the work has to happen. And also, you know, when there's rumors going around, "Oh, this guy did this, or this woman did this," rarely is it a woman, but there are, at least one out there, maybe just one. That we don't just sweep it under the rug, under the crooked, uneven rug in the Mysore room in Pattabhi Jois's studio.

We need to empower women in so many ways because ever since I was born, I was taught, "Oh, men are like that. That's how men are." So you just, you dodge 'em when you can and you just make the best of it.

For me personally to be able to remember or learn maybe for the first time that my body is a temple, you know, that's a big step that I might not make in this lifetime, but I'm working towards it. From that perspective, I might be like, "Get the fuck off of me!"

I guess there's a part of me that wants everybody to be happy, all the time and I want everybody to like me all the time. And one of my biggest challenges is speaking the truth when it's uncomfortable and I know I'm not alone in this, so that's the big challenge for me is to figure out how to ... how to be fully myself even when it's uncomfortable. So one of my best skills is to squish myself into whatever shape is necessary to keep everybody peaceful and keep everything quiet.

[MR] *Like being adjusted.*

[TH] I have been in adjustments that were so painful that I was just quietly crying, never spoke out, never called out, never said anything. I guess that's the freeze part, isn't it? Flight or freeze.

There's the belief that this person who's your teacher must know more than you, right? So maybe it's a good thing, right? Probably a great thing and then you realize, "No, wait. There's a muscle ripped. Or no wait. My heart is broken."

PERSONAL PAIN, STRUCTURAL HARM

There is no way of telling how many women in total were assaulted by Jois over his three-decade-long international career. As Jubilee Cooke points out, he might have committed tens of thousands of individual criminal acts.

These crimes, of course, are in the past. At the time they were shielded from accountability by group dynamics and an unfamiliar or uninviting policing system in Mysore. Now they are legally eclipsed by statutes of limitations and the death of Jois. Many of them were committed against students who were only briefly involved with the group, or who have since moved on. What relationship do they have with the much larger global population of people who continue to love and practice Jois's yoga? Should current students who are doing just fine in the present care about the past? Are *they* responsible for something? Isn't Jois dead and gone? Aren't the experiences of Karen and Tracy vanishingly rare in terms of intensity and impact? Aren't they really just private nightmares, after all, that they should work out in therapy?

Part Three of the book will show how those private nightmares were both enabled and reinforced by social mechanisms, in ways that stretch far beyond the personal betrayals evident in the material we've just covered. Simply put: Jois would not have had the power he exerted over Karen and Tracy and many others were there not a support structure that rendered him beyond reproach. That support structure included the intimate networks of relationships that, in places, exhibited cultic qualities. It also included an outer layer of market legitimacy, broadcast through reams of literature devoted to the promotion of Jois's method and wholesomeness. That literature remains in place today, largely unchallenged, intersectional with other industry discourses that can manipulate the credulity of practitioners for profit. I'll be using the term "propaganda" to describe aspects of this genre.

How does the typical Ashtanga practitioner relate to the propaganda of the core community, from the media stars who describe Jois as a saint, to the videos that claim his method will cure diseases, to the books that assert his method is unchanged from ancient times? It's hard to say.

Consider the group of practitioners that gather every morning in a room close to London Bridge to be guided through the sequences by Scott Johnson. Scott arrives before dawn and lights incense and a candle in front of a picture of his late co-founder, Ozge, who died in a tragic accident. Students file in in silence, unroll their mats, and start to breathe and move as the light gathers. They come from all over: Europe, the Middle East, Asia.

Scott teaches them what he's learned from his own teacher, who was certified by Jois in the 1990s. But Scott has never been to Mysore and has no plans on going. Intuitively, he has learned over the years that gentleness should be the guiding principle in the application of adjustments. There was no formal discussion of consent when he began, but now the culture is buzzing with it. As his work with the new training cooperative "Amayu" shows (p. 237), he's taking it in, and taking action on it.

There's no bookshop in his rented space and nothing on his website that references Jois, although the daily classes are called Ashtanga yoga Mysore classes. Many of his students won't have heard of the method's founder, nor would they care about him. They're there because they love the movement, the room, the way it starts and centers their day, and Scott's affable presence.

If Scott's students' main connection to Ashtanga yoga comes through their relationship with him, does the propaganda of the Ashtanga inner core impact them at all? Not consciously, perhaps. But materially, it might. Whether they know or care about who Jois is, Scott's students have a place to come in large part because of the cultural power broadcast by Jois. And if they ever come to be interested in the source, it will be close at hand, just a few web-browser clicks away.

Consider also the rank-and-file practitioners who study with authorized or certified teachers who keep commitments to the memory of Jois that Scott doesn't. These students may have as little interest in Jois as Scott's students have. But they are in a strange position. Through their teachers, their fees are effectively tithed to Mysore, inasmuch as the teachers must maintain their positions by traveling regularly, at great expense, to study with Sharath Rangaswamy. People don't have to be emotionally invested in a high-demand group with an unresolved abuse history to be financially supporting it.

Perhaps the loosely self-identified Ashtanga practitioner is to Mysore as the typical consumer is to the abuses of global capitalism. Until you really look at where your food comes from, you'll just consume and enjoy it. Part of waking up to the reality of the world and our relationships—if that's what yoga means to us—would be starting to ask questions about where things come from, and why they have power, and what are the hidden costs of consuming them.

Dimi Currey is one of those Ashtanga practitioners who caught the Ashtanga wave after Jois died. Reading Karen Rain's testimony, however, made her think deeply about why she had been able to encounter Ashtanga yoga at all, and what her responsibilities might include, moving forward. "These women's suffering," she wrote on Facebook,

> is as much a part of why we have Ashtanga today, as David Williams', or Norman Allen's contributions. [Williams and Allen are early Jois students.]
>
> If these women had filed charges back then (and there were some that wanted to), maybe the system would not have spread as it has? These women suffered through it, in some ways sacrificing themselves for what seemed to be a greater cause. And the system has lived on.
>
> Now those women who were hurt, would like the wrongs done to them to be recognized. It doesn't seem like any of them are out to publicly shame others regarding the situation. Only that their suffering be recognized, so that steps can be taken to insure that others are not hurt as they were.
>
> I think there should be some action—very clear action taken to recognize this. I think it should become part of the history of the lineage. It is the truth. History is supposed to be factual.
>
> So, maybe we should know the faces and names of these women who were hurt by P. Jois, but carried on the lineage? Because, it is in part due to their suffering that we have Ashtanga today. Maybe instead of his picture in studios, on altars, etc. maybe it is their pictures that belong there.[60]

"History is supposed to be factual," Currey writes. Regretfully, that is often not the case, as those writing history can have their own biases or agendas. **Part Three** of the book will clarify some aspects of Ashtanga history, which, like the stories of the women, have been distorted to serve the group. The analysis is offered in the belief that one cannot mature—intellectually, psychologically, or spiritually—if one is being lied to.

Refuting the claims of a high-demand group relies on critical sources that come from outside of the group. **Part Three** will examine the wider circle of deception cast by Ashtanga literature by measuring its claims against scholarship and reports from those who have no investment in Jois's legacy.

PART THREE

Developing Discernment

The world is full of falsehood, deceit, and exploitation. A yogi has the power to correct this and to attract people of the world to the right path.

— *Pattabhi Jois*[61]

My God, everybody knew.

—*Beryl Bender Birch, author of Power Yoga, remembering Jois assaulting women in 1987*[62]

"NO ONE JOINS A CULT"

Whether loosely or tightly-bounded, temporary or long-lived, every high-demand group thrives on deception.[63] The high-demand group can be deceptive about what its intentions are, and what its leader and core followers are doing. It can be deceptive about the origins of its teaching content. It can be deceptive about money, and the benefits of its programs. It can be deceptive about its history.

Understanding how this deception works can vastly reduce the amount of shame and guilt associated with cult awareness, recovery, and analysis. Like reclaiming the word "victim", emphasizing the deceptive strategies of the high-demand group can help the group member assign responsibility where it belongs as they transition to the outside world. The fact is: one is never to blame for being deceived.

"No one joins a cult," says Cathleen Mann. "They delay leaving organizations that misrepresented themselves."

Mann's MIND model[64]—**m**anipulation, **i**ndoctrination, **n**egation, and **d**eception—describes many of the group dynamics we'll see at play in this part of the book: how a group manipulates and manages the impressions that members have of it, how it fudges its facts and history, how it denigrates the ego and assures conformity to a teaching without question, how it denies the reality of members' experiences, how it wears down resistance through changes to diet, sleeping patterns, and physical activity. Deception, however, is the lynchpin.

"Without deception," Mann writes, "no one would affiliate or stay. Termed the true hallmark of a cult, deception prevents critical thinking and good decision making. Deception is not prevented by intelligence or rational thought, but is maintained by emotions, fear, and isolation."

To take the position that accepts the narratives of "New Religious Movements" in their own terms only *could involve ignoring or even indulging a means—deception—by which the group maintains its potentially harmful control over members*. It might miss the possibility that members are only members in the first place because they have been deceived. This position may be good for reporting on what a person says they felt about their practice of Ashtanga yoga under Pattabhi Jois in Mysore, while having nothing to say about whether those feelings were manipulated. It tells us little about whether faith has been allowed to evolve in good faith.

When I was in a Buddhist cult, I tolerated all kinds of social dysfunction and abuse because the leader misrepresented himself and his material. A critical mass of followers, including me, was deceived. I believed he was teaching a rare and precious truth about human life that had been passed down in an unadulterated form from medieval Tibetan sages. I did not enter the group with any of the tools I would have needed to evaluate that belief. The leader convincingly presented himself and what he taught as authentic, and I believed him. I lived that belief passionately. It directed my daily experience, and was reinforced by practices like "guru yoga", in which I was to meditate on the enlightened nature of the lineage—and the leader himself—in rituals repeated several times per day.

Interviewing me back then as a member of a "New Religious Movement", a researcher basing their study solely on a member's internal experience might have gathered rich information about how these beliefs, reinforced by group practice, affected my work, finances, diet, political will, relationships, sex life, and even dreams. But they may not have considered that they could study how this web of commitments was simultaneously harming me through emotional, financial, and labor manipulation. They would probably have assumed that I was freely participating in a movement that spoke to my needs and values. But the truth is that the group spoke to my needs and values only because it had convinced me that it did.

In fact, the group actually *programed into me* needs and values I didn't previously have. Only six months into my relationship with the group, I firmly believed that I was working my way out of a meaningless, mundane existence towards successive levels of enlightenment, and that my progress would be accelerated to the extent that I viewed the leader and his inner circle as divine beings that were guiding me. Further, any negative experience I had in relation to them was the projection of my own delusional mind. It took me three years to remember my pre-indoctrinated state, and to see that beneath the trappings of religious authenticity, the leader was an intellectual, emotional, and sexual manipulator.

No one is free when they are being lied to. I'm much freer and happier with my critical thinking restored, but there has been a cost. My psyche remains heavily armored against the possibility of being deceived. This makes it difficult to remain open to the intuitive, aspirational, and imaginary aspects of life.

This is what I think of when I hear the term "spiritual abuse". I lost six years of my life to the high-demand groups I was in. I suffered physical, economic, emotional, relational, and cognitive deficits for years afterwards. But the thing that hurts the most to this day is the wound of cynicism, ever-present, like a door standing perpetually open to distrust and melancholy.

When I close that door, I can feel a cozy innocence return in flashes. It happens quite clearly in relation to echoes of my childhood self, as I engage with my sons. As I read things like *Harry Potter* to my eldest. I'm safe joining him in J.K. Rowling's fantastical world, which asks nothing of me but attention and wonder. She uses fiction, transparently, to tell a truth. Spiritual abusers use truth manipulatively to bend their followers to their will.

The uncertainty I may share with some former students of Jois and other abusers in the yoga world regards whether and how spiritual abuse can be prevented, if it cannot be repaired.

DECEPTION AND ITS ROLE IN "BOUNDED REALITY"

Deceptions about Jois and the Ashtanga technique helped to create and maintain power over those he abused. His disciples described him along a spectrum of idealizations ranging from spiritual teacher to Tantric master to fatherly caregiver. Many said that his physical touch was healing. His method was "traditional" or "ancient", and governed by the sacred etiquette of the teacher–student (*guru–shishya parampara*) relationship. The Sanskrit here implies a lineage of teacher (*guru*)–student (*shishya*) transmission that links back (*parampara*) to a source of prehistoric wisdom. These beliefs formed a strong part of lived experience for many Ashtanga yoga practitioners. They granted certainty, a sense of validity, of the tried-and-true. To this day, they continue to invoke safety and trust for many.

What is the status of beliefs that arise out of deception? What are we to do when we find out that the marketing of a practice as "ancient" and "traditional" is not true—or worse, has manipulated us? What are we to do when we find out that a community believes in the wholesomeness of its founder because the founder's key disciples have suppressed the fact that he was sex offender? What are we to do when we start to see that that suppression may have been part of what allowed those same disciples to build lucrative careers?

People are harmed when they are deceived. They put their bodies into positions they otherwise wouldn't, they give their money and time and emotional labor to people they'd otherwise stay away from, they endorse and even campaign for worldviews that they would otherwise reject. Some will even learn to harm underlings as they climb the ladder of influence. The more they are deceived, the more harm they may tolerate, and inflict.

When interpersonal deception scales up to a systems level as an organizing mechanism of a high-demand group, it becomes difficult for members to gain access to alternative points of view. Add charismatic authority, a transcendent belief system, systems of control, and systems of influence—the four ingredients that researcher Janja Lalich describes as being at the heart of cultic dynamics—and the member's reality becomes smaller still. "Leaders and members alike," writes Lalich, "are locked into what I call a 'bounded reality'— that is, a self-sealing social system in which every aspect and every activity reconfirms the validity of the system. There is no place for disconfirming information or other ways of thinking or being."[65]

Lalich agrees with most researchers who suggest that one of the most powerful ways in which members can break out of this self-sealing feedback loop is to expose themselves to outside influences who can provide a reality check against the ways in which they have been misled. For Jubilee Cooke, whom Jois assaulted repeatedly in 1997, a space away from the deceptive, "bounded reality" of the Lakshmipuram shala was provided by local friends she made in Mysore, friends who had zero investment in Jois as any kind of special person.

LISTENING TO MYSOREANS

Jubilee Cooke traveled from Seattle to Mysore in the same year that Tracy did, after learning the Ashtanga method at the same Seattle studio. In July 2018, she published her detailed, first-person account of being assaulted by Jois in many of the same ways reported by Karen Rain and T.M. I edited the piece for publication on the independent blog site *Decolonizing Yoga* after the managing editor at *Yoga Journal* showed initial interest, but ultimately turned it down. This is an important detail to be taken up later, because, as we'll see, Cooke specifically cites a 1995 issue of *Yoga Journal* as a key encouragement for her trip to Mysore. That part of her story points to a crucial, if unconscious, collusion between mainstream yoga media platforms and systems of abuse and silencing.

Cooke's account is remarkable not only for its breadth and clarity but also because she takes pains to fill in an important gap: How did local Mysoreans regard Jois? How would they respond to reports of his abuse? Did any of the apologist remarks around "cultural differences" creating misunderstanding between Jois and his women students hold merit?

Cooke's stance on the issue flows from her cultural immersion in south Indian culture. She had spent years studying Hindustani music with Indian teachers on her way to attaining a PhD in ethnomusicology. She hung out with local folks when she wasn't at the Jois shala.

"After yoga practice", she writes,

> I would spend most of my afternoons at a small shop that sold writing supplies. The shop was run by a family that my yoga teachers [from Seattle] had befriended. My teachers had told me that this family could help me find a Hindustani music teacher. The parents were originally from northern India. Both the father and an adult son were amateur musicians. I also met the mother and two other young adult daughters. Since I had studied some Hindi at university and made a trip to northern India for further language training a few years earlier, I was able to have basic, slow-paced conversations with the mother who did not speak English, but could understand it. On most days, I would visit with the family for hours and was scolded when I did not show. One day I shared with the family how Pattabhi Jois was adjusting me, touching my breasts and genitals. The mother became very upset. In Hindi, she began, "You tell him…" Then, for the first and only time I ever heard her speak English, she said emphatically, "Don't touch my body!" I was not brave enough to comply with her imperative and confront Pattabhi Jois, but her words made a deep impression that gave me vital inner protection.
>
> That summer Pattabhi Jois was charging over $300 per month for the morning classes, and the price continued to rise. When I shared the amount with the family at the shop, they were shocked. To give some perspective, the Mysuru family told me that if I worked full-time for them, I would be lucky to receive the equivalent of $1 per day.
>
> This little stall-like shop was a regular meeting place for many friends. During my afternoon visits, I met several local professional musicians and others, including a banker and a journalist for the local paper. One day, the journalist stopped by, and the family shared with him how Pattabhi Jois was touching me and how much he was charging for lessons. The journalist left the shop with a new mission, saying, "I'm going to write an exposé." That was the last I saw of him, and I doubt he ever wrote the article, given that I was his only informant. Please note, however, that no one at the shop

> defended Jois's behavior or told me that I didn't understand what he was doing because of cultural differences or suggested that I had somehow "asked for it" by not wearing enough clothing. In fact, all of these residents of Mysuru condemned it.

***

Jubilee's Mysore friends weren't the only locals who condemned Jois. His next-door neighbor, Dr K.R.I. Jagadish, had a lot to say as well. His apprentice, Cyril Martin, heard about my research and reached out with his own stories about the Ashtanga students who would come to see his boss, known as Dr. "Jag".

From 2009 through 2014, Martin apprenticed at Jag Therapy, a physiotherapy clinic in Lakshmipuram. Martin said that the clinic treated KPJAYI students for broken vertebrae, shoulder and hip tears, and, in one astounding case, a vaginal tear similar to those that can occur during childbirth. Martin was continually flummoxed that the patients seemed to want treatment only so that they could get back to the shala and practice their extreme contortions.

Jagadish is in his eighties, and doesn't mince words.

"Pattabhi Jois was my neighbor in Lakshmipuram," he said. "He became famous when Madonna became his student. His students came to me right from the beginning. The ashram, the yoga shala was right next door to me."

In 1994, after 30 years of studying traditional medicine throughout South Asia, Jag returned to his home city of Mysore and opened his clinic. In 1996, he moved to a location across the street from Jois's Ashtanga Yoga Institute. Jag explained that he knew Jois well through his grandmother, whom, he said, also studied yoga with Krishnamacharya back in the day. Jois's students came to him for soft tissue massage and physiotherapy. He was very concerned about the injuries.

"In fact, I went to see Pattabhi Jois about this when he was alive and I just spoke to him," says Jag. "I said: 'This is really ridiculous. Creating Ashtanga yoga is a gimmick. You are destroying the beautiful art of our yoga, turning it into something which is very vicious and causing so much injury.'"

"So you just said all of that to your neighbor?" I asked.

"Yes. And you know what the answer was to me? 'You give me that money, and I will stop teaching.'

"He was charging about $600 per student per month, and there are 60 students in one class with one instructor. How do you expect safety of the patients, safety of the students?"

"Do you think he was joking with that answer?"

"He was getting a lot of money. He said 'People want this kind of hardness, and I am providing it, and they are paying me. If you provide me that money, I will stop teaching.' So he was a greedy man."

I wondered if that was the only conversation they had.

"That was the only conversation I had," Jag said, "because there was no point in arguing with such a bad man, who was so stubborn. I respected him a lot before I knew him doing his Ashtanga because he was one of the authorities on yoga. No doubt about it, Pattabhi Jois was a genius, but perverted. His depth of knowledge about yoga was unparalleled."

I asked Jag whether he'd heard of Jois touching women inappropriately.

"Oh yes, a lot. That is true. I have a lot of stories of women who came to me after his way of teaching. They were very unhappy, and at the same time, they became almost like slaves to him."

Jag got particularly prickly about what he saw as Jois's blatant disregard for the health of his students. He claimed that his daughter's sister-in-law had gone to Jois for lessons, and that he'd injured her spine by sitting down on her while she was in a posture.

"He never asked any student of his whether they were fit to do the yoga. He never examined them, he never consulted with them, no physical or medical examination was conducted. For everyone he said, 'You continue practice and it will all disappear.'"

I asked Jag if he felt that Jois was unaware of the value of medical care, or if he should have known better.

"He was unaware, and he should have known better. If he sent half the patients [for examination], they would not come back to him as students. It was greed. He was a master of yoga. Beyond that, nothing else."

Was there any local authority to which he could have reported Jois?

"This man could not be sued. In India, anyone can become a 'Guruji.' The mob mentality doesn't help. I went to see him with the intention of making his mistakes known to the public, but it was a failure."

I asked Jag what would have happened if a complaint had been made to the Mysore police. He described one incident in which another Mysore yoga teacher had been accused of sexual assault. He was arrested and charged. The case went on for three years, and the teacher was found not guilty.

"The police do take action. The problem is: where are the students who go there? They become slaves of him. I don't know whether it is due to mesmerism or a hypnotic approach. Students would go when he was alive and bow down and kiss his feet and all sorts of nonsense. Nobody expects such treatment."

I asked whether Jois was shown such deference outside of his own ashram. Jag said that out in the market he would have been treated as an ordinary man, except by a Western student, who would have bowed down. I asked if this would that be a source of embarrassment to him in front of fellow Mysoreans?"

"No, he would think that was his greatness. He would think he was almighty. Depressing to see that such a wonderful art is being distorted, and created demons out of it."

YOGA BELIEFS, YOGA MARKETING, YOGA KNOWLEDGE

Claims about the healing powers of yoga teachers and their methods are by no means unique in the modern yoga scene. Yet they've been a key feature of an exploding, unregulated, global industry, fueled by the wellness aspirations of seekers, and the projected mystique of charismatic masculinity.

B.K.S. Iyengar's *Light on Yoga*, originally published in 1966, features unsubstantiated medical claims on almost every page.[66] By the time he was in his seventies, he was offering "Medical Classes" around the world, despite having received no formal medical education at all.[67] Disciples of Bikram yoga say that his 26 postures can heal many diseases. Swami Satyananda implied that his practice of "Yoga Nidra" was derived from ancient texts.[*68] Yogi Bhajan claimed that his Kundalini yoga method recovered the lost yoga of Sikhism.[69] John Friend of Anusara yoga claimed that he'd discovered or synthesized five "Universal Principles of Alignment".[70]

Factoids are fascinating, but they shouldn't distract from the basic impact of deception. "People are free to believe what they want," cult expert Cathleen Mann says. "Beliefs are not the point. The point is how people use beliefs to treat each other. Cults can be political, secular, or religious in nature. The content doesn't matter."[71]

Mann asserts that the beliefs held by high-demand or cultic groups are inconsequential compared to the *mechanisms* by which they assert control over members. To focus on the content marketed by a high-demand group is to indulge a mirage. It sensationalizes and distances the group's activities from so-called "normal" observers. "Focusing on the beliefs," Mann writes, "reinforces the 'not me' syndrome."

There are two other things to be clear about. First—and to repeat—an

* It most likely was not.

examination of whether something is deceptive does not speak to whether that deception is intentional. Dead or alive, the inner lives and intentions of Jois, Iyengar, Choudhury, and the rest are forever uncertain. They may or may not earnestly believe in their claims and the helpfulness of those claims. What matters are the impacts that their claims have on the credulity of their followers, and how that credulity can be manipulated.

Secondly—and what makes things tricky—is that the credulity of yoga practitioners can also be mobilized in *helpful* ways that an unrelenting skepticism or demand for empirical proof might overlook. We have to look carefully at where inspiration is spurred on by myth or hyperbole, and allow for the fact that this works for some people. The answer to the fact that magic can be manipulated cannot be to outlaw magic.

Many practitioners, disillusioned with the depersonalization of contemporary science and medicine, are earnestly drawn to the "pre-modern" values and techniques of traditional yoga cultures. They long for transcendent promises and ways of knowing. So when, for example, Iyengar fills his books with unsupported promises of cures, his apparent overreach reflects aspects of aspirational teaching that may irritate scientists, but attract those who recognize that scientific knowledge is only one way of understanding reality.

By claiming that a certain posture treats diabetes or strengthens the liver, for instance, a figure like Iyengar may be drawing on a cultural knowledge that has been repeated so often it doesn't need to be traced back to any source. The source—and implicitly the validity of the claim—is established not by citation but through an older form of peer-review: a heritage of communal sharing. Additionally, some modern Indian teachers may have been employing an old convention of emphasis that used flowery rhetoric and hyperbole to provoke the student to reach beyond the mundane with images and commands they are unlikely to forget. An oral culture staple, this technique can be more performative than definitive, used to break lethargy and inspire action at a critical initial stage of personal development.[72] Iyengar would have absorbed this way of teaching through many sources, including the style of his own teacher Krishnamacharya, who openly claimed that certain postures could cure "all diseases",[73] but demurred from the more fantastic claims of medieval yoga literature, in which certain breathing techniques were said to make a yogi 16 years young again,[74] and specialized asanas sublimate subtle energies towards the goal of immortality.

In contemporary terms, there is an aspirational element to older forms of yoga pedagogy that is not only historically authentic but might also be benign. Overreaching claims might play a positive role in fostering the placebo or "meaning" effect, in which patients, clients or students feel more positive about their lives and therefore report better health outcomes because they have been held in a sphere of hope and possibility.[75] The difference between promise and poison may only be a matter of dosage.

So to be clear, focusing on the deceptions of certain claims made in the name of Ashtanga yoga does not imply malice or deny the power of the hopeful aspiration. It is to find those places where aspiration crosses the line into dishonesty and where magnanimity crosses the line into grandiosity. Like a well-dispensed sugar pill, things that are untrue can be helpful, for a while, within circumstances of care. But untrue things can embolden and justify those parts of a culture that are not committed to care so much as to marketing and income.

Some of the analysis that follows might seem academic and nit-picky. That's part of the problem: endless discussions, usually between men, about the origins and authenticity of not only Ashtanga yoga but also many other modern yoga methods have effectively distracted practitioners and researchers from more obvious things, like reports that Jois assaulted women in public spaces for decades with impunity. Taking the time to show the web of white lies, overreaches, fudges, and deceptions—whether aspirational or grandiose—helps us to understand how Jois's assault victims were intellectually groomed. By showing a common pathway by which victims were inducted into credulity, it is possible to see why many students like T.M. found it hard to push back against being told that Jois's groping was "not sexual".

The following zones of deception concerning where Ashtanga practice came from, the "tradition" that it was transmitting, and the values it offered do three things.

1. They set the student up to accept abuse under the guise of an authentic spirituality and proven history of care.
2. They make the abuse itself something more likely to be denied by both members and victims in order to lessen cognitive dissonance.
3. They surround the enabling culture with a halo of credibility, which makes the denial of abuse more effective.

THE STRANGE CASE OF THE *YOGA KORUNTA*

"Guruji has often spoken about a text called the *Yoga Korunta*, an ancient manuscript on Ashtanga yoga, which had been the basis of the practical lessons on yoga taught to him by Krishnamacharya." So writes Jois disciple Eddie Stern in the Foreword to *Yoga Mala*, Jois's signature practice manual.[76]

> Attributed to the sage Vamana, it was one of the many texts taught orally to Krishnamacharya, which he learned by heart during the seven and a half years he spent living with his teacher, Rama Mohan Brahmachari. Korunta means "groups," and the text was said to contain lists of many different groupings of asanas, as well as highly original teachings on vinyasa, drishti, bandhas, mudras, and philosophy. Before Krishnamacharya was sent off into the world to teach, around 1924, he was told that he could find this text in the Calcutta University Library. According to Guruji, who has never seen the text and doubted that it still exists, Krishnamacharya spent some time in Calcutta researching this book, which was badly damaged and had many missing portions. When Guruji began his studies with Krishnamacharya in 1927, it was the methods from the *Yoga Korunta* that he was taught. Although the authenticity of the book would be extremely difficult, if not impossible, to validate today, it is generally accepted that this is the source of Ashtanga yoga as taught by Pattabhi Jois.

Independent researcher and yoga practitioner James Dylan Russell summarizes the legend. "In the mid-1920s … Sri T. Krishnamacharya went to the Calcutta library accompanied by a young and earnest student named K. Pattabhi Jois." Together they found the ancient *Korunta*, and saw that its banana/palm leaves were:

> bound with an ancient edition of the *Yoga Sutra* of Patanjali (a 2000 year old treatise on the psychological technology of yoga). This system is known as Ashtanga Yoga (meaning eight-limbed yoga) … the two systems were therefore intended to be practiced and studied together. Hence the name 'Ashtanga Vinyasa'.
>
> Having deciphered the text, Krishnamacharya taught the method to Pattabhi Jois. The final part of the story is that the *Korunta* soon-after disintegrated, and/or was consumed by ants (not implausible in

> the Indian climate): never to be seen again by anyone other than Krishnamacharya and Pattabhi Jois. It is thought to have been a unique copy.[77]

Ashtanga Deep Throat muddies the water further. By email, he reports asking Jois sometime in the 1980s about whether he'd seen the original *Yoga Korunta*. Jois replied that he had. But Amma, Jois's wife, scolded him into a fuller disclosure. Jois reportedly backtracked to say that Krishnamacharya had copied the text by hand in the Calcutta library, and that was the copy that Jois had seen. Jois in turn had copied that copy, and Jois's copy was still extant in his voluminous library above the yoga shala, although he'd never shown it to anyone.

The accounts show how hopes and dreams can overcompensate for a fragmented history. Stern is invoking ancient Vedic times when he cites "Sage Vamana". But the most recent scholarship shows that that there is no available scriptural, architectural, or artistic evidence to suggest that the sequences of Krishnamacharya existed prior to the 20th century.[78]

The assertion that Krishnamacharya learned his method from Ramamohana over seven and a half years is challenged by the investigations of yoga scholar David Gordon White. White shows that even if Ramamohana existed, it is impossible that Krishnamacharya spent that amount of time with him (in Nepal, Tibet, or Tamil Nadu, depending on who Krishnamacharya was telling the story to), given the distances he must have traveled on foot, the seasons in which he must have traveled, and claims made about simultaneous other travels in conflicting biographical notes.[79]

Russell's telling would have us believe that at the age of the twelve, having just met Krishnamacharya, Jois journeyed with him for over 2,000 km from south India to find the text in Calcutta. Jois himself says nothing about any such research adventure in any autobiographical account I'm aware of. Through Russell, we are also meant to think that finding the asana instruction manual anachronistically bound with a copy of Patanjali suggests that the books are as intrinsic to each other as lock and key. The binding suggests the meditation insights of the *Yoga Sutras* cannot be accessed without the practice of the flowing postures of the *Yoga Korunta*, and vice versa. But the two books might have simply been owned by the same person who at one point bound them together for convenience.

Does, or did, the *Yoga Korunta* exist at all? Sankritist Jason Birch has spent the last decade undertaking an exhaustive review of the medieval *hathayoga* literature to which the modern yoga movement appeals for its sense of antiquity.

He notes that the *Yoga Korunta* is cited by Krishnamacharya's most famous students, including his son and grandson, as well as B.K.S. Iyengar and Jois. But "despite the prominence of the *Yoga Korunta* in this lineage," he writes, "no one has produced a copy of it. My research has not located a name similar to *Yoga Kurunta* in any catalogue of an Indian manuscript library."[80] Birch does, however, link the book to an undated—likely 18th century—compilation of practice instructions that Krishnamacharya most probably knew about through a 19th century compendium. The unpublished manuscript, which is called the *Hathabhyasapaddhati*, is attributed to a writer named Kapalakuruntaka (a possible source for the word "Korunta" in *Yoga Korunta)*, and details 112 postures. It does not mention vinyasa or the sun salutation (both crucial to the Jois method) but "there are what one might call 'linking' postures," writes Birch, "a strong emphasis on movement in the asana practice and postures similar to the up and down dog poses."[81]

"*Yoga Korunta* is one of a number of 'lost' texts that became central to Krishnamacharya's teaching," summarizes yoga scholar Mark Singleton, politely. "Sri Nathamuani's *Yoga Rahasya*, which Krishnamacharya received in a vision at the age of sixteen, is another.... It is entirely possible that the *Yoga Korunta* was a similarly 'inspired' text, attributed to a legendary ancient sage to lend it the authority of tradition."[82]

That lending has been so successful that senior Jois students like Guy Donahaye are able to speak about the book as though they have not only read it, but compared it to similar texts. But this is impossible, given the specialized education and access to unpublished manuscripts such a claim would require. "There are several unique features to the system presented in the *Yoga Korunta*," writes Donahaye, "especially insofar as it integrates philosophy and practice with detailed explanations of how the practice of asanas and pranayamas should be performed."[83]

"Texts such as the *Hathabhyasapaddhati*," write Birch, "do teach the practice of many asanas and pranayama with unprecedented detail. However, they do not integrate philosophy."[84]

Is there a relationship between the asana instructions reportedly contained in the *Yoga Korunta* and the *Yoga Sutras*? Singleton suggests that:

> such assertions can be better considered as symptomatic of the post hoc grafting of modern asana practice onto the perceived "Patanjali tradition" (as it was constituted through Orientalist scholarship and the modern Indian yoga renaissance) rather than as historical indications of the ancient roots of a dynamic postural system called Ashtanga yoga. In accounts such as these, a talismanic Patanjali provides the source authority and legitimation for the radically gymnastic asana practice that predominates modern yoga today. Indeed, it is telling that according to one Mysuru resident who studied these practices with Pattabhi Jois in the 1960s... the name "Ashtanga Vinyasa" was applied to the system only after the arrival of the first American students in the 1970s. Prior to this, Jois had simply referred to his teaching as "asana."[85]

Singleton and other scholars have faced considerable backlash over their research. In social media flame wars, they are regularly painted as misinformed neo-colonialists out to debunk the historically authentic transmissions of Indian masters.[86] But the late T.K.V. Desikachar, Krishnamacharya's second of three sons, once told an interviewer: "My father never acknowledged that he discovered anything even when I have seen that it was he who discovered it." Desikachar was an innovator himself, having almost single-handedly inspired the now-globalized yoga therapy movement based on the work of his father, but also influenced by his cosmopolitan and interdisciplinary cohort of followers.

"[Krishnamacharya] has discovered postures," he said,

> but he would say that it was his teacher who taught him. Rarely had he said that it was his "original work." At the same time, I have seen him—because I am his son also—composing some verses and correcting those verses for the *chandas* [meter of verses in Sanskrit poetry] and all that and finally saying—"This is what Nathamuni [a mythical sage in the family's religious heritage] is saying and this is what my teacher says!" I tend to think that Nathamuni's *Yoga Rahasya* that he taught us is quite likely to be a combination of his own commentary and the lessons he received, though he would not accept it.[87]

ON THE ANTIQUITY OF "VINYASA" AND THE SEQUENCES

If the source of Jois's teaching is as symbolically powerful as it is historically unclear, what can we say about its content?

"In the ancient treatise," writes Ashtanga teacher Gregor Maehle, referring to the *Yoga Korunta*,

> *vinyasa* refers to every counted movement, accompanied by breath and focal point. The vinyasa count is a format in which the Rishi Vamana recorded the Ashtanga practice. Each movement that is needed to enter and exit a posture in the traditional way is counted.[88]

The work of Sanskritist Jason Birch and yoga scholar Jacqueline Hargreaves, which draws on an exhaustive survey of the Sanskrit literature, casts doubt on this presentation.

> The term vinyasa rarely occurs in medieval yoga texts. However, it does appear more frequently in the ritual sections of medieval Tantras. Nonetheless, never does the term vinyasa mean the movement that links breath with postures (asana) as is the case in modern yoga.[89]

AG Mohan, one of Krishnamacharya's most venerated students, writes that

> A special feature of the asana system of Krishnamacharya was vinyasa. Many yoga students today are no doubt familiar with this word—it is increasingly used now, often to describe the "style" of a yoga class, as in "hatha vinyasa" or "vinyasa flow." Vinyasa is essential, and probably unique, to Krishnamacharya's teachings. As far as I know, he was the first yoga master in the last century to introduce this idea. A vinyasa, in essence, consists of moving from one asana, or body position, to another, combining breathing with the movement.[90]

Some researchers of Krishnamacharya suggest that he used the word *vinyasa* to refer to the "arrangement" of the postures into series. "This is a valid meaning of the word," writes Birch by email, "but nonetheless does not occur in premodern yoga texts with this meaning in the context of asana, as far as I know."[91]

If textual support for the historical validity of Jois's Ashtanga yoga is difficult to find, and the centerpiece of his method—the vinyasa as a counted series of movements connecting one posture to another—is a 20th century invention, what about Jois's series, or the ordered groups, increasing in difficulty, in which his postures are meant to be practiced? Some of Jois's prominent students believed that the series had remained unchanged from Krishnamacharya's day.

"He is constantly referring to scriptural evidence," Nick Evans told an interviewer, "almost as though he is simply a vessel for the teaching that he received from his guru and his family guru. He's very clear that he is simply passing on methods and techniques that were passed on to him unchanged."[92]

Some of his oldest students endow the series with even more antiquity. "As I understood it," David Williams told an interviewer in 2001, "this series can be chanted move by move, breath by breath in Sanskrit. It's an exact formula that goes back thousands of years and has been time-tested to be the most efficient way that one can get themselves fit." Williams is one of Jois's oldest non-Indian students. He's practiced the Ashtanga method daily for over 40 years. This is possibly longer than Jois himself practiced it.

"After practicing more and more years," he says,

> I realize the perfection of the ordering of the postures. I say now that it's like a combination lock. If you do the numbers in order, the lock will open. If you just do any numbers, nothing happens. I feel this is the way with yoga practice. If you do the yoga practice in a certain order, your body and your mind open up. If you just do random yoga like is taught in so many places, it's much less efficient. So the greater amount of times I practice, the more I appreciate the order of the series. When I teach people, I try to teach them exactly the way I was taught and try not to modernize it in any way.[93]

Indications point to Williams being more faithful to an imagined antiquity than Jois ever was. As yet, there has been no definitive scholarship that tracks the evolution of Jois's series in response to the demands of his first job at the Mysore Yoga Shala under the supervision of Krishnamacharya, and later the needs of his non-Indian students. But according to Ashtanga historian Anthony Hall, Jois made no fewer than ten key changes to the series he learned from his teacher.[94] Of those ten, half involved shortened breath or fewer breaths and shorter stays in each posture. The changes trimmed the length of the average practice time. Many senior students say that these changes, along with an increase in standardization, were intended to relieve congestion and simplify teaching responsibilities in the increasingly lucrative Mysore shala, as traffic exploded in the 1980s and 1990s.

IS ASHTANGA YOGA A PARAMPARA?

"When I teach people, I try to teach them exactly the way I was taught and try not to modernize it in any way." With this, David Williams is pointing towards the archetypal concept of *parampara*, a mechanism of sacred preservation, transmission, authorization, and exclusion in Indian wisdom traditions. The Sanskrit term is most often translated as "lineage", a word used to describe everything from a distinct spiritual heritage to a collection of branded techniques. Sharath Rangaswamy lays out the concept of *parampara* in detail on the Institute's website, which has recently changed its URL to *sharathjois.com* to reflect Rangaswamy's adopted name.

> *Parampara* is knowledge that is passed in succession from teacher to student. It is a Sanskrit word that denotes the principle of transmitting knowledge in its most valuable form; knowledge based on direct and practical experience. It is the basis of any lineage: the teacher and student form the links in the chain of instruction that has been passed down for thousands of years. In order for yoga instruction to be effective, true and complete, it should come from within parampara.
>
> Knowledge can be transferred only after the student has spent many years with an experienced guru, a teacher to whom he has completely surrendered in body, mind, speech and inner being. Only then is he fit to receive knowledge. This transfer from teacher to student is parampara.
>
> The dharma, or duty, of the student is to practice diligently and to strive to understand the teachings of the guru. The perfection of knowledge—and of yoga—lies beyond simply mastering the practice; knowledge grows from the mutual love and respect between student and teacher, a relationship that can only be cultivated over time.

> The teacher's dharma is to teach yoga exactly as he learned it from his guru. The teaching should be presented with a good heart, with good purpose and with noble intentions. There should be an absence of harmful motivations. The teacher should not mislead the student in any way or veer from what he has been taught.[95]

Rangaswamy makes three main points. First, *parampara* is both knowledge and the means of transmitting it. (The word is like "yoga" in this sense, indicating both a state and a practice.) Secondly, a *parampara* is strengthened through its longevity, which ensures it has been tested by time and relationship. Thirdly, the flow of *parampara* is accomplished through the younger generation surrendering to the older, while the older generation surrenders to the ancient ways. The content of the lineage is unchanging, and bred in the bone. It's like spiritual DNA.

Rangaswamy does not say how any of these ideals actually apply to his own organization. Dedicating a page of his website to the term under the subheading "The Practice" lets the notion that Ashtanga yoga is a *parampara* hover at the level of strong suggestion.

It's not just a suggestion for inner core disciples. The idea has acquired such gravitas in the global community that second-generation, non-Indian students of Jois and Rangaswamy have begun curating their own life stories, signaling their insider status, and strengthening the disciple's view on a site called *ashtangaparampara.org*. The site currently hosts 48 interviews with authorized and certified Ashtanga yoga teachers, mostly American, mostly under 50. Each page leads with an artful photograph of the interviewee in a difficult posture.[96]

But is calling Jois's method a *parampara* accurate? Brief discussions of the likely fictional *Yoga Korunta* and the maverick biography of Krishnamacharya have weakened the claims that the Jois physical yoga method has remained unchanged, or has historical roots that predate the 20th century. If Sharath Rangaswamy is suggesting on his website that it's his grandfather's physical yoga technique that dates back over millennia, he's stretching the truth.

To be fair, the usage of *parampara* may be an overflow from other aspects of Jois family identity. Their *Smarta* Brahmin religious heritage, dedicated to preserving the teachings of the non-dualist philosopher Adi Shankaracharya, dates back to at least the ninth century. And while Jois's physical yoga training came from a largely secular gym program he attended while a schoolboy, he was also part of a *parampara* in the family practice of *jyotisha* or Indian astrology. ("Jois" is a contraction of *jyotisha*.) This field of study, in which practitioners are said to be able to predict births and deaths and everything in between, leaked out into the lives of disciples, imbuing the family with an aura of mystical, fateful knowledge. One American student remembered Jois spending the afternoons reading astrological periodicals in his receiving room, while his wife, Amma, would sit on the front stairs combing her long hair.[97]

It is further likely that Pattabhi Jois engaged other Sanskrit studies under a *parampara* system. So Sharath Rangaswamy may be using the term in a generally accurate sense with regard to how his grandfather understood the deepest parts of his education. But if Jois was enmeshed in one or more *parampara*, it was not one that taught physical yoga. Very few of his non-Indian students would have known the difference, and the Jois family has made no known effort at clarification.

As we'll see, a *vinyasa* of meanings, in which *parampara* is associated with the teacher or the content they teach, becomes useful to disciples when either the teachings or the teacher falls short of expectations. Students like Diane Bruni, who suffered physical injuries related to practicing the Jois method, were encouraged to trust the wisdom of the teacher. But when Diane was told that Jois was assaulting women, she was encouraged to trust the wisdom of the teachings.

Going further, is the Jois method an exclusive expression of a line of teaching? Typically, *parampara* refers to not only the historical longevity of a teaching practice, but also its exclusivity. Jois disciples use the word in interviews and advertising materials to describe the purity of their method, and to position their authority in yoga matters as descending directly from Krishnamacharya, and, by implication, Krishnamacharya's teachers. This signals that Krishnamacharya initiated Jois as primary successor and inheritor of his lineage. However, Krishnamacharya graduated several prominent students, each of whom went on to promote very different methods, each of which trace their authorization back to him.

The Jois brand is not alone in formally claiming *parampara* status in relation to Krishnamacharya. Krishnamacharya's grandson Kausthub Desikachar uses the term "lineage holder" and has claimed copyright over one of the guru's methods, known as "viniyoga", which is very different from Jois's method.[98] Desikachar protects the power of his position by controlling access to allegedly secret teachings by offering them only through in-person retreats.[99] In 2012, he was accused by several Swedish students of sexual harassment and misconduct during a series of these retreats. Reportedly, he told one of his alleged victims that if she wore the ring he inherited from Krishnamacharya while she had sex with him, she would receive spiritual benefit.[100] The allegations have never been tested in court. Desikachar continues to teach, after having published a "Legal Closure" statement.[101] His website now features references and testimonials to his therapy work as being effective for trauma survivors.[102]

The Jois brand enforces its *parampara* claim by requiring all students who wish to officially (i.e. recognized by KPJAYI) claim they are teaching Jois's Ashtanga yoga be directly authorized by Sharath Rangaswamy in person. A key ingredient of that authorization is bodily contact with Rangaswamy in the form of adjustments. This authorization-through-touch modernizes a medieval form of transmission and blessing. But it's not a one-time affair. Authorized teachers are required to return to the Jois shala in Mysore regularly to maintain their status.

Sharath's writing on *parampara* also suggests that the system fosters love and intimacy. Scrutinizing this begins to bridge the gap between structural and psychological expressions of power, framed by who is in the Jois inner circle or family, and who wants to be.

There is no doubt that many of Jois's students loved him. In an interview, senior student Brigitte Deroses confesses tenderly:

> There is not one day when I do not think about him. His pictures are everywhere in my *shala*, he is like my father, somebody very important who transformed my life, who truly helped me a lot. And I experience always the same emotion when I see him… I always have a lot of emotion.[103]

Karen Rain has mused about whether such feelings were one-sided. "When I hear my former colleagues talk about how much they loved him, I always wonder: 'Did he love you back?' He never seemed to be feel bad when he injured somebody. 'Did he think about you when you weren't there?'"

Some students, like T.M., felt no reciprocity. "I'm not even sure he knew my name," she said. "I didn't get any sense that I was an important student that he was transmitting something to."

TEACHING THAT FLOWS FROM ONE EMPTY VESSEL TO ANOTHER

No one can know whether Sharath Rangaswamy is using the word *parampara* to inspire, include, exclude, or manipulate students. That it can do all of these things is what makes the word so charged within Ashtanga communications.

Further, its power increases by arcing between two unspoken visions for how learning takes place. In the *parampara* model, the student receives teaching from someone who acts as *the empty vessel* through which the content flows. Alternatively, the teaching comes through *an intimate bond* with the nature and personality of the teacher. In his online description, Sharath Rangaswamy ties these two together. But it's good to see how they operate individually.

Parampara translates literally as "one after the other". As Sharath Rangaswamy explains, it indicates a stream of teachers who deliver unchanging teaching content from generation to generation. One of its more archaic forms survives into the present day through the labor of Brahmin priests who teach their sons to memorize hours or even days worth of mantras for the administration of temple rituals. Men use a call-and-response technique by which boys as young as four learn to reproduce each vowel timbre, consonant placement, and rhythm with perfect fidelity. Jois likely learned the prayers of the family puja in this same way. He reports that his earliest education consisted of chanting the verses of astrological scripture with his father.[104]

In traditional Indian pedagogy, as well as in other cultural contexts, faithfulness to the original is key—important enough that, as we've seen in the example of the *Yoga Korunta*, the "original" might have to be invented to facilitate faith. This means that the sounds of the mantras must be reproduced with perfect fidelity. The reciter of Vedic liturgy in the present day, ostensibly, sounds identical to those first sages who repeated what they heard from the cosmos in their deep trance states, way back when. If the pronunciation is marred in even the slightest way, the sacred power, which can be used to bless everything from harvests to weddings, is null and void. The sounds can be written down, but writing is considered a degradation, an insult to the power of collective memory.

Perhaps this is why it's entirely plausible from Jois's perspective that his own copy of the *Yoga Korunta* can gather dust in his house without anyone seeing it. Yet some students believed it was his source, because he ostensibly quoted from it regularly. This recalls the saying that the Veda does not exist unless it is being recited in the present moment. The highest student, therefore, is one who can sacrifice their individual speech to literally repeat exactly what they have been told, or can remember, rather than interpret what they read in books. You can keep the book for back-up, but its truth exists in sounds made by your body.

The order of operations in this learning regime is to do first, ask questions later. Should students understand what they are doing? Maybe—at the end. Boys who learn to recite the Veda are not taught what the mantras mean at first. Discussing meaning would inevitably lead to interpretation. Interpretation, it is believed, is liable to distort the original.

Similarly, the non-Indian students of Jois often reported being inducted into the asana method without any preamble, philosophy, or explanation. They were simply given the postures—which many of them presumed were ancient—to memorize and perform. The idea was that meaning would come later, and more fully to the extent that the student remained empty of their own ideas and motivations. Or—and this is where the non-Indian fetishization of postural performance may have gotten an extra push—*meaning was to be found in the moment of performance itself.*

Wherever meaning was found, it did not come from personal expression, but through faithful reproduction and repetition. So when David Williams says that he tried to teach his students "exactly the way I was taught and try not to modernize it in any way," he's identifying himself as the ideal "empty vessel", the Vedic metaphor for the perfect student and eventual teacher, through which an eternal knowledge can flow, unchanged.

PARAMPARA AS "INTIMATE BOND"

But *parampara* implies more than a series of empty vessels through which knowledge flows. Ideally, it also forms—or is formed from—an intimate bond. In a separate interview, Sharath Rangaswamy ties *parampara* relationships into notions of bloodline. "The longer you spend with your guru," he writes, "the more you understand him and his knowledge and his teaching. So it becomes like a father-and-son relationship."

Saraswati Rangaswamy is Sharath Rangaswamy's mother, the daughter of Pattabhi Jois, and a lead teacher of the Mysore home base. She learned yoga in the same way that Jois did with his teacher, Krishnamacharya.

"My father took me to so many places when he was lecturing on yoga," she tells an interviewer.

> I would do the demonstration of the asana as he spoke of the particular benefits. He would call the vinyasa and I would demonstrate, say, *kurmasana* [tortoise posture]. My father was a big man, maybe eighty kilos. He stood on my back and then started to lecture, explaining the benefits of the asana. Maybe he was talking for one hour while standing on my back. My mother would tell my father, "Don't talk too long." My father would say, "Only five minutes, that's all." But then when we got there, he would do the same—one hour! It didn't hurt; I was very small, very happy, so many people were seeing me.[105]

Saraswati Rangaswamy's tolerance was likely aided by the intimate bond between learning and love. "Guru—that is mula [root, base]," she says.

> If you don't give that respect there is not coming God. That is very important. Some people change it, but it is just their ego. Think who is the best teacher, and go there. If you keep changing teachers, it is not correct. You will get confused. When your mind is strong, you stay with one teacher. You go everywhere and try, then when you find one, you follow that one person. When you meet the right one, you will know in your heart.[106]

The intimacy of this paternalistic learning duet (which, as we will see, reaches deep into the psyches of some of Jois's students) is further reinforced by a structural theme in yoga literature descended from the tradition of Vedic call-and-response. In both epic and philosophical yoga texts, sons sit at the feet of fathers, gurus teach disciples, and deities teach each other as husbands and wives. This mirroring between teacher and student is often positioned as both foundational to and produced by love. In the *Bhagavad Gita*, perhaps India's most beloved compilation of yoga philosophy and instruction, Krishna can help the warrior-hero Arjuna plumb the depths of selfhood not only because Krishna discloses his divinity, but also because they have been friends since childhood. As if obeying some law of eternal return, generations of teachers convey yoga by conversing with students, lovingly, about loving conversations that ancient teachers once had with ancient students.

The intimate *parampara* bond is reinforced by the unchanging essence (*atman*) it is meant to transmit and explain. Most versions of yoga seek to help the practitioner access, remember, and contemplate the unchanging perfection of the *atman*. *Parampara*, therefore, is not just a matter of religious protocol; it is where the message of eternal intimacy intersects with the messenger with whom one must be eternally intimate.

In this paradigm faith in the content and its method becomes inseparable from faith in the man. Distorting the content would mean breaking relationship with the father. Forgetting your metaphysical source is indistinguishable from forgetting your biological source. If this works, the teaching bond might become a strong example of what Alexandra Stein would call a "securely attached relationship", by which the student is empowered by the knowledge that the teacher will provide a constant source of love and protection. This would enable the student to develop agency and autonomy. In **Part Four**, we'll see how the reality of relationships between Jois and many of his students fell short of this security.

Through *parampara*, the teacher is now many things at once: the vessel through whom an ancient, unchanging lesson flows; the parental object of devotion through which the student can absorb that lesson; the granter of life and livelihood; and the home of the soul itself made visible. All possible bases are covered, and then reinforced by teaching strategies like rote memorization that discourage independent thought. The combination of these virtues will always trump the failure of one, and always transcend the teacher's personality and foibles.

But as much as the notion of *parampara* connects the teacher and teaching, it can also separate it, should one or the other fail. Both factors of the equation are so powerful that either can stand on its own, which allows devotees to excuse or forgive from many different angles when things go wrong.

Throughout the year before he died in 2017, I corresponded with T.K. Sribhashyam, Krishnamacharya's middle son. Our dialogue reveals how the empty vessel and intimate bond threads of *parampara* can be untangled when emotionally necessary.

Sribhashyam taught yoga in France. I'd reached out to him with delicate questions about how B.K.S. Iyengar and Pattabhi Jois described his father physically and emotionally abusing them as boys. Did he believe their accounts were true, or exaggerated? Had he ever experienced anything similar to what they described? How might we understand such stories in light of his own memories? His responses were diplomatic.

"In Hinduism," Sribhashyam wrote,

> we owe a debt of recognition to our Masters—spiritual, music, dance, science.... We receive from them an invaluable knowledge, we live with and on this knowledge, often we obtain renown and God willing we also become Masters. We keep in memory of what all we learnt from him (or her) or them and every day we invoke them before we practice what he (she) or they taught us. They are considered as God. What they taught us is more important than how they taught. We strive to make them eternal by thinking of the precious knowledge they imparted and by transmitting their teaching faithfully.
>
> In my humble way, I follow these principles. So much so, I plead my inability to respond to your questions. I wish you all the best. May God be with you.[107]

***

The empty vessel and intimate bond threads of *parampara* can also be untangled when *politically* necessary. This enabled some adherents of Ashtanga yoga to venerate Jois before the #MeToo crisis, but after #MeToo made that veneration unsustainable, they could pivot to defending the practice, and their businesses. In 2012, senior Jois student Kino MacGregor had the following to say about her guru, in the mode of the "intimate bond".

> He was a person that in his presence I experienced transformation... Just because he was in the room, I was inspired to be a better person, I was inspired to make changes. I was inspired to live in accordance with his model. And one of the things that's given me faith and inspiration throughout the years of my practice is that he was a person whose integrity on certain levels were absolutely unquestionable.... In no uncertain terms there were lines that Guruji would have never crossed. And the consistency and the dedication that he devoted to this practice, and the presence that

> he brought into this practice is what gave me faith to practice.[108]

But in her 2017 response to the Jois revelations from Karen Rain and others, MacGregor abandoned this position to adopt the "empty vessel" stance.

> It would be a grievous misunderstanding of the yoga tradition to throw out the entire lineage of Ashtanga yoga because of the mistakes of one man (whose actions have been largely accounted for and removed from the system of Ashtanga yoga). Ashtanga yoga is also based in Patanjali's *Yoga Sutras*, not only the physical teachings, but the spiritual lineage.[109]

To summarize, Sharath Rangaswamy's usage of *parampara* might be appropriate to the description of his commitment to his family's Brahminical rituals, or to his grandfather's relationship to astrology. But is it appropriate for the entrepreneurial business model through which the Jois family's non-Indian students have taken it up, and through which they now claim authority in yoga matters? It's not an accurate term to apply to Jois's asana innovations. And while some students felt the intimate bonding aspect of it, others felt the opposite.

Bottom line: Ashtanga yoga marketing deploys a powerful term of self-definition and exclusivity that carries rich cultural and historical influences and has bolstered and justified the faith of its adherents. Depending upon the shifting social and psychological needs of the person using it, it either defines an exclusive relationship to a person, or a dedicated relationship to a practice.

If Ashtanga yoga isn't a technical *parampara*, it might be something equally communicable and heritable, but much, much simpler: an idea so compelling it needs neither ancient anchors nor magical transmissions. An idea about care, expressed through breath and movement and concentration and discipline and repetition and sweat—all rolled up into a morning ritual that regulates time while hinting at the eternal.

ARE ADJUSTMENTS "TRADITIONAL"?

It's impossible to know how many Jois disciples were attracted to his method and swayed by the claim that his sources were both ancient and sacred. Did anybody choose to invest life and limb solely based upon believing that *vinyasa* was a traditional technique recorded in the *Yoga Korunta* and conveyed by a legitimate *parampara*? These would be pieces—often unconscious—of the larger deception puzzle that groomed some students towards being victimized. But they are only pieces. Confusingly, they may also function for many as relatively benign aspirational beliefs, no less useful than articles of faith held by adherents of mainstream religions.

Physical adjustments and their purported healing properties, however, are so integral to the Jois method, as well as the professionalization process of KPJAYI authorization, that without them, and without the intimate care and attention they are said to convey, Ashtanga yoga and its global derivatives—Power yoga, Jivamukti yoga, Vinyasa yoga—would look very different.

Formal authorization to teach Ashtanga yoga has always been dispensed through contact with the bodies of the Jois family. The only way to officially qualify as an Ashtanga teacher is to have gone to Mysore for years on end—the number of years is unspecified—to take classes with Jois, his daughter, or his grandson. For the first several decades of his international career, Jois signed the homespun Authorization certificates himself. Sharath Rangaswamy has inherited that responsibility. Getting that paper requires crossing "threshold" postures, such as the dropbacks which must be completed before more postures are assigned. No one progresses through dropbacks in Mysore along the KPJAYI authorization track without being physically assisted by a member of the Jois family or inner circle. This same practice has been routinized by Jois's students who repeat it with their own students thousands of times every morning, in every time zone around the world. The homogeneity and predictability of these exchanges helps support the notion of "tradition", which is deeply embedded in Ashtanga discourse.

The word "traditional" can also be code for "the way Jois used to do it in the 1970s and 80s." If you prod some Ashtanga practitioners, they'll likely reveal a belief that Jois's adjustments were inherited from Krishnamacharya. They may be right about that, but if they go further to imply that Krishnamacharya inherited postural adjustments from a prior *hathayoga* lineage, they are on thin ice on two counts: neither adjustments nor an attitude of forcefulness is traditional within the practice and teaching of yoga.

To date, Jason Birch hasn't found any textual evidence describing one person assisting or adjusting another in any yoga practice. Some, including defenders of the antiquity of adjustments, will argue that an absence of textual evidence does not rule out that adjustments were happening; they just were not written down. The sole piece of material evidence, Birch notes, is an illustration in a copy of a 19th-century "royal compendium" called the *Sritattvanidhi*. The book was commissioned by Mysore's Maharaja at the time and "covers many topics that interested the royal family, from board games to temple deities," writes Birch via email.[110]

The illustration shows one practitioner placing his hands on another's knees as the latter performs a posture called *Viratasana* (described below). The textual description refers to neither an assist nor an adjustment.

> Placing the shanks and back on the ground and positioning the thighs on the calves, [the yogin] should touch his backbone [on the ground] again and again. [This] is the pose for one who has ceased [from worldly activities].

Birch explains that the compiler of the *Sritattvanidhi* borrowed the posture and its description from the *Hathabhyasapaddhati*. "Therefore," Birch writes, "the idea of receiving an assist in this posture was introduced by the artists who illustrated the *Sritattvanidhi*, and not the yoga tradition from which it was borrowed."

> It is possible that the artists of the *Sritattvanidhi*'s asanas had a practical knowledge of the asanas. They do add details to other asanas that are not in the Sanskrit descriptions and many of these additional details make good sense. We were under the impression that *Viratasana* could not be performed unless someone was holding down the thighs of the yogin in the pose, because the yogin is supposed to lift the torso up and down and this usually can only be done if the knees are secured. But we have recently seen teenage yogins in Khed and an Ashtanga yoga practitioner in London do it without assistance.[111]

Birch's colleague at the Hatha Yoga Project, Dr James Mallinson, is also a Sanskritist who specializes in *hathayoga* texts. His education owes a large debt to his decades-long apprenticeship to Sri Ram Balak Das Yogiraj, his guru in the ascetic yogi lineage of the Ramanandi Tyagis, who live mainly in North India. When Mallinson wanted to learn yoga postures, he had to specifically ask Ram Balak, who instructed him in a way that is likely to be far more continuous with older *hathayoga* traditions than anything that came out of the influence of Krishnamacharya's group classes.

There was no group class, for starters. The guru described a selection of postures orally, and told Mallinson to go off and practice them for several months. Then he was told to come back and report on his progress. The guru gave no demonstration, nor asked for a demonstration from his student. There was no physical contact.

"TRADITION" AND "FORCE"

Many Ashtanga practitioners use a whisper network to categorize the adjustments of teachers in their communities and help each other to find those with the right touch. For example, here in Toronto, one senior Ashtanga teacher is known for a liberal and exploratory approach to teaching, often breaking down postures for closer examination. Accordingly, their adjustments are said by many to be "sensitive". But when students speak of adjustments given by this teacher's former protégé, who is more closely aligned with KPJAYI than his teacher, they use terms like "traditional", "strict", or "old school". These are all code words for "forceful" or "intense". They often seem to carry conservative or religious undertones, and echo of one of Jois's favorite aphorisms: "with heat, even iron will bend".[112]

But if the word "traditional" is not appropriate to use in reference to the practice of adjustments, what about that sense of "traditional" that is used by Ashtanga students to mean "forceful", and to justify the brutal manipulations by Jois? Does this bear any relation to the history of *hathayoga* practice and pedagogy prior to the 20th century?

Jason Birch also addresses the broader question of "force" in the historical practice of *hathayoga*.[113] Birch shows that the perception that *hathayoga* should be intense or "forceful"—a notion upon which much of the allure of Ashtanga yoga hangs—arises out of the complex and historically shifting meanings of the term itself. The compound term translates literally as "yoga of force". But up until about the 15th century, "force" in *hathayoga* texts did not refer to stress applied to the body or through bodily effort. Rather, as Birch explains, it pertained to the effect of its techniques in "forcefully moving vitality... up through the central channel." The "central channel"[114] here refers to the energetic body-within-the body that the yogi is attempting to activate, through posture, focus, and breathwork, towards a stone-like state of stillness called *samadhi*.

Birch explains that a few systems of *hathayoga*, which were recorded in texts composed after the 16th century, began to incorporate some austerities as asanas. Examples include asanas that resemble holding one arm up (*Urdhvabahu*) and hanging upside down from trees (*Tapakara asana*). These were known and expected to injure the practitioner's body. It's not unreasonable to think that tree pose (*Vrksasana*) in the *Gherandasamhita* (2.36) was inspired by the practice of the Khareshwari, an ascetic who stands in this position indefinitely, aided by ropes and slings, until their lower legs and feet were permanently swollen and ulcerated. However, the late texts on *hathayoga* extol the healing benefits of their asanas, so it is likely that tree pose was held only for short periods of time by *hathayoga* practitioners.

This intersection of *hathayoga* and asceticism was further tangled by the interpretations of 19th-century European scholars like Monier-Williams, who compiled the first Sanskrit–English dictionary. Monier-Williams, Birch explains, was aware of the ascetic influence upon *hathayoga* from the ethnography of his time. But he conflated this ethnography with texts like the 15th-century practice manual called *Hathapradipika*. This text does not advocate for austerities.

Birch reasons that if, in the older literature,

> the name *hathayoga* was based on the notion of forceful effort, one would expect to find injunctions to forcibly... perform its techniques.... In fact, the qualification *sanaih sanaih*, which specifies that a technique should be performed gradually, slowly, or gently, depending on the context, occurs frequently.

He also notes that the *Hathapradipika* lists "exertion" as "one of the six factors that ruin *hathayoga*."[115]

It seems that a more "traditional" idea we can recover from *hathayoga* about how practice should be carried out has been largely overlooked by Jois and his disciples. Traditionally, the practitioner would not be *forced* into any particular position or experience. Rather: the gentle, careful, and diligent practice of postures and breathing are meant to create the conditions through which the yogi cannot help but to awaken to the deeper mysteries of life. If the yogi is "forced" towards an awakening, it is in the same way a bulb is forced to sprout when surrounded with warmth and moisture.

At least some of Jois's students got this older memo. "Opening your body is like opening an envelope," David Williams told *Yoga Journal* in the same 1995 issue that drew Jubilee Cooke to Mysore. "You can rip it, or you can steam it open without a trace.... Concentrate on your mula bandha and your breathing, and you will open like a flower—not through tearing the flesh, but through stretching it."[116]

THE "MULABANDHA ADJUSTMENT"—OR SEX THAT IS NOT SEX

Content warning: *This section cites rationalizations for sexual assault that might be retraumatizing for sexual assault victims to read.*

If it's clear that unicorns don't exist, it might be a waste of breath arguing that purple unicorns are especially non-existent. If there really is no such thing as a "traditional" yoga adjustment (let alone a "forceful" one), we shouldn't have to spend much effort showing that there's no such thing as a yoga adjustment—also framed as traditional—in which a teacher digitally rapes his students.

Nonetheless, a few points on what was often called the "*mulabandha* adjustment" will be useful to show how some Ashtanga practitioners spoke with such a blend of earnestness and bypassing that a basic deception was obscured. Ostensibly, they are referring to how Jois would "help" women find their "root lock" (*mulabandha*), a reference to the perineal musculature that helps control genital and anal function. He would "find" it for them via groping or digital penetration. As with the usage of terms like *vinyasa* and *parampara*, "*mulabandha* adjustment" carries a mixture of historical echo and rationalization.

You can hear Richard Freeman wrestling with this mixture, while adding in a touch of modesty—or cynical euphemism—in that podcast with Kathryn Bruni-Young.

> He was obsessed, I know, with *mulabandha*. With the pelvic floor. And somehow, through some kind of self-delusion he had, or through some cultural gap between the liberal western world and the medieval provincial orthodox world, he started doing this occasionally. And he would do it, and people would complain, and he would stop. But somehow he would start again.[117]

The way the term "*mulabandha*" has been used mirrors a disorienting spectrum of assertions about Jois, ranging from the puritanical to the libertine. It allowed T.M. to be told by her colleagues that Jois assaulting her "was not sexual." Meanwhile, Marisa Sullivan was told that the women he was assaulting "have sexual issues, and he's healing them." Even more outrageously, Ashtanga Deep Throat insisted that Jois and his women students were engaged in consensual exhibitionistic sex. He claimed that some of the women told him that they'd had the best orgasms of their lives through the hands of Jois.

Through the fog of terms like "*mulabandha* adjustment", Jois was either a celibate priest officiating over a solemn ritual of yoga postures, a therapist for traumatized women, or an orgiastic liberator. All three of these characterizations share two deceptive qualities. They place his identity above his behavior, focusing on his intentions rather than his impacts. Secondly, they dubiously connect Jois to a stream of legend. For centuries if not millennia, the yoga master has been conceived of in India as a master of sex, but also beyond it. This is evident in the literature describing sexual practices in *Tantra* and *hathayoga*, by which the masterful yogi is encouraged to indulge in sexual activity so long as the bliss of their encounters is sublimated for spiritual purposes.[118] The phrase used by Indologist Wendy Doniger to describe Siva—to whom Tim Miller compared Jois—is apt. She calls the primal yogi, known for alternating between millenia of celibate meditation and millenia of sexual sport, "the erotic ascetic".[119]

Whether in earnest, or under the influence of group-think, modern Ashtanga literature presents this conflict in an unprocessed form. In her memoir, *Sacred Fire: My Journey Into Ashtanga Yoga*,[120] Kino MacGregor recounts meeting Jois for the first time. She'd discovered his book *Yoga Mala* during a period of soul-searching. It became her "bible", she writes. "I read only at night when my day was finished so that Jois's words would be the last thought on my mind before I fell asleep."

When she finished the book, Jois appeared to her in a dream.

> He appeared as a redemptive figure who rescued me from the arms of an angry Shiva and placed me on a peaceful cruise ship bound for the dawn. The salvific feeling of the dream left me breathless and I awake from this fantasy with a life-changing thought on my lips. I opened my eyes, panting, and whispered aloud, "I have to go to India."[121]

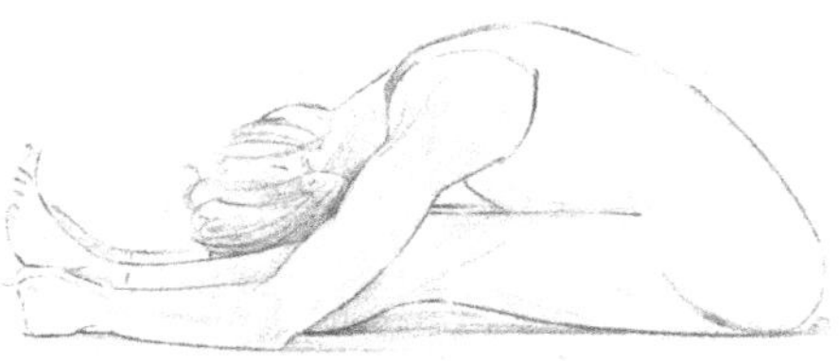

Figure 7: Paschimottanasana

MacGregor describes the ensuing expectation around her first practice with Jois in erotic terms.

> The first yoga practice in India is like losing your virginity. It is a moment you spend hours fantasizing about, and when the fateful moment comes, it is over before you know it and you are left wondering what happened, contemplating the details and replaying the event over in your head."[122]

The edge sharpens as she describes being touched by Jois for the first time, but MacGregor is also careful to frame the moment as chaste.

"As I dropped from my last backbend," she writes,

> my hands were on the floor and my eyes drifted towards my feet. I could see my new yoga teacher's toes standing at the edge of my mat. Guruji placed his hands on my hips and said, "You go back." I went back, barely breathing, shaking to have his attention directly towards me. After three times he said, "You catch" And I released my fear in the arms of my teacher and before I could say yes or no my hands were on my knees. Peaceful in a wordless, thoughtless unity I opened my eyes and surrendered into the hug that Guruji gave his female students after deep back bending. Breathing together in an intimate space that was not defined by gender but by humanity, my heart opened even more. The tender ache inside me cracked open. He guided me to the floor for the counter stretch, forward bending, called *Paschimottanasana* [*see* Figure 7, above]. Laying his full weight on my back, tears that I

> had been holding back for lifetimes flowed freely. In his joyful spirit he said, "Good good, best. Thank you very much."[123]

ABUSER, MAGICIAN, STEWARD OF TRADITION?

For some, a conflict between Jois the abuser and Jois the sexual magician becomes explicit. In his response to the #MeToo comments of Karen Rain, senior Jois student Steve Dwelley not only firmly decries Jois's sexual abuse, but also asserts that he was a "tantric master" whose real sin was in not being able to navigate the risky demands of his role.

"I'm not using 'tantric' in the sense of sexual master," Dwelley clarifies,

> but rather as one who understands various dimensions of bodily based subtle energy and who can work with the material aspect of the yogic endeavor, understanding something of how the material is connected to the subtle, ie: an accomplished hatha yogi. They actaully [sic] exist.
>
> As such, Pattabhi Jois pioneered an unpredictable dimension in the history of yoga: the intimate adjustment. It did not play out in his shala as "corporal punishment"; there is a reason so many powerful teachers were drawn to him, including women. Wonderful things happened in his room, events I have yet to see replicated. The world of shared professional intimacy must not die with MeToo, and I don't believe women are asking for that. This is the whole, truly wonderful universe of yoga, bodywork, even Orgasmic Meditation. Pattabhi helped open that door. Unfortunately, he personally was inadequately equipped to manage some of its temptations.[124]

Such rationalizations can take subtler and more modest forms. Though Jois disciple Richard Freeman's life and teaching partner Mary Taylor has more clearly denounced Jois's assaults, Freeman also muddies the water by claiming that Jois comes from a Tantric lineage, implying that he designed his method to work on mystical bodily energies. "If we look at the different texts of Tantric yoga," he said in a video posted to social media,

> we get a different definition of Tantra than is popular. We discover that Ashtanga Vinyasa yoga is definitely a very concentrated and pure

> Tantric practice. And this does not mean an interest or obsession with sexuality. It means a movement of *prana* into the central channel and this movement of *prana* is a use of breath body and you know, the manifesting world in a way that reveals that the world itself is this delightful, pure radiance of consciousness. And so the lineage that Pattabhi Jois is in is the *Sri Vidya* Tantric lineage, which was practiced by the great philosopher, Sri Shankaracharya, and these many Tantric schools in no way contradict many of the other schools that support you know, more, let's say, understandable and less esoteric practices.[125]

This statement, posted seven months after Freeman minimized Jois's assaults on two podcasts, is riddled with idealizations and factual errors. Strictly speaking, whether something is a "Tantric practice" or not is defined by whether the practitioner has been formally initiated into it via a religious ceremony, and whether the practice itself is described in a scripture understood to be part of the Tantric literature. Ashtanga Vinyasa yoga is *not* a Tantric practice by textual authority or any known extant transmission mechanism. The 8th-century non-dualist philosopher Adi Shankaracharya predates Sri Vidya, which is a heritage of formal Tantric practice lineages. He could not have been a practitioner of it.[126] Whether they pass muster or not, Freeman's views are interpreted as authoritative in many yoga circles.

More important, perhaps, is how such statements distract the accountability discussion that should follow abuse revelations.

"I guess that for Freeman, the experience of the "delightful pure radiance" of consciousness overrides that Jois sexually assaulted and raped some of his students," writes Karen Rain in response to Freeman's statement.

> To Freeman, and most other Ashtanga yoga teachers, the value attributed to Jois's lineage is more important to discuss and outweighs the legacy of abuse. This was the exact behavior and attitude that enabled the abuse in the first place. Teachers who knew of the "weird adjustments," otherwise known in legal terms as sexual assault, kept silent and continued to glorify and profit from their association with their "Guruji," while other people were violated and injured.[127]

"NO PRECEDENT"

Jacqueline Hargreaves is a yoga scholar who gathers ethnographic data on contemporary yoga culture in India and Asia. She has also played an active role in analyzing how other yoga organizations—namely Satyananda Yoga—have dealt with revelations of abuse.*[128]

In an online response to obfuscations from Jois students about the "*mulabandha* adjustment", Hargreaves is unequivocal.

> There is no precedent for the mulabandha adjustment (as given by Jois) in classical, medieval or pre-modern yoga. Nor is it replicated in any other lineages which extend from Krishnamacharya (i.e., Iyengar, Desikachar, Ramaswami, Mohan, Devi, etc.). This practice appears to have started with Jois and to suggest that there is a yogic teaching in this method is unjustified.[129]

Hargreaves also responded firmly to the widely repeated comment that Jois's women students provoked him with scanty clothes. This isn't a fringe attitude. It was mainstream enough to appear in the wake of Karen Rain's #MeToo statement, in the belly of a blog post response from Mary Taylor. Taylor is a senior Jois student, Richard Freeman's wife, and was co-host of the events where Charlotte Clews and Katchie Ananda were assaulted in 2002. In the blog, she dismissed the idea that "scantily clad or overly effusive women were at fault for the sexually inappropriate adjustments"—but only after suggesting precisely that.

"I can say that my experience," Taylor writes,

> was that he began doing these adjustments after foreign female students came to practice with him wearing very revealing Western-style clothing. To a provincial, orthodox Brahmin from a tiny village, who knows what these women looked like? Certainly they probably didn't appear to be chaste or well bred. Around the same time, Western students stopped bowing to his feet in appreciation for class and instead began hugging and kissing him as a demonstration of gratitude. I am certain both of these things were mixed messages to him culturally.**[130]

* Satyananda Yoga has exerted tremendous influence over the modern yoga world through hundreds of translations and commentaries on medieval texts, issued under the auspices of the Bihar School of Yoga.

** Taylor seems to be conflating direct experience with group narrative here. She cannot have had direct experience of Jois's treatment of Indian women prior to the arrival of non-Indian women students. Taylor began studying with Jois in 1988; non-Indian women students were training with Jois in Mysore as early as 1976. Jois had been on tour in the United States in 1975 so had seen how women dressed for yoga at that time.

Hargreaves dismissed this argument.

> To suggest that Western-style dress was the provocative cause of Jois's behavior completely diminishes the power he held in his position as guru. It also displays a limited understanding of the constant threat to women's safety that is experienced when living and traveling in India, regardless of what one wears! It is never acceptable for an orthodox Brahmin to inappropriately touch and/or adjust a woman regardless of their age, race, caste or clothing, and such an offender would be well aware that this type of action is improper and provocative. If anything, the cultural differences would mean that these adjustments by a provincial Brahmin are even more inappropriate.[131]

Another problem with the argument that Jois was provoked to assault by scantily clad women is that there are two photographs that show him assaulting men in much the same way.[132] In the first photo, Pattabhi Jois is seen sexually assaulting a male practitioner in reclining hand-to-foot pose (*Supta Trivikramasana*, also called *Supta Padangusthasana*; *see* Figure 1, p. 28). Jois is seen sexually assaulting Karen Rain in the same posture in a similar photo she published in a widely circulated article.[133] The photo with the male practitioner was taken in the old Lakshmipuram shala, and so dates from before 2003.

In the second photo, Jois is seen assaulting a male practitioner in a forward fold. A source says that the photo was taken in 2003 in Encinitas. This would be the latest date for which there's evidence for Jois's assaults.

The identities of the practitioners are unknown. They remain anonymous because their faces are hidden. I published them to my blog with the awareness that the practitioners might dispute that the photographs depict sexual assault.

However, victim testimony alone does not define sexual assault. Other factors can include whether: there was full consent; the alleged victim was capable of granting full consent at the time; the alleged victim was in a position or condition of submission; the contact was administered under the false premise of medical treatment; and/or there was a significant power imbalance between the alleged assaulter and the victim.

Karen Rain commented on these photos in a thread on Facebook.

> I've heard a couple stories about P Jois sexually assaulting men,

> including one story of a male digital rape. I know that the AY community likes to say that what he did to women wasn't sexual assault because he did the same thing to men. This is the most nonsensical argument. Imagine if we used that reasoning with priests: they did the same thing to young girls as they did to young boys, so therefore it isn't sexual abuse(??). It's important to understand that sexual abuse/assault is about power not about sex. Unfortunately, males are perhaps, even more than females or non-binary people, conditioned in ways that prevent recognition and disclosing of sexual assault. So much for the argument that P Jois was tempted by effusive, scantily clad western women.[134]

If Jois's sexual assaults on men were more difficult to recognize and disclose, this may have increased the tendency, especially among the senior male students, to ignore or rationalize assaults against women as well.

"OPENINGS" OR RATIONALIZING INJURY AND INTRUSION

"You see," wrote Tracy Hodgeman, "in Ashtanga loud clunks and 'strong sensations' are commonplace, our guru Sri K. Pattabhi Jois calls them 'openings.'"

The word "opening" has been used in Ashtanga circles for decades to reframe injuries as positive possibilities. As we see in T.M.'s case (**Appendix 1**), it can even be applied to an injury caused by the manhandling or clumsiness of Jois or one of his students. The word has been ubiquitous throughout the interviews I've conducted on yoga injury. There are synonyms for it: "releasing"; "surrendering"; "shifting"; "realigning"; "rearranging"; "growing pains". The general meaning is that the practice, or the teacher, is taking apart the flawed body—and personality—in order to reassemble it according to a higher order.

This category of euphemism has at least three ramifications.

1. It helps students to resolve the cognitive dissonance of pain being associated with a practice meant to give physical and spiritual healing.
2. It can suppress a fear of the intrusive teacher.
3. It can also inhibit students from seeking medical treatment when they are injured.

Tracy Hodgeman didn't seek medical assistance for her injured shoulder for nine months. She was encouraged to continue to come to practice, and to do whatever postures she could, in the belief that the practice that had harmed her would also heal her. This resistance to medicalizing the injury made the interpretive authority that Jois and his devotees hold over his students' bodies that much stronger. Who was going to argue with Jois himself calling an injury an "opening"? Dissuading students from medical care, however, is a form of isolation.

Finally, using "opening" for "injury" has a deceptive and social grooming ring to it when we see it as continuous with the usage of "*mulabandha* adjustment", the code phrase that allowed Jois's sexual assaults to be either reframed as a esoteric healing technique, or minimized with a nod and a wink.

"OPENING" AND ITS DISCONTENTS: AN ANECDOTE

In many forms of yoga, the term "opening" is used to describe a slow and delicate process of increasing psychosomatic flexibility. The idea is that as your range of motion increases, your personality will soften, become more receptive, less reactive. Muscular stiffness is associated with emotional or spiritual defensiveness or armoring. You want to "open" wherever you can. Through the "release" of muscular tensions, psychospiritual knots can be unraveled. Apparently, this is especially true for the hips. Many yoga teachers commonly claim that you hold repressed emotions in your hips. They say you know it is true when you cry silently in "hip-openers" like pigeon pose or reclining butterfly. It isn't pain you are feeling, but release and opening.

In my personal case, all of this felt true, at least for a while. Staying present to the fluid stretching and breathing in the postures challenged a certain rigidity within me that wasn't just about my tissues. Within a few months of starting practice, I found myself more relaxed in stressful situations, more able to find a long, smooth breath. I became more receptive to my own feelings, and to other people. Less got under my skin, because it seemed my skin had become malleable, permeable. I learned how to physically surrender.

I associated such feelings with moral virtues like forgiveness, and attributed the improvements to the technique. But in retrospect, the intensity of my practice at that time might have provoked these sensations from a more mundane direction. Exercise in general—which I had been lax with prior to starting a yoga practice—is well known to lower stress responses. I also wonder whether my sessions, which at their peak could exceed two hours per day, simply exhausted me.

Over time, I became addicted to the sensations and potential benefits of stretching. But the returns diminished, and eventually began to reverse. My hip and spinal joints got loose. Strange pinches, pulls, and aches cropped up and wouldn't go away. I had to concentrate harder on holding myself upright with lax spinal muscles. Gradually, I began to admit that I was in chronic pain, which, paradoxically, I could temporarily relieve through yet more stretching. I didn't understand that all the "opening" had actually destabilized my musculoskeletal system, and that I needed to rebalance things with weight and resistance training.

More problematically, as a teacher myself, I had assumed that everyone else would share my (initial) positive experience with "opening". I was ignorant of the fact that people come to yoga with a huge spectrum of joint mobility and ego strength. Not everyone needed to become more flexible, or receptive. "Openness" was a principle that I thought would offer peace and health to everyone, but some people just didn't need it. The hypermobile might need to muscularly engage, and those who struggled with boundary issues or who had been victimized by power imbalances didn't need further lessons in surrender.

A lot of Ashtanga teaching language, regardless of the individual needs of students, has likewise turned "opening" into a gospel of universal salvation. It's also given the word a new emphasis. "Opening" is used to not only describe a process, but a sacred event. When T.M. feels a "tree branch snap" in her hamstring, or Diane Bruni hears six gunshot sounds come from deep in her hip as she executes a simple forward fold, or Michael Kazamias, an Ashtanga practitioner from Germany, describes hearing two of his spinal discs pop and hiss like tires being punctured—these moments are framed as "openings" along a general pathway of breaking down bodily resistance. The practitioner is said to have passed through a threshold experience, a rebirth, an initiation into a new self.

The opening process with which I was familiar was only really a novice version of the Ashtanga event of opening. Their use of the term implied something far deeper than the softening that came through building a tolerance to stretching. The Ashtanga opening event expressed an outright confrontation with the harder tissues of the body, viewed as the solid cause of suffering. In its most extreme forms (we'll see an example from the testimony of Jois disciple Brad Ramsey in **Part Four**), it implied that the flesh was a kind of prison, and the bones and ligaments represented the bars of ego. The body is the scar tissue of personal history, seen as dull, unresponsive, needing to be broken up, and mobilized. The hard tissues must be heated, stretched, stressed, and even ruptured for the student to experience freedom.

With heat, even iron will bend.

"OPENING"—ANCIENT AND MODERN

Where did this obsession with "opening" come from? On one hand, Jois was perpetuating a physical performance requirement for simple flexibility inherited by all of Krishnamacharya's students. As a boy, Jois would have proven his worth as a student of yoga—and later, a junior teacher—through the intensity of his contortions. Yoga historian Elliot Goldberg suggests that Krishnamacharya's teaching must have been influenced by the contortionistic circus training that was gaining popularity at the time.[135] Jois's colleague B.K.S. Iyengar concurs.

"One of the duties I was often called upon to perform in this period of my life," writes Iyengar in his final autobiography,

> was to give demonstrations of yoga for the Maharaja's court and for visiting dignitaries and guests. It was my guru's duty to provide for the edification and amusement of the Maharaja's entourage by putting his students—of whom I was one of the youngest—through their paces and showing off their ability to stretch and bend their bodies into the most impressive and astonishing postures. I pushed myself to the limits in my practice in order to do my duty to my teacher and guardian and to satisfy his demanding expectations.[136]

These performance demands to "stretch and bend" also carry a spiritual meaning insofar as they resonate with ancient metaphors that painted the material world as a site of bondage. "Ropes and knots; binding, loos[en]ing, and cutting," writes David Gordon White in *The Alchemical Body*, his study of medieval Tantric views and practices.

> It is in these terms that India has perennially portrayed the conundrum of existence. Creatures ... are bound to a phenomenal world that is a tightly stitched net of magic or a veil of *maya* [illusion]; and when this life ends, it is the noose carried by Death himself that ensnares them. In such a world of bondage, what term could better describe liberation and salvation than *moksha*—which pre-

> cisely means the loos[en]ing or releasing of the knots and webs and snares that fetter all creation?[137]

In the Ashtanga world, as well as many other forms of contemporary physical yoga, the body is ground zero of the knotted web. The postures are meant to help you to sever those bonds. For some, Jois's manipulations were not seen as injurious but as an attempt to speed up the breakdown process.

"He'd see a blockage or had a sense of you being stuck in some way and then would help to break that," says senior Jois student Guy Donahaye, as he interviews his elder colleague Nancy Gilgoff, who first went to Mysore in 1973.

"The energy does get blocked in the body," Gilgoff affirms, "and that can be from injuries and emotional things that keep coming up. There is a way to unblock it through heat and breath, and that's what the Ashtanga series seems to do."[138]

"I felt like I was being dismembered," said the late Jois devotee Brad Ramsey, describing the sensation of being adjusted by Jois.[139] He describes giving the pain up to God. Ramsey's stark view, examined more fully in **Part Four**, points to the intersection between spiritual and relational meanings carried by the word "opening". Opening to the postures equals opening to unknown experiences, which in turn can mean opening to the will of the teacher.

"You had to surrender to his adjustments, and then you would be safe," New Zealander Peter Sanson told Donahaye.

> If you tried to resist anything you were in serious trouble. Many times I could hear things tearing in my body—like the sound of sheets ripping—I thought I was going to be finished. But in the end I would just let go, and surrender up to him, and allow him to take me into the different asanas, and then I was safe.[140]

In another Donahaye interview, Jois devotee Tomas Zorzo connects surrender back to opening.

"When I went to Mysore, I had this aspiration of an opening. You open to the guru and you allow the guru to work on you."

"What sort of attitude does the student need toward the guru?" asks Donahaye.

"Humility and trust and opening to him, to receive from him—the capacity to learn."[141]

LETTING THE MASTER INTERPRET THE BODY

Ramsey, Sanson, and Zorzo opened themselves up to learning the postures, the breath counts, how to be adjusted, and how to adjust. They learned everything the practice had to offer their different bodies and minds, everything that would have been inevitable to learn through the collision of their personal psychologies with Jois and his community. But they also learned a further meaning for the concept of "opening". They opened themselves up to Jois's interpretation of—and authority over—their body and reality.

"Jois saw the body in a totally different way that no-one will ever completely understand," says Dr. John Doyle, a student of Jois and Iyengar who has taught the medical modules of the "Masters of Yoga" graduate program at Loyola Marymount University in Los Angeles.

"He walked out of medieval times into the 20th century," Doyle told me. "He wound up teaching all of these counterculture, outlier Westerners, who wanted to see what he saw."

A key part of how Jois saw his students was through a stern distrust of contemporary medical knowledge. In *Yoga Mala*, he declares that medical treatments for congenital diseases are "like a thorn in a leg that is removed by another thorn,"[142] and that

> diseases that cannot be cured by medicine can be cured by yoga; diseases that cannot be cured by yoga cannot be cured at all. That is definite.... Indeed, the practitioner that keeps faith in and practices the limbs of yoga can achieve anything in the world. He can even redo creation.[143]

On the shala floor, Jois reportedly ignored any medical evidence brought by his students that would challenge these articles of faith. To illustrate, Doyle related a story that's taken on legendary status in Ashtanga circles. A burly practitioner once brought Jois an x-ray taken prior to starting practice in Lakshmipuram. The image clearly showed the hardware holding his joints together after a rough and tumble life, and multiple surgeries.

"Guruji: look at my bones," said the prospective student. "This means that I won't be able to do deep backbends and twists."

As Dr. Doyle tells the story, Jois looked quizzically at him and said, "Bone? What bone?"

Brad Ramsey told Donahaye that he believed that "Guruji was looking at energy fields instead of the body."

> What he was seeing wasn't "If I step on this guy's knee, he's going to scream and he's going to be out of action for a couple of weeks." He was seeing energy circuits... and I believe that sometimes he was not conscious of the physical dynamic at all. That wasn't what he was looking at and that's the way it's supposed to be with a guru.[144]

Zorzo also suggests that Jois could transcend medical imaging with a kind of "divine eye", as found in Indian epic lore, empowered to peer into both material and moral bodies. "He was looking through ... to the heart of the person, not how they were appearing," says Zorzo. "I realized that when he seemed to be treating me harshly, it was the result of something not clean inside of me. He was reading my state of mind."[145]

Zorzo went so far as to allow Jois to read his bloodwork.

"The first time I went to India I got very sick with amoebic hepatitis," he told Donahaye.

> I had been close to death. On my second trip I was afraid to fall sick again. No mineral water, toilet paper, etc.—it was difficult to travel in India. First, I went to do *vipassana* [meditation] in Bombay and then on to Mysore. But on the way to the vipassana course I got dysentery, so I could not sit the course. I was very sick with a high fever and I was thinking it was amoebic hepatitis again.
>
> Then I went to Mysore, but I was still very sick. I met Guruji and told him how sick I was. He said, "Oh, you remove all these medicines." I had all these medicines which the hospital had given to me, about fifty tablets of different colors. "You just throw these out and just practice, practice, practice. This will clean the liver and other internal organs and you will be just fine."[146]

Zorzo discarded the pills and practiced. He recovered, and later attributed his fortune to Jois's wisdom.

MIRACLES AND LETDOWNS

Ashtanga discourse is not unique in recording and promoting miracle stories. The literatures of Iyengar, Bikram, and Yogi Bhajan are likewise filled with accounts of mystical healing: cancer reversals, diabetes cures, scoliotic spines straightened, the effects of childhood polio reversed. People describe being cured of addiction, depression, of leaving lab-coated doctors and their medications behind as they find health solutions that are indistinguishable from religious conversions.

These stories are woven throughout yoga literature and marketing. They share the mixed qualities of folk knowledge: they are enormously inspiring, but also anecdotal, and never confirmed. They also rarely show an awareness of the mechanisms of projection and transference, or the power of groupthink.

Overall, we have seen how "opening" in a general sense describes the process—pleasurable for many—of becoming less rigid in body and mind. In the Ashtanga world and elsewhere, it is elevated to the level of a critical imperative, ultimately indicating a moment in which the body cracks or is forced open to reveal a new identity. This meaning is mingled with the ideal of opening oneself to not only the physical intrusion of the teacher, but also their interpretation of your experience. Along this journey, any harm is often interpreted as a boon.

Many interviewees have managed to close themselves off to the intrusions of not only overstretching and adjustments but also to the interpretations that made their bodies into marionettes of the teacher's ideology. They tell the opposite of miracle stories—about how through some critical mass of pain and disillusionment, the idea of "opening" began to ring hollow. Further, they suspected that Jois or his students were using a dubious framework for healing to mask their ignorance.

Near the end of Karen's stay in Mysore, she approached Jois one day after class. He was sitting on his stool. She asked him why she had back pain. She felt nervous asking the question. He said he didn't know. Then he told her to eat *ragi*. Ragi is finger millet, which is mixed with water to form dumplings called *ragi mudde*. It's a staple food amongst the farmers of the Mysore region.

Michael Kazamias told me about reporting his spinal disc injuries to Sharath Rangaswamy in 2011. Jois's grandson referred him to the Institute's own branded "No Pain No Gain" gel, on sale in the retail shop. Kazamias opened his wallet to buy a jar for five hundred rupees. He got back to his hotel and opened the jar. It was repackaged tiger balm, available in the local pharmacy for fifty rupees.

Rangaswamy did not respond to requests for comment.

"YOGA THERAPY"

Much of the above points to a subtle, vexing, and far-reaching confusion within not only Ashtanga language, but also in modern yoga marketing in general. It's a confusion that can sharpen and escalate into a type of cultural deception that manipulates the conflicting aspirations of students. A prime example of this can be found in the Sanskrit title given to Jois's Primary Series, *Yoga Cikitsa*, which translates as "Yoga Therapy".

It's not clear when this clinical-sounding name first came into use. In his 1962 *Yoga Mala*, he uses the words *cikitsa* and *shodhana* to loosely describe qualities of certain postures, but not as names for distinct series. The Second Series eventually became known as *Nadi Shodhana* or "Purification of the Subtle Channels".

Whether Jois used the terms explicitly or not, Ashtanga devotees to this day commonly describe the Primary Series as being "healing" or "therapeutic". They will struggle, however, to find a physical or occupational therapist, sports medicine doctor, or kinesiologist who would look at the Jois method and affirm it's any more physically "therapeutic" than any other exercise. At least, not in the way it is promoted and commonly taught: often the same way to everyone, ideally performed six days a week, in the same order every day, often to the exclusion of all other activities, indefinitely.

Most sports medicine experts agree that while any exercise is better than none, exercise in general should be varied and not repetitive. Some also criticize the Ashtanga method for having too many forward folds to be generally good for spinal health and for doing little in terms of cardiovascular fitness. It also omits actions like hanging and pulling that are integral for the upper-body integrity demanded by the advanced arm-balancing postures that factored into Tracy Hodgeman's shoulder collapse.

Authorized Ashtanga teachers have been discouraged from teaching other forms of yoga or movement. And yet some of these very forms might mitigate the above weaknesses in the method. As of 2018, they're *contractually obligated* by the new KPJAYI Code Conduct to refrain from teaching anything but the method as taught by Rangaswamy.[147] The authorized Ashtanga teacher who wants to teach anything outside of the method risks losing their listed status. If they have built their finances around the job of leading morning Mysore-style practice program, losing their listing could be a real hardship. The new Code also forbids teachers who sign it from teaching in the more popular and lucrative workshop format without approval from Rangaswamy.

If an authorized Ashtanga teacher wants to be sensitive to the injury liabilities of the repetitive practice, the best they can do is to slow down a student's introduction to the postures and encourage an attitude of relaxation and non-achievement. The common claim is that this personalized approach is "more traditional" with regard to Jois's Mysore style, even though Jois led at least some of his first American students through all of the series at breakneck speed. David Williams learned the first four series in just four months in Mysore in 1973.

Ashtanga teachers who have trained for authorization at KPJAYI work with a further educational deficit: at no point are they required to formally study anatomy or physiology, nor any evidence-based manual therapy techniques. They have inherited a pedagogy based less in anatomy than in the premodern reality of energy circuits. As Ramsey described, this energetic focus may have been more important to Jois than whether or not he injured students.

Whether traditional, grandiose, or simply unhelpful, this attitude towards anatomical realities extends out into Ashtanga satellite shalas around the world. In Finland, where Jois's work ethic has found kinship with the national virtue of *sisu*—a white-knuckled, gritty determination to overcome all odds—it wreaked havoc on the spine of Eija Tervonen. Eija started practice in 1997 in Helsinki. During her Ashtanga honeymoon, she felt elated by the effects of the postures. The breathwork was entrancing. Her instructors noticed her natural flexibility in conjunction with her bodily proportions (torso to leg), and enthusiastically pushed it to its limits with intense adjustments.

Her forward folds were spectacular. When seated with her legs outstretched, she could touch her big toes with her nose. When standing, she could touch her forehead to her ankles. Backbending, however, was another story. Her teachers encouraged her to do all of the typical backbending postures, up to catching her ankles from behind while standing. Within 18 months, Eija began to develop spinal pain. It escalated steadily. She went to chiropractors and physiotherapists for treatment.

Eija recalled, "I was trying to explain to everybody: 'I can't do the practice. It's something about me, about my spine. My spine can't take the practice.'"

Eija's teachers told her that it would eventually resolve. They said that the pain was all in her mind and could be worked through. "And you believe that you are doing something so dramatically good for you. I believed 150%."

As she kept up her practice with faithful determination, Eija also injured her hamstring tendon and her shoulder. When Jois himself came to Helsinki in 2001, her yoga injuries were so acute she could not practice. But she observed his classes.

"I saw his ways of adjusting then," she says, referring to his sexual misconduct.

When the pain finally became intolerable, Eija began her own research in anatomy and biomechanics, and eventually went for diagnostic imaging, which made the damage clear: three disc protrusions in her lumbar spine, all going in different directions. This explained why every movement of her spine—forward, back, and side bending, and also rotation—was extremely painful.

"I was in pain being upright and lying," Eija says, "but any movement in any direction caused serious pain, like leaning over just a little to wash my face or brush my teeth. All normal daily activities."

But the imaging also showed something atypical. Eija was born with six lumbar vertebrae, a congenital oddity that occurs in as many as 3-4% of the population. Her natural skill at forward flexion resulted from the combination of her unique anatomy, including her torso-to-leg length ratio, and her enthusiasm. But when she went into backbending, no amount of enthusiasm could move that extra vertebra out of her way.

It *was* something about her after all.

WHEN "HEALING" AND "THERAPY" BECOME DECEPTIVE TERMS

After years of faithfully practicing the Primary Series, Diane Bruni began to develop severe knee pain.

"I was telling myself that this method was going to heal me and that the knee pain was part of the process of healing," Bruni said.

"I thought that what I needed was to go through that pain to re-align my structure, so that I would be in better alignment, more optimal alignment."

The worldview behind this thought is striking. It is like the body is being used as a metaphor for the unconscious, and that the postures are a form of exploratory surgery meant to look for and eradicate a mysterious disease. Practitioners are using postures to hunt for karma, hidden in the body.

"I believed that practice found the problem, and practice would fix the problem. It did not even *occur* to me that practice was the cause until the pain got so bad it started waking me up at night and I started getting nervous about it."

Diane thought she had a meniscus injury, "like everyone else in Ashtanga had," she said. She made an appointment to have an ultrasound, which revealed a cyst deep in the joint. The doctor speculated the cyst had developed to prevent cartilage damage. She recommended castor oil packs and to stop doing poses that were creating friction in the joint. Bruni followed the advice, and felt better after a month. But when she returned to regular practice, the pain returned and she realized she had to stop.

Diane turned to her lineage mentors for advice. These were some of the top direct students of Pattabhi Jois.

"They told me my knees were in pain because my hips weren't open enough." They prescribed a regime of hip-opening postures that eventually led, Diane believes, to her catastrophic hip injury.

A senior Jivamukti teacher told her that she would have to "break her knees" in order to do the postures. As we'll see in **Part Five**, the Jivamukti Yoga School is an offshoot of the Jois community.

"I wanted to believe it. I wanted to believe in the practice."

"Was this a therapeutic belief, or a spiritual belief?," I asked.

"It was a spiritual belief. But it got confused with a therapeutic belief."

Tracy Hodgeman had a similar experience. She'd been practicing for 13 years when her shoulder collapsed in 2007.

"I was used to my body being rearranged on a regular basis," she wrote in a 2010 blog.

> A sore back, sore sacrum, sore shoulder, sore wrist, sore knee, sore neck—I saw all of these as normal, necessary—even honorable phases through which we all must pass on the way to the perfect yoga body/mind, one finally free of resistance and pain. Growing pains, that's how I thought of it. "Do your practice and all is coming" is another quote from this wise old man.[148]

The work ethic in Tracy's community encouraged her to continue coming to practice and doing what she could. She was advised to stick to the Primary Series.

"In that culture," Hodgeman told me, "any not practicing is seen as avoiding your *dharma* and not doing the work, and slowing down the process of evolution in yourself."

(*Dharma* translates here roughly from the Sanskrit as "social and spiritual duty".)

> I thought: "It's my body rearranging," It happens all the time in yoga. You give yourself these chiropractic adjustments. You twist, and the cracking can roll up the spine, and your spine changes. I've even had ribs come out. I thought "O well, my shoulder will go back." And it didn't go back. For nine months it didn't go back, and I couldn't use my arm. I called it "my broken wing." I had the belief that if I just kept going, yoga would correct all of the problems in my body.

The Primary Series makes strong demands on the shoulders. As a fallback practice for the person with a shoulder (or spinal) injury, it's both ineffective and humiliating. The humiliation aspect encourages some Ashtanga students to use such setbacks as opportunities to interrogate their pride, and to re-position themselves in deference to their teachers.

Michael Kazamias ruptured two of his spinal discs during practice at his home shala in London, England, and was immobilized at home for a full day and a half. He was assisting his teacher, a certified Ashtanga teacher, during that time. For two years prior, he had arrived at the studio long before dawn to do his own practice before helping his teacher adjust the long procession of students who trickled in every morning.

"I had such an obligation to go back and assist him," he told me, "because I was so scared of losing that place. I was so scared, and obligated, and I wanted to do my practice.

"I went back and my teacher said 'Oh, just do sun salutations.' It was ridiculous. I was raising my hands and then crawling on my knees back and forth."

Like T.M., Tracy Hodgeman, and many others, Kazamias kept practicing, and didn't seek medical treatment until much later. He went for massage and acupuncture. His recovery took nine months.

"People said to me: 'It happens to everyone. You just have to go through that.'"

THE CONUNDRUM OF PAIN, THERAPY, AND TRANSCENDENCE

A famous 1977 *Yoga Journal* article by American yoga innovator Joel Kramer coined a phrase that many practitioners now use to describe a treasured goal at the heart of physical practice.[149] "Playing the edge" is the phrase, and the name of the article. We'll see that it works in conjunction with the now-familiar principle of "opening". The "edge", according to Kramer, is where the practitioner can challenge and then open themselves to greater physical and mental capacity.

> Hatha yoga stretches and strengthens one physically so that one has a stronger and more flexible body. Similarly Jnana yoga [the practice of contemplation and meditation] stretches and strengthens one mentally so that one can use the structures that thought builds creatively and harmoniously, and yet not be bound by the limits that thought places on life.
>
> Mental edges are similar to physical edges in that they are marked by resistance to movement and opening. In the mind, fear is the indicator of resistance as pain is in the body. Fear circumscribes the structure of personality or ego. The ways you think about yourself or the world are the basic building blocks of personality and they are very rigid. When these structures are challenged, fear arises. Fear often expresses itself through attack and defense as a means of alleviating the pain that fear brings. Attack and defense are a way of shoring up (protecting) the challenged structure and burying fear in what is called the unconscious, giving you the illusion of not being afraid. Fear is a great teacher since it is a key to finding out the nature, depth, and degree of your attachment to various thought structures.
>
> In Hatha yoga, as you awarely play the edge of what is physically possible, your edge moves. What is possible has changed—you have changed. There is more flexibility, more openness in the tissue, and correspondingly more energy. As Jnana yoga plays the edges of mental resistance, the very doing of this moves the edge, enlarging the limits of what is possible. This is really what expanding consciousness is all about.

The theme of pushing against bodily limitations to stretch the boundaries of self-perception, expressed succinctly here by Kramer, has been a dominant theme in the teaching of India's most popular modern yoga evangelists, such as Jois and B.K.S. Iyengar. But over time, it has also highlighted a conundrum, especially as those same figures have preached the physically healing and therapeutic values of their methods. The simple reason is that the "edge" is defined by pain. One of our most subjective and incommunicable experiences, pain can be developmentally valuable on the road to recovery, as anyone who has done physiotherapy to rehabilitate an injured joint can attest. Of course, pain can also be the sign of injury or harm. In the most complicated situations (as in some cases of self-harming behaviors), pain can also signal a returned sense of embodiment to the traumatized person who has relied on dissociation to survive. In the Jois events described in this book, pain as harm was too often disguised by the premise of pain as progress, with no attention given to the extraordinary range of meanings the person feeling pain—or whatever they might call it—might give it.

Kramer's approach to pain is careful. He writes:

> ...the body's edge in yoga is the place just before pain, but not pain itself. Pain tells you where the limits of physical conditioning lie. Since the edge moves from day to day and from breath to breath (not always forward), in order to be right there, moving with its often subtle changes, you must be very alert. This quality of alertness which is a meditative state is at the heart of yoga.

By contrast, both Jois and Iyengar seem to invite pain as a critical growth experience. "Pain is real," Jois told a student in one conference, suggesting it indicated an increase of purified blood flow. "First you suffering pain," he says. When asked for how long, he replies: "No time ending."[150]

Iyengar's attitude resonates. "When you begin yoga," he told Noëlle Perez-Christiaens, who in 1959 became one of his first Western students, "the unrecognized pains come to the surface. When the *prakriti* has ascended to the level of the soul, then the hidden pains are dispersed."*[151] He also told her: "There should always be a certain amount of pain; then only will you see the light."[152] Then: "What is pain if it enables you to see God?"[153] And, most ominously: "Pain is your guru."[154]

The interviews in *Guruji* seem obsessed with pain. The word appears 118 times over 460 pages. Guy Donahaye asked almost every one of his interviewees about how they dealt with pain in practice. Many gave voluminous philosophical answers about its therapeutic and spiritual necessity, setting the stage for a new generation of readers to surge towards the "edge".

* Here prakriti refers to material, biological nature. Iyengar is suggesting that asana practice brings the body into a purifying relationship with the soul.

CHASING PAIN

"On the one hand," Diane Bruni said about her elite Ashtanga experience,

> practicing asana made us very aware of our bodies. But it also taught us to dissociate with our bodies. It teaches us how to be okay with pain. You're stretching out, you're tearing connective tissues that are meant to be stable structures. The postures hurt! But we keep doing them. The teacher might say, 'Don't let it hurt.' But no one's going to get their leg behind their head unless they have a congenital condition of hypermobility. The average person is going to work really hard for a really long time to try to get their leg even close to behind their head. It will hurt. And they deal with it. Even when I tore my hip apart, I knew how to deal with pain.

"That can be really useful," I offered.

> Absolutely. In childbirth, you know how to deal with pain and you know how to breathe. Or you fall off your bike and you're in a lot of pain, you can keep your head straight and get your phone out and make a call. It comes in handy, but it's also so... what are we doing? Why are we training ourselves to... well, because we had a goal. The goal was extreme postures.

Was that actually the goal? Or was the goal to encounter pain, with the posture serving as proof of survival?

"There's some kind of connection between pain and endorphin release," said Diane.

> Getting high from getting into those postures would linger for hours afterward. That's why it's so hard to give it up when it starts to hurt you. We're all craving that buzz—our own opiates! We associate that feeling with spiritual well-being.
>
> Over time, you need to feed your craving. Otherwise you won't be happy. You're not going to get that rush unless you're pushing past the edge again. Once you've stretched out those connective tissues, and it doesn't hurt anymore, what will you do? The tissues gradually become dysfunctional. How far will you need to go in order to get the pain response that you're craving?

CONFLICTING DESIRES

Many yoga researchers have worked tirelessly to define the modern yoga movement through its postures, techniques, lineages, and entrepreneurs. But the accounts of Diane Bruni, Tracy Hodgeman, Michael Kazamias, Eija Tervonen, and others point to the possibility that something else is at play in holding it all together: a tension between the need for therapy or self-care and the drive towards transcendence, or overcoming the limitations of the self altogether. That tension is both communicated through and confounded by various interpretations of pain. At the best of times, the interplay allows practitioners to explore where everyday life meets the unknown. They can pursue "mundane" goals such as injury repair or emotional self-regulation, while also exploring, against the test of pain, existential questions like *Who am I?* and *What is this body?* But this same tension can allow the harm that a teacher commits on physical or emotional levels to be reframed as spiritual care.

What does the confusion between the desires for therapy and transcendence feel like in the body? Let's consider a basic sensory unit of a physical yoga practice: the humble muscle stretch.

Does it feel pleasurable? For how long? Why are you doing it? Is it improving circulation or "lengthening" the muscle, or is that bad science? Are you, rather, entraining your nervous system to accept a greater ranger of motion for that joint?[155]

Will mobilizing your fascia translate into a deeper capacity for "openness" in your spirituality? Where do your tissues meet the mind? Does bodily flexibility symbolize something that lies beyond the body?

And what about the actual joint? Is this movement healthy for it? How far should you go? How do you know? What happens when you go farther? What happens when you have to go farther to experience the same sensation, because the sensation has receded in intensity? If some stretching is healthy, is more stretching better?

When do you hear your internal language go silent with pain? Is there pleasure in that silence? Peace? Did pain bring you peace? Or are you trying to build tolerance for "breaking through"? Did someone tell you that pain was the voice of the ego's self-imposed limitations? Does the sensation—now pain—change back to pleasure when you release the stretch? What does this all tell you about yourself, locked into what Leonard Cohen calls our "tangle of matter and ghost"?[156]

Broken down into such questions, it's clear how tangled physical and metaphysical drives can be.

As we'll see in **Part Four**, many of the interviewees in *Guruji* complicate these questions by considering them in the context of Jois pushing them into their stretches, or touching them in disorienting ways. Was he nurturing them? Correcting them? Healing them? Testing their boundaries? Taking them beyond their limits? Did they know what their limits were? Did Jois? Did Jois care?

Dedicated yoga practitioners can express a basic conflict in desires, which teachers like Jois are able to exploit unconsciously or consciously. They might want yoga to help them to take care of themselves, but also to take them beyond themselves. They may crave the clinic and spa, but also the austerity of the mountaintop. They may use yoga to foster acceptance of where they are, but also to reject the ordinary lethargy of the selves they know. They may want to accept their bodies, but also reshape them, and sometimes dissociate from them all together. Yoga gives them nurturance, but also deconstruction. They may use postures to put themselves back together, but also to pull themselves apart.

CONFLICTING MEANINGS OF HEALING

In the *Power of Ashtanga Yoga*, Kino MacGregor writes with conviction about the "healing" properties of Jois's method. Her eloquence depends in part on giving the word "healing" many meanings. In some cases, her focus is on physical or therapeutic aspects, but there are also side hints at aesthetic goals.

"The mere practice of the asanas has a healing effect," she writes.

> Forward bends purify the midsection of the body of any excess fatty tissue and help to optimize digestive function. Twisting the torso wrings out the body like a towel from the inside, encouraging the digestive system to work more efficiently and facilitating the removal of stored weight. The gentle pressing of the organs helps any accumulated toxins find their way out of the body.[157]

Whether "traditional", scientific, pseudo-scientific, aspirational, or all four, such notions are common in popular yoga literature and marketing. They also amplify the body-image concerns of the book MacGregor regarded as her "bible". In *Yoga Mala*, Jois describes a forward fold as curing "a number of afflictions, including: body fat; water retention; thighs swollen out of proportion to the size of the body (elephant leg); piles; and sciatica. It also makes the body symmetrical."[158]

But in other usages, MacGregor uses "healing" to refer to the spiritual level of being. The net effect is that "healing" in the Ashtanga world becomes as flexible and potentially manipulative a term as *parampara*, or "opening".

On one hand, the flexibility of the term emphasizes holism. Practitioners who sense that their physical, emotional, and spiritual well-being are all linked together receive powerful validation. On the other hand, a term used in too many ways can lose meaning altogether, and strand the student in the position of never being able hold the teacher responsible to a reasonable and agreed-upon standard of care.

Conflicting meanings of "healing" can be played off each other in such a way that perpetuates a student's confusion, and may lead them to literally chase pain. These problems intersect in Ashtanga stories from people like Diane Bruni, Tracy Hodgeman, Michael Kazamias, and Eija Tervonen that describe an addictive feedback loop in which yoga causes physical pain that is reframed as "opening". If practice is implicated in physical injury, it also promises to heal that injury. If the yoga doesn't heal the injury it likely caused, the practice will be said to have addressed emotional and spiritual levels that are more important than the body anyway. Through all of this, the teacher can be positioned as a shaman of the student's physical experience, interpreting pain and injury according to a metaphysical narrative that only they can discern. The student is encouraged to rationalize harm as care. As we'll explore in **Part Four**, this is a key way in which a cultic organization can foster disorganized attachments amongst its members. It drives people into the paradox of actively seeking out harm from teachers, under the belief that it is care.

The spiritual level to which the teacher appeals is impossible to define. It is not the object of targeted therapy with defined goals so much as a zone of endless toil. This suits the high demands and indefinite timeline of the higher-level Ashtanga commitment. MacGregor and her colleagues both practice and advocate the austerity they learned from Jois: six days of class per week, with two further days off per month on the new and full moons. Whether daily intense practice was a spiritual value of Jois's, or a necessity of the short-term stays of yoga tourists, many of the dedicated students I spoke to corroborated T.M.'s statements about how physically and cognitively exhausting the pace could be. In Mysore, injuries related to intensity and lack of rest were commonplace. When Guy Donahaye interviewed one of Jois's first American students, Norman Allan, Donahaye offered that most people end up crying at some point in the yoga practice.

Allan agreed. "That's true. I did. Usually after, when I was trying to get into the bathtub. Crawling in."[159]

"As we used to leave the shala," replied Donahaye,

> there was a lady who cooked for us, Nagarathna, perhaps after your time. These healthy Westerners used to come to the shala and then we used to just stagger out and limp over to her place for breakfast. A trail of us at dawn, the sun was rising and one was holding a hip, another a knee, the other a shoulder.

"March of the invalids," jokes Allan.[160]

Donahaye's reminiscence not only suggests that injury was common and well-known, but that it was repeated and normalized. It's as if the "health" of said Westerners was the actual problem they had come to heal. This can only make sense within a system of transcendent—as opposed to therapeutic—values, in which the desire for (or pride taken in) bodily health might be framed as a source of delusion and attachment.

WELLNESS GOALS VERSUS ENDLESS GOALS

There are many forms of painful post-operative rehabilitative therapy—like those that follow joint replacement surgery—that require daily effort. But most such tasks are goal-oriented or time-limited. Longer-term psychotherapy is understood to have a natural arc and ending-point, often marked by the resolution or exhaustion of a particular tension for which the therapist has held space. The era of five-sessions-per-week psychoanalysis is virtually over.

But the ultimate aim of the yogic effort for many—spiritual union—is ineffable and unboundaried. It might be considered therapeutic, but only in an existential sense that attempts to untie the knot of the body and resolve the mysteries of the human condition. This means that yoga practice can never really end. It's not something one does for a few years to sort something out. There's always more to do, more to improve along an arc of increasing difficulty. *Practice and all is coming.*

Most contemporary understandings of the professional term "therapy" are not coherent with intensive daily liturgies undertaken to achieve metaphysical goals. But it's easy to see how the two things might be confused by nostalgia, projection, or glossing over the intensity factor. Many Ashtanga practitioners speak of daily practice in ritual terms. The consistent time of day, the candle-lighting, the sequences, the rhythmic breath and adjustments become reliable sacraments. These things might give disciples a secure and therapeutic space.

In part, the tension between therapy and transcendence has ripened out of a rift in the history of what yoga has meant for its practitioners, as well as how its teachers have operated as public figures. Krishnamacharya's career marked the 20th-century shift from the yoga master as a wandering eccentric with a few dreadlocked disciples to something more like an evangelical gym teacher, charged with whipping teenaged boys into shape as paragons of health and nationalist courage. Commissioned by wealthy, Western-educated political reformers, Krishnamacharya's generation modernized yoga to invigorate the body politic of the Indian Independence movement. Central to their concerns were the public health values of "therapy" and "wellness". They plucked yoga out of its medieval heritage to construct an indigenous form of character-building fitness that would prepare the nation for modernity while retaining its connections to the past.[161]

In that past, many yogis indeed craved freedom from disease, and to bolster their immunity using energetic medicine—but not primarily because health was the highest goal.[162] They weren't interested in becoming more productive citizens or adapting to the stresses of urban, industrialized, or middle-class life. They often viewed themselves and were viewed as living outside the joys and troubles of family and business life, focused exclusively on spiritual practice. The general idea was that practice required great vitality and that it took a long time to bear fruit. Yoga was a fire that would eventually consume the yogi. His goal was to make the radiance sustainable, so it could light the way to a new form of existence.

Wellness in premodern yoga was a step towards attaining the deathless realm, where it would then be irrelevant. Along the way, the yogi might get glimpses of enlightenment through practices specifically designed to generate altered states through which he could contemplate or transcend death. *Pranayama*, for example, literally translates as "breath control". In its most extreme usage, it is said to lead to the goal of *utkranti*, or "yogic suicide", by which the yogi uses breath retention techniques to project his life-force out through the crown of his head and into immortality.[163] But in the 20th century, *pranayama* has typically been translated as "breath regulation", and reconfigured according to more worldly health goals. Today, it's studied in relation to things like vagal nerve theory by those who are hopeful that it can lower blood pressure, balance glandular function, or even heal trauma.[164]

Echoes of this historical spectrum of drives contribute to the tensions that increase the allure of the modern yoga movement. The confusion between therapy and transcendence resonates with other paradoxes that can be manipulated: Is yoga ancient or modern? Spiritual or religious? Indian or universal? Patriarchal or progressive? Is the teacher an empty vessel, or the source of an intimate bond?

As the questions echo, an undefinable practice shimmers into view. We can struggle to parse it all out. But that struggle, like friction, seems to increase the charge. Indeed, yoga's power as a practice and culture seems wrapped up in the fact that no one can quite say what it is. This creates both opportunity and vulnerability. The opportunity lies in yoga's capacity to break down and intermingle our typical categories of knowledge and experience, nudging us to swim in the river between the banks of art and science, tradition and innovation, heart and head, sensation and thought, intuition and evidence, religion and medicine.

But swimming can be disorienting. There's little to hold onto. Negotiating an undefined freedom can be scary and exhausting. Perhaps it stimulates a yearning for authoritarianism, to find someone with all the answers. In the absence of the institutions, regulations, scope of practice, and informed consent policies that might define yoga in solidly modern terms, the charisma of individual teachers can easily play an outsized role in answering that need. Some river guides might be pirates.

THERE IS NO TRANSCENDENT SCOPE OF PRACTICE

Those attracted to the Ashtanga yoga space because disciples claim that it is physically healing, or because the Primary Series is called "Yoga Therapy", would need highly attuned filters to truly understand what these claims really mean. The modern consumer of wellness or therapy generally expects certain standards of care. If the modality they are engaging treats musculo-skeletal health, they might expect basic training and proficiency in anatomy and biomechanics. They might expect the practitioner to be able to accurately assess the presenting issue and offer a treatment plan according to a defined scope of practice. Above all, the relationship would be governed by policies like informed consent and collegial accountability that promote transparency and egalitarianism, protect the consumer from fraud or harm, and protect the provider from malpractice claims.

Transcendent or metaphysical models of yoga teaching resist all such regulation. What anatomical training could be relevant to the master who either ignores or doesn't understand what an x-ray is showing, and who sees circuits of energy instead of joints and ligaments? What diseases was Jois *not* qualified to hold forth on, if he was able to advise Tomas Zorzo to give up his hepatitis medication? Why did he shrug off Karen Rain's questions about the back pain that his postures and manhandling likely contributed to? Setting aside the crime of sexual assault—to what college of Jois's peers would Karen appeal if she felt that Jois was injuring her spine?

The starkest differences between the expectations of the modern wellness seeker and the realities of what Jois had to offer are found in the categories of *scope of practice* and *informed consent*. Jois's status among devotees as "guru" meant that there were few if any areas in which, regardless of what they knew about his training, they didn't defer to his vision. In afternoon conferences held in Lakshmipuram and later in Gokulam, students would ask him questions about yoga philosophy, diet, ethics, relationships. "He was an almost God-like figure," as Karen said. "He was all-seeing, all-knowing, all-powerful, and all-loving."

What would limit the scope of practice of such a person? This basic mystique has had broad implications for the entire culture. At the time of writing, no yoga organization in the world has yet formulated a widely accepted scope of practice description for what a yoga teacher can and cannot do. On one hand, this reflects the indefinability of yoga itself and encourages teachers to find work and meaning in the spaces between more institutionalized forms of wellness service. On the other hand, it is also an open door through which the grandiose may walk to exploit the credulity and aspirations of students who want basic care, but also something more.

The possibility of *informed consent* is uncertain within the transcendent mode that hovers in the backdrop of the Ashtanga language of therapy and healing. By definition, the student cannot be informed of the transformation through which they are ostensibly about to be put. It's not like Tracy Hodgeman having her shoulder repaired through surgery or Diane Bruni having her hip put back together with the help of physiotherapy exercises. If the student could understand the mysterious levels upon which the teacher would "heal" them, there'd be no need for practice. But enlightenment can be presented as something the "ignorant" and often unwilling student must be pushed into. Like an extreme posture.

A basic premise of spiritual transformation is that it transcends mundane understanding. The teacher cannot inform the student about what it is before it happens. This makes consent problematic. Spiritual transcendence is not just about rising up out of physical and emotional tension and turmoil into another realm. It potentially involves the abandonment or even destruction of that part of the person that could consent to any process at all. The unenlightened, after all, are bound by their ignorant wills and choices. The limited, fearful, egoically concerned person who would be deciding whether or not transcendence was desirable is exactly the person that the practices of transcendence, and relationships to transcendence-mode teachers, would deconstruct.

To sum up, we can consider the words of Nick Evans, interviewed by fellow Jois student Guy Donahaye. Evans describes coming to Jois in Mysore in 2000 after a youth of punk rock and compulsive behaviors, and a perilous recovery from an aggressive cancer. In his hymn of praise below, many of the above themes begin to coalesce and illustrate how a rich spiritual poetry can both inspire practitioners, but also provide opportunities for—and disguise—abuse. "Healing" is associated with transcendence when it doesn't have a concrete physical referent. The therapy Jois offers surpasses all understanding. It is hands-on. It can only be accepted when the student gives up their resistance.

"Do you see Guruji as a healer?" Donahaye asks Evans.

"Yes."

"What qualities does he embody that lead you to say that?"

> When I look at his face and when I'm in his presence, I think he knows that there is one eternal infinite power living in us all and making all this happen and grow and move. It's making the sun go up and making all the galaxies not fall into themselves. In his tradition, they call it Ishvara. Not only Guruji and his guru but his family have spent generations and generations and generations acknowledging and working with this power and understanding that this power is what's real, and what we perceive to be reality is a covering, or the clothes that this power wears. When your primary contact is with this power, with this source of being, and that's something that you've inherited in the work that your parents have done and the work that their parents have done and their parents have done and the work that the entire culture has done—regarding that as the way life works. Not that we are

> all separate people striving for our own. And I think that light shines through you, and I think that light shines through him. I think he knows. He says, "All is God." He makes no bones about it. In *Yoga Mala*, he says, "Nothing is achieved." I can't remember the exact quote, I don't want to misquote him. I think the quote is something along the lines, "Nothing in the universe is done by individual will alone, that is definite.... All is God. Practice, practice and all is coming." And I think there is less between him and that understanding than other people and that understanding.

"How does that play into his healing powers?" asks Donahaye.

> Because when he puts his hands on you, when he smiles at you, when he is with you, that's what's with you. That understanding, that firm belief, established understanding, knowledge, is what pours out of him. And of course it's everywhere all the time, but because we are so enmeshed in our bodies and our histories and resistance and fear, we don't contact it. We don't make a connection with it. But when he touches us, it is like light flowing from him into us. Healing love, knowledge, power, forgiveness, kindness. You are already perfect. He knows it, we don't know it. He knows it, he touches us, and with absolute certainly [sic] he knows that to be the case. We don't. We go, "Oh yes," but arrogance and personal self-preservation get in the way.[165]

THE DECEPTION OF *GURUJI*

So far this book has cited well over a dozen passages from the book of interviews that Guy Donahaye co-edited with fellow American Jois disciple, Eddie Stern, himself one of Karen Rain's co-demonstrators in that famous 1993 video. Donahaye has since distanced himself from the book, writing in a post that:

> Since his death, Guruji has been elevated to a position of sainthood. Part of this promotion has been due to the book of interviews I collected and published with Eddie Stern… which paints a positive picture of his life and avoids exploring the issues of injury and sexual assault. In emphasizing only positive stories it has done more to cement the idea that he was a perfect yogi, which he clearly was not.

> By burnishing his image, we make it unassailable—it makes us doubt the testimony of those he abused. This causes further harm to those whose testimony we deny and to ourselves.
>
> I would like to offer my sincere apologies to all victims who were harmed by Guruji or by his teachings as passed through his students for my part in cultivating this image of perfection that denies the suffering and healing of many.[166]

In light of this admission, the book's online advertising copy now rings hollow. "It is a rare and remarkable soul," it says,

> who becomes legendary during the course of his life by virtue of great service to others. Sri K. Pattabhi Jois was such a soul, and through his teaching of yoga, he transformed the lives of countless people. The school in Mysore that he founded and ran for more than sixty years trained students who, through the knowledge they received and their devotion, have helped to spread the daily practice of traditional Ashtanga yoga to tens of thousands around the world.[167]

The collection of 30 interviews—24 with Jois's non-Indian students, three with family members, and three with Jois's Indian friends and colleagues—has become a staple of Ashtanga literature. On *Goodreads,* 90% of over 240 ratings show four stars and above. In her five-star review, an influential Ashtanga blogger writes that the book is "a profound treasure-trove and I read sections of it over and over again to absorb its inspiration." In 2014, the blogger made the book the subject of a Sunday discussion group for students at her yoga shala.[168]

Only a few online reviews express skepticism about the general tone of the book, or its haloed subject.* This is despite the fact that the photograph showing Jois groping the genitals of two women at the same time was in circulation from 2009 and Anneke Lucas's disclosure about being assaulted by Jois had been published in 2010.

Guruji can be categorized as a classic form of hagiography: an account of the nature, virtues, and miracles of a saint. As a literary form, hagiographies in this style date back to the early medieval period in Europe and even earlier in various parts of Asia. Its purpose is to uncritically elevate the subject as a

* 79% five-star review rate on *Amazon*; 86% four-to-five-star review rate on *Goodreads* as of 11/15/2018.

focal point of spiritual power and inspiration. Stories about saints are given pride of place in the life of many religious communities. The books they are printed in sit on altars. Readings from them can lend content to homilies and color to rituals.

A hagiography stimulates, supports, and validates faith while extending the reach of a community. But it can also delay or even suppress the possibility of other views about that community, and its leaders from forming and appearing. The book you are reading now does not take an anti-hagiography stance because it is not making claims about Jois's inner nature or character. Focus remains on his behavior, and the purported network of care associated with him. This behavior, and that network, harmed many people. This book is built upon stories that the reader of *Guruji* alone would not have access to.

The voices of these stories have to fight for air and space in relation to the stories told in *Guruji*. They face all of the typical rape culture mechanisms of silencing, customized for the yoga world. Karen Rain and the others have to speak out against a decades-old, well-practiced, and continuous chorus of idealization and sentimentality. They have to compete with Donahaye's interviewees, many of whom professionally and socially benefit from having their views platformed in his volume. Donahaye's interviewees didn't have to perform complex emotional calculations around how much more they would lose by being interviewed, how they might be further marginalized or minimized by speaking out. They didn't have to gird themselves against the violent questions to which Karen Rain responded in one of our final interviews:

"Why did you stay if he was abusing you?"

"Why didn't you resist?"

"Weren't you getting something out of it?"

"How could what you're saying be true, if Jois was such a healing teacher for so many?"

On page after page, Donahaye and Stern lob softball after softball, and wait for each disciple to hit it out of the park with the bat of devotion.

Yet the book is not implausible for the prospective Ashtanga student who knows nothing of Ashtanga's real complexities. The *Guruji* interviews may be strongly filtered through an adulation towards Jois, but the voices are diverse enough that the aforementioned blogger, in her review, conveys the impression of a well-rounded picture. She writes of "the varying degrees of professed certainty about the tradition, throughout the text", and "the different explanations subjects give for the transformative energy of SKPJ: some say he's magic, some say he's an archetypical-mythic healer, some say he's a therapist for psyche and soul, some say what he transmits is discipline and science." The blogger points to the humanity of the interviewees—"the brittle certainties of Brad Ramsey and Annie Pace"—and even to the troubling structural dynamics at play: "the hidden influence of the caste system and gender norms."[169] This attentiveness to detail obscures a far more obvious reality, hiding in plain sight. The book's *apparent* subtlety, spot lit by reviews like these, both reinforces and markets the Jois idealization.

Arguably, *Guruji* crosses over from hagiography into a soft form of propaganda. "Soft" because it was published after Jois's death, and so could not be technically said to be drawing prospective recruits directly to him. However, the majority of online reviews show that the book has had a galvanizing effect upon group faith in the practice and Jois's certified and authorized teachers.[170] It would be impossible to thoroughly assess how this faith translates into commitment to the group, nor how that commitment translates into financial returns for Jois's students or the KPJAYI. Nonetheless, these are questions worth considering. *Guruji* is not only representative of the group's aspirations and mythology; it can't help but to contribute to the consolidation of its social and physical capital as well.

"The group's propaganda," writes cult researcher Alexandra Stein (drawing on Hannah Arendt),[171]

> must serve to prevent the recruit from examining too closely its actual practices and history and instead must sway them through overwhelming their critical thinking with superficial and emotionally arousing information and experiences. Through deception it engages recruits by presenting the group in a non-threatening light. It begins to introduce the language of indoctrination in preparation for consolidating the recruit as a group member.[172]

Stein goes on to distinguish the plausible and digestible propaganda of a cultic organization from more radical and hidden forms of indoctrination.

> Few would willingly join an organization that ends up controlling every element of life, but many might be interested in charitable works, or developing themselves spiritually, politically or socially. Few women would deliberately enter a relationship in which they are to be beaten. They are wooed into it. Propaganda serves this initial wooing function.[173]

In *Guruji*, you will not read about assaults being rationalized as healing touch, or about women being told point-blank that "it's not sexual." You will read "ideas, messages, images and narratives that are used specifically to communicate with the outside world," in the words of Stein. She explains that propaganda is "delivered through the front groups that form the outer shell and entry point for many totalist groups." Following Arendt, Stein suggests that front groups "serve as transmission belts between the internal world of the cult and the external world." Indoctrination follows upon propaganda, and takes root once the member has been isolated from other points of view, and is able to consider the truth of the group's beliefs without being repulsed.[174]

The idealizations and omissions upon which *Guruji* is built can be seen as preparatory to the indoctrination of Jois's victims being told that their injuries were part of a spiritual process, or that his groping "wasn't sexual." These details were as hidden from both the general public and casual Ashtanga practitioners as the voices of the victims themselves.

WHO KNEW, HOW MUCH, AND WHEN?

By nature, propaganda is deceptive. Stein's analysis carries the strong suggestion that it is intentional: that the cultic organization has carefully crafted its public message for the purpose of recruiting new members. In the case of *Guruji*, the intentionality and motivations of the interview subjects and the editors are unknowable. The facts, however, are clear.

The book was first published in 2010 from interviews dating back to the 1990s. Anneke Lucas says that she told Eddie Stern about Jois assaulting her in Manhattan in 2001. Stern confirmed this by email. A colleague of Stern's who wishes to remain anonymous describes meeting with Stern and two other senior Jois students in Mysore in 1993. At that meeting, Jois's assault behavior was openly discussed, but no commitment to addressing it was formed.

In response to a question about Jois and assault sent in October 2016—before his distancing statement—Donahaye wrote: "As far as inappropriate touch is concerned—I have heard the same rumors and stories as you."[175]

In a follow-up email he wrote:

> I am not interested in gossip or bad talking people. The *Guruji* book was a celebration of his life, which was made during his

> lifetime and with his family's collaboration. There were a few moments where the interview subject kind of chuckled and said "well, you know, Guruji loved the girls..." But no more stories about inappropriate touch.[176]

There is only one moment in the book that comes close to what Donahaye describes. Nick Evans, whom the blogger-reviewer writes has a "raw, warm, attractive honesty," is quoted as telling Donahaye that before he met Jois, "I heard all sorts of funny tales, that he liked gold and he kissed the girls."[177] Donahaye did not respond to a question which I put to him in May 2018 about whether there were similar quotes from other interviews which had been edited out for the book.

"It was in the air," said *Details* journalist Larry Gallagher about Jois's behavior, remembering his assignment to Mysore in 1995. "Pretty much anyone who was there for any length of time knew about it."

Dozens of interviews with senior students, the vast majority of whom insisted on staying off record, confirmed Gallagher's statement. Bryan Kest, who went on to coin the term "Power Yoga", and apply it to his interpretation of Jois's method, read an early draft of the article this book expands upon, and made the following statement: "I can confirm that everything mentioned did happen, and even if I didn't see it happening to the specific persons named, I saw these things happen to others, and I saw a lot more than that."

Beryl Bender Birch, another Power Yoga pioneer, echoes Kest. "My, God, everybody knew," she told yoga teacher and podcaster J. Brown in a revealing interview about the Jois's summer tour of southern California in 1987.

> By the time the end of that summer came around, you know, every single town we were in, somebody, uh, there was some uproar about a woman being, uh, you know, molested, abused, mishandled, um, having, you know, hands put in inappropriate places.
>
> And I remember this woman came up to my husband and me and, and we were studying with Pattabhi Jois, uh, at Richard's studio in Boulder, came up to us in the, in the Co-op after the class and crying, saying, "Oh, he put his finger up my [inaudible]. Do you think that's clinical?" My husband burst out, cracking up. He goes, "Uh, no, it's not clinical."

...

> **[Brown]:** Well, I want to ask you, because you've mentioned that you didn't, you didn't consider yourself a devotee. Um, and you, you just told us the, and I've heard this before, that people knew that stuff was going on, like everybody, everybody says it was obvious...
>
> **[Birch]:** Oh my God, everybody knew!
>
> **[Brown]:** Why do you, why do you think nobody said anything? Was it just like the dynamic around him and the power differentials at play, and essentially some kind of cult dynamics at work? Why, why nobody questioned that that was happening. Like right in front of everybody?
>
> **[Birch]:** I asked the same question like, how come nobody, but you know, I mean in Santa Cruz was it say, yeah, Santa Cruz, this man stood up and he said, "I have a", we were all in rest or anything. We're about 25 people in that class, maybe 30 and, he stood up at the end and um, he says, "I have an announcement to make. I like to say that I'm very disappointed. My wife was molested in this class," and you know, everybody's going, Oh my God. Oh shit. Oh no. And you know, hiding in the corners and um, and you know, and Pattabhi Jois just feigned complete ignorance. Like "What are you...? I don't speak English. I don't know what you're talking about." Um, People, someone called the police on him, and I forget if it was Boulder or Encinitas. Tim* every time Pattabhi Jois came to Encinitas. Tim was trying to [inaudible ... the heat] just calm everything down.[178]

Birch traveled with Jois in 1987. Kest was in Mysore in 1989 and 1990. The accounts of Mysore travelers Kiran Bocquet (1983), T.M. (1996), Marisa Sullivan (1997), and Maya Hammer (1997) all strongly suggest that the behavior was widely known. Jubilee Cooke (1997) writes that she strongly suspects that the senior students all knew.

Donahaye started his interviews in 1997. While neither he nor Stern

* Birch is referring to Tim Miller, who took over the Ashtanga Yoga Nilayam in Encinitas, California, from Brad Ramsey and Gary Lopedata in 1980. Miller's shala is now called the Ashtanga Yoga Center, and it's located 10 miles away, in Carlsbad.

may have been aware of the *extent* of Jois's assaults—and certainly not their impacts, as the impacts of sexual assault are hidden from most men—the odds that they were completely unaware of them must be small. Even if the allegations existed for both of these editors between 1997 and 2010 only in rumor form, it would arguably be the responsibility of anyone committed to the premise that yoga practice requires honesty and truthfulness to seek out those voices and ask them what they know. If *Guruji* sought to present truth, it presented one version of the truth that excluded and silenced many others.

The promotion of Jois continues, both in Mysore and Jois satellite shalas worldwide. At the time of writing, a life-sized black and white portrait of Pattabhi Jois, taken in the 1980s hangs on the wall overlooking the practice floor of Eddie Stern's well-appointed Brooklyn Yoga Club. He sits in full lotus on a striped cotton mat, his head tilting downward. His closed eyes bless the current generation of twisting and sweating aspirants below. In the retail space, they can relax after class, sipping smoothies and browsing copies of *Guruji*.

Part Four

Disorganized Attachments

[Disorganized attachment] responses occur when a child has been in a situation of fright without solution. Their caregiver is at once the safe haven and also the source of threat or alarm. So, when the child feels threatened by the caregiver, he or she is caught in an impossible situation: both comfort and threat are represented by the same person—the caregiver. The child experiences the unresolvable paradox of seeking to simultaneously flee from and approach the caregiver. This happens at a biological level, not thought out or conscious, but as evolved behavior to fear. The child attempts to run TO and flee FROM the caregiver at one and the same time... *However, in most cases the need for proximity—for physical closeness—tends to override attempts to avoid the fear-arousing caregiver.* So usually the child stays close to the frightening parent while internally both their withdrawal and approach systems are simultaneously activated, and in conflict.[179]

—Alexandra Stein

We don't need non-attachment. We need better attachments.

—Diana Alstad, personal conversation, August 2009

OVERVIEW

Part Three showed that Ashtanga yoga has on occasion promoted itself through deceptive means, which is a foundational cultic technique. Jois, his family, and his senior students have consistently endorsed or used inflated or exaggerated terms, claims, or legends to attest to the longevity and spiritual authenticity of the method. They have used ambiguous terms like "healing" and "opening" that have confused students about the nature and benefits of the postures and the injuries they cause. They have silenced or suppressed other points of view. Some have gone beyond propaganda into the territory of indoctrination, using euphemisms like "*mulabandha* adjustment" to describe sexual assault.

Following *deception*, a member's *dependence* upon the group and their *dread of leaving* round out the classic cultic triad. This part will begin with a survey of other basic models from cult analysis literature that can help us to understand the self-sealing nature of toxic group dynamics.

Following that, a review of Alexandra Stein's work on attachment patterns in high-demand groups will outline how systems of undue influence actively confuse members about the nature and meaning of love and care. Members get caught in a seemingly endless loop of running towards a leader to give them their money, their bodies, and their hearts, even as the leader harms them. Examples from Jois-centered literature will show this in action.

CULT ANALYSIS MODELS: STARTING WITH "DECEPTION, DEPENDENCE, DREAD OF LEAVING"

Cult analysis literature offers many models for exploring how the behavior of Pattabhi Jois was enabled for close to 30 years, while his community grew in numbers, financial strength, and cultural impact. **Part Three** covered a feature that all of these models share in common: deception. A high-demand group deceives the public and its members. Deceiving the public is affected through propaganda, while members are deceived to the point of difficult return by processes of indoctrination. The two other steps in the famous model of Michael Langone, who updated studies from the late 1950s of victims of Korean War "brainwashing" techniques, are that the group fosters a sense of *dependence* within the member, and then instills them with a *dread* of leaving.[180]

MIND MODEL

Cathleen Mann's MIND mode begins with ***Manipulation***, a series of "techniques used by cults to ensure compliance by using undue influence." Mann writes that manipulation

> involves several other elements such as: impression management; lying about facts and history; assuring conformity to a teaching without question; betraying of confidences; denying reality; and changes to diet, sleeping patterns, and overactivity.
>
> The ***Indoctrination*** phase features deliberate changes to a person's environment without consent, knowledge, or awareness .... begin[ning] with recruitment, binding an individual to the group through ritual and secrets, creating a sense of specialness, and replicating family bonds....
>
> ***Negation*** is next...a process of devaluing the individual and their past through sustained criticism often labeled as feedback or disengagement. All successful cults downplay the ego and consider it the ultimate enemy.

In this light the continual degradation of the "ego" in some yoga discourses merits close consideration.

Finally, cults use ***Deception*** in Mann's model to foster a temporary betrayal of self without awareness of the reasons driving it. "Deception occurs in a pyramid fashion where those above know more than those below, and leaders at the top restrict knowledge through the use of loyalty tests to climb higher in the pyramid."[181]

BITE MODEL

Steve Hassan spent two and a half years as a lieutenant in the Unification Church, aka the "Moonies" (after its founder, Sun Myung Moon (1920–2012)). He's since become an anti-cult activist, best known for what he calls the BITE model. Hassan argues that the mechanisms employed by cults seek to control members in four areas: behavior, information, thought, and emotion.[182]

The members' ***Behavior*** is controlled through work, rigorous daily schedule commitments, and isolation from other forms of relationship. This is something to consider in relation to the commitment of the devoted Ashtanga member to practicing a regime six days per week that demands reorganizing family and work schedules, often leaves them preoccupied with diet and sleep, and with recovering from exertion or injury. At middling-to-advanced levels of commitment, members will sometimes practice in excess of two hours per day. Here we can recall how Tracy Hodgeman reports that at the time of her shoulder collapse, she was practicing up to three hours per session, and having to visit her chiropractor weekly to help her continue.

After behavioral control, Hassan says that the amount of ***Information*** the member of a high-demand group receives is limited to that which will support their relationship to that group. To see how this maps onto the Jois community, refer back to the omissions and deceptions detailed in **Part Three.**

The ***Thoughts*** of the member are controlled through various means, such as instilling black-and-white thinking, using "loaded language" and "clichés" to overwrite the rational mind, and reject the value of critical analysis. Here, the common Jois mantras come to mind, which were typically offered in response to questions: "Practice and all is coming," and "Yoga is 99% practice and 1% theory." Recall that T.M. remarked that critical thinking was also inhibited for her by physical exhaustion and the low-protein diet—one example of the ways in which control mechanisms overlap to reinforce each other.

The ***Emotions*** of the member are controlled through instilling a fear of leaving, outlawing anger or other emotions that might resist the leadership, doling out praise and love when the member excels at the program, and shutting the member out when they fall off. These are all detectable in stories emerging from the inner Jois world, but looming large over all of them is the monolithic love and devotion both embodied and encouraged by books like *Guruji*, and the prominent placement of Jois's photograph—and sometimes veneration—in virtually every studio in the world that teaches his method.

"TRAUMATIZED NARCISSISM" AND "PROPHETIC CHARISMA"

Technical models can be really useful for instantly naming and reframing group behaviors in a new light. There are also slower, warmer types of analysis.

The American psychoanalyst Daniel Shaw, a survivor of the yoga cult of Swami Muktananda (1908–82),[183] has produced rich work on the inner landscape of the cult leader, which he describes as being one of "traumatized narcissism."[184] He describes the typical cult leader as someone who has never healed from a childhood trauma that disrupted the capacity to feel like a functional self. Subsequently, they cannot help but to sociopathically exploit the emotional energy of their followers.

Len Oakes, another cult survivor (yes, it's a theme), operates through a similar frame in his examination of several cult leaders who exhibit what he calls "prophetic charisma", a narcissism that expresses through self-isolation, a burning desire for autonomy, a tendency towards grandiosity, and a skill for manipulation.[185]

Writers like Shaw and Oakes add to the insights of theorists who study the power of loaded language, bounded choice, group trance and other means of silencing critical thinking and isolating group members while conveying the impression of loving unity. I personally found their ideas to be very useful for me at a beginning stage of my cult recovery. The psychoanalytic concepts are contested by more scientifically oriented psychologies, but their poetry is compelling. Beginning to imagine the inner world and feelings of the person at the top of a high-demand group seemed to hit closer to home than the abstractions of the more clinical frameworks. They allowed me the time and space to reflect on how I'd related to cult leaders I'd known, how they presented certain moods or wounds or behavioral patterns that I found attractive or familiar to me.

Analysis focused on the personality traits of group leader can be limited in two ways. First, the correlation between traumatized narcissism and the likelihood that someone will become a cult leader can be weak. Likewise, charisma expressed through grandiosity and even manipulativeness is not a predictor of cult leadership. Plenty of traumatized narcissists, charismatic or not, don't become cult leaders.

Secondly, analysis of the inner life of the *leader* may bias the reader towards asking questions about the inner life of the *follower*. This can detract from the structural analysis of group power that more accurately measures the effects of the cult as a *system*, and can lead readers up to and often over the edge of victim-blaming territory. The inner lives and motivations of both Pattabhi Jois and Karen Rain are immaterial to the crime of sexual assault and the social forces that enabled it.

The cult analysis language of "deception, dependence, and dread of leaving", however, is intense and impersonal. The picture it forms is harsh; the reasoning aggressive and seemingly bulletproof. At a feeling-level, it seems to mirror the problem it tries to untangle. This is not surprising, since so much of this research comes from the study of military-grade thought reform techniques employed by hardline Maoists against POWs during the Korean War, or, if the theory is reaching back to Hannah Arendt, from an analysis of Nazi and Stalinist totalitarianism.[186] Additionally, it matured in a panicked rush in the 1980s in response to the extreme cult disasters at Osho's

(1931–90) Rajneeshpuram community in Oregon in the mid-1980s and the massacre at Jim Jones' (1931–78) People's Temple at Jonestown, Guyana in 1978. The result is an often alarmist and dark literature that presents the cult as psychopathic machine wreaking unspeakable horror.

But to insiders, cult life often does not feel this way. My own cult experience consisted of a messy series of complex relationships, experienced up close and personal, one or two at time, through infinite micro-moments that recorded themselves into my feeling-body as deeply and subtly as childhood experiences. "Brainwashing" or "mind control" sound too technocratic to describe what this actually felt like. I may have been "rewired" by my cult experiences, but it happened in the same way that family or romantic partnerships happened. It happened through closeness and contact that felt indistinguishable from love.

CULT ANALYSIS: HEART AND MICRO-MOMENTS

The work of British social psychologist Alexandra Stein bridges the crucial gap between exposing structures of oppression and explaining the feelings through which they are built in moment-by-moment relationship. She humanizes and normalizes the cult experience by using a potent tool of contemporary relational psychology called "attachment theory" to show how the cult or high-demand group exploits the common human tendency to form bonds through trauma.

Stein agrees with Langone, Mann, Hassan, and others that cults definitely deploy the tactics of deception, dependence, and dread. They propagandize, manipulate, indoctrinate, and negate the agency of the individual. They seek to control behaviors, information, thoughts, and emotions. Stein's innovation is to suggest that the primary means through which cults perpetrate all of these abuses against members—who not only do not leave, but also seem to become advocates and defenders of their precarious condition—is to foster a series of relational responses that attachment researchers define as "disorganized". "It is, in fact," Stein writes, "the primary task of the totalist system to effect this change: to gain control of followers it must, in fact, rewire attachment behavior and utterly reconfigure followers' attachments."[187]

I highly recommend reading Stein's book for a comprehensive introduction to attachment theory in relation to cult dynamics. The following summary will be enough to frame her work as a powerful lens for studying yoga culture in general, and the Jois events in particular. It will allow us to focus on the non-verbal micro-moments of intimate contact between teachers and students as the basic medium for how power is either shared or abused.

Feeling into those micro-moments is not easy. The interviews that form the backbone of this book tell us a lot, but it's often prohibitively hard for people to slow down their memories to the granularity of sensation—especially when the memories are traumatic, and even more so when they are talking to a writer they may not entirely trust.

The bodily context for how Jois's touch was harmful or assaulting is just such a granular phenomenon. When we talk with a person about being assaulted, listening to the words is critical, but just as critical is tuning in to the wordless moments driving those stories. I have learned so much, for instance, from just driving in a car with Karen Rain, or meditating on a grainy photo of Jois groping an unnamed woman in a California shala, bearing witness to the eerie dissociation on her turned-away face. We have to understand that most peoples' relationships with Jois—and in the next generation, with his senior students—developed in silent gestures and pressures that the theoretical language of yoga cannot really capture, and most language of cult analysis seems to "murder to dissect", in the words of Wordsworth. [188]

Like mindful yoga movement, attachment theory gets us right down into the sensations of relationship, where both harm and healing are first made known.

ATTACHMENT THEORY PRIMER

Attachment theory has its roots in the work of the British psychologist John Bowlby, who in the late 1950s—likely inspired by the separation stresses of his own war-torn childhood—plunged headlong into the study of what happens when children are separated from and then reunited with their caregivers. Bowlby had an early fascination with the work of researchers who studied the way baby monkeys and goslings imprinted themselves with a primal sensorimotor link to their mothers. Later, he was deeply influenced by his mentorship with the old-school Viennese psychoanalyst Melanie Klein, and through his collegial relationship with British child psychoanalyst and developmental theorist DW Winnicott.

Both Klein and Winnicott were pioneers in revising the individualistic and overly theoretical legacy of Freud. Up until that point, psychologists had primarily speculated on the internal dynamics of a person's development, extracted from the pervasive relational influences that surround and inform them. Klein, through her granular focus on mother-and-infant dynamics, zeroed in on the human personality as a relational phenomenon, rather than something essential, inborn, or solitary. Legend has it that Winnicott took this theme to its logical conclusion by standing up at a meeting of the British Psychoanalytical Society in the 1940s and shouting, "There is no such thing as a baby!" His point was that it's impossible to understand the experience of the infant—and by extension, the adult—without understanding the relationships through which we emerge. There is no baby, according to Winnicott, but there is an all-important "nursing couple".[189]

Klein, Winnicott, and Bowlby grounded their theories in highly detailed clinical observations of how parents and children interact with each other non-verbally: through eye contact, mirroring, facial expressions, body positions, and signs of arousal or relaxation. (These are all elements at play in full force in a high-intensity yoga classroom.) Their practice of close study threaded its way forward through the work of analysts like the American Louise Kaplan, whose 1979 book *Oneness and Separateness* innovated a breathtaking poetry for how the parent and child become themselves in relation to each other through the push and pull of discovering they are neither unified when with each other, nor truly separated when apart.[190](Kaplan's book reads like an extended meditation on yoga philosophy.) This same attention informed Mary Ainsworth's 1965 "Strange Situation" experiments, in which babies and toddlers were closely observed for their bodily reactions to being separated from and reunited with their caregivers, after an intervention by a stranger who enters the laboratory to offer comfort.[191] Daniel Stern picks up this thread of close observation in his work on the "Motherhood Constellation", in which he meticulously tracks the smallest changes in bodily orientation between parents and children as they attempt to attract or avoid attention and connection.[192]

In different ways, all of these clinicians studied what observably happens when an infant, toddler, child, or adult experiences separation from their primary caregiver or partner. In response to that stress, the child exhibits an "attachment behavior" that seeks to regain the protection of the caregiver. The specific behaviors are many and overlapping, and people can exhibit more than one pattern as they pass through different situations and times of life. The differences between them are said to be reflective of the quality of attunement that the person has experienced in relation to their caregiver, the subsequent levels of trust they feel, and the confidence they have that their needs will be met. The person who has had the repeated experience of a caregiver soothing the stress of separation and meeting their needs with empathy—but without being overbearing—will have one attachment "style", while the person who had the repeated experience of not being appropriately soothed and cared for will develop another.

Within the spectrum of attachment behaviors, several main categories emerged from Ainsworth's and Bowlby's research, and have gone on to fuel a rich literature.

SECURE ATTACHMENT

In ideal circumstances, a person metabolizes the stress of separation or unfamiliarity with an ease that comes from entrained trust and confidence that the caregiver will return to them, be recognizable to them, and give them familiar support. This not only means that their experience of relationship in general is one of grounded kindness, but that the security built up by repeated trusting experiences allows the person to exercise their independence with confidence and curiosity. This person has the profound advantage of being able to turn off their attachment behaviors or strategies whenever they return to their assured safety.

"INSECURE" ATTACHMENT

In less ideal circumstances, the person has not benefited from enough repeated and predictable nurturing experiences to have been able to fully build trust. This means that separation or the stress of the unfamiliar amplifies an ongoing sense of relational anxiety. Their attachment strategies are said to be "insecure". Whereas the securely attached person might simply note a new circumstance of aloneness or unfamiliarity as a novel landscape to explore with confident prudence, the insecurely attached person is instantly triggered by the stress of separation, and will begin to execute one or a mixture of the following two anxious strategies in an attempt to quell stress and restore order. These two groupings of insecure attachment behaviors reflect an emphasis on one or the other main forms of attaining safety: when under stress, people tend to both *approach* potential sources of help and *withdraw* from causes of harm.

"PREOCCUPIED" ATTACHMENT BEHAVIOR

Those who exhibit more of the *approaching* strategy often present what is called an "preoccupied" attachment style. They will hover and seem to be constantly craving the presence and attentions of their caregiver. But because they don't completely trust the caregiver, being close to them isn't fulfilling or reassuring. This is why the word "ambivalence" is often used as a descriptor here. The person is expressing the need to be close to a caregiver whom they know may not fulfill this need.

"DISMISSIVE" ATTACHMENT BEHAVIOR

On the other side of the insecure spectrum, those who exhibit more of the *withdrawing* strategy are often said to present a "dismissive" style of attachment. In this more self-isolating scheme, the person pre-emptively cuts the emotional losses they expect to experience in relation to a caregiver who has repeatedly failed or neglected them. They develop a skill for detachment, but may lag behind in the capacity to ask for help.

These two types of attachment behaviors are thought to become patterned. Because the relationship to the caregiver is not fully trustable, the person will always be somewhat vigilant, and that vigilance will color the entire relationship, and perhaps amplify within it over time.

The preoccupied and dismissive styles pose personal and social challenges, but because they are more or less predictable and manageable, they are said to be "organized". This means that the person who wants to work on these tendencies in therapy with the goal of becoming less clingy (preoccupied) or less aloof (dismissive) has a good shot at making sustainable progress. The preoccupied person can work with a range of techniques to self-regulate, and the dismissive person can work on their resistance to reaching out. The theory suggests that because a person's life experience is rooted in these relational strategies—again, the categories are porous and we all employ some of each—understanding these core patterns of how one relates to caregivers will have far-reaching benefits.

"DISORGANIZED" ATTACHMENT BEHAVIOR

When a person's experience in relation to caregivers has become unmanageable, they might begin to display bouts of what researchers call "disorganized" attachment behavior. This is thought to be the result of the caregiver not simply being undependable or prone to irritability, depression, or neglect. Here, the caregiver was abusive and manipulative to the extent that the person's approach and withdrawal mechanisms have been locked into constant high arousal and conflict. The person must approach the caregiver, who, if it is a parent, will help them stay alive. But they also must flee from the rage and the danger. The resultant attachment style is neither preoccupied nor dismissive, but a volatile oscillation between the two, taking both to extremes. It is "disorganized" because it is mirroring the unpredictability of the caregiver, and also because it is the result of the collapse of more functional, "organized" strategies.

The disorganized category was identified through research in which children were, as Stein reports,

> unpredictably frightened by their caregivers—whether directly as a result of frightening behavior by the caregivers, or indirectly resulting from the caregivers themselves being frightened. These children sometimes showed the typical secure and insecure (pre-occupied, dismissing) strategies described above, but they also displayed brief but disorganized and disoriented behaviors including signs of confusion, fear, freezing and strange movements.[193]

Films of children presenting disorganized attachment responses are almost unbearable to watch. "He or she makes movements to approach the frightening or frightened parent," observes Stein, "at the same time as trying to avoid the fearful stimuli coming from the parent."[194] The child looks lost and glassy-eyed. Their movements and gestures might be repetitive, as though caught between wanting to communicate something they cannot, and wanting to rock or soothe themselves with something predictable. They look isolated, cut off.

A POTENTIAL CONFUSION OF DISSOCIATION AND MYSTICISM

At a certain pitch of "confusion, fear, freezing, and strange movements", the child either is dissociating, or on their way there—although the dissociative state is literally *nowhere*. That is, they surrender the attempt to cognitively understand an unintelligible situation. Their mind goes quiet and numb. If there is emotional or physical pain, they may absent themselves from the feeling-body. This can feel like *depersonalization*: floating above the scene, or standing beside themselves, watching something happen to someone who vaguely resembles them. It can also feel like euphoria, simply because an unmanageable identification with an assaulted body has been momentarily relieved.

How these sensations might emerge in relation to abuse in a yoga or spiritual setting are crucial to understand, because every one of them can be reframed by the priest, teacher, or even the indoctrinated person themselves as a sign of spiritual attainment. The person's thoughts have stopped, and they may have disidentified from their body and emotions. This can feel euphoric. According to a manipulative reading of several yoga philosophies, it could be said that they've attained a kind of liberation.

Stein suggests that understanding dissociation as the end-limit of disorganized attachment behavior provides a master key for understanding group trance and manipulation in high-demand settings. A basic deference of the follower to the organization can be reinforced through dissociation. Followers can be brought repeatedly into a state of cognitive and emotional collapse through the stress of disorganized attachment. The empty, isolated feeling of having lost all capacity for resistance can be framed by the group as surrender, devotion, or love.

"Along with giving up the struggle to fight against the group and the fear it has generated," Stein writes,

> the dissociated follower comes to accept the group as the safe haven and thus forms a trauma bond. This moment of submission, of giving up the struggle, can be experienced as a moment of great relief, and even happiness, or a spiritual awakening.[195]

MY EXPERIENCE AT ENDEAVOUR ACADEMY (2000–3)

How does this all work on a daily basis, in a group context? How does it actually feel? As I slowly started to absorb Stein's analysis, a key embodied aspect of my own cult experience came into startling focus. I'll describe some of it here to show how and why I've made this connection.

My sharing is also guided by Stein's own reflection that often the most effective way for a high-demand group member to see what they're wrapped up in is to see how the dynamics are working in another group. Even though the teaching content of Endeavour Academy was influenced by a mashup of yoga-like ideas, we didn't do yoga there, *per se*. Nonetheless, the group activities mirrored those in many yoga groups where daily rhythms and devotions are tightly choreographed. The teaching *content*, we should remember, is irrelevant in relation to the *structures* through which a high-demand group functions.

Our daily lives at Endeavour Academy revolved around a morning group ritual called "Session". Charles Anderson (1927–2008), the *Course-in-Miracles*-thumping charismatic leader, would come down from his staging room in the old hotel the group had taken over for its "school" at about 8am. You could hear him preaching from down the packed hall where hundreds of us stood in ecstatic expectation, waiting for a touch, a dirty joke, a hand gesture, or whatever crazy-wisdom *koan* burst out of his mouth. He was in a trance state, and we mirrored him, and each other, raising our arms in the air, some of us jumping up and down uncontrollably to both generate and manage the sensation that God was expressing a mixture of love and chaos within us.

For all the talk of absolute love and peace, the space wasn't safe. We would crush together, many of us speaking in tongues. Our language centers were already off-line. Someone would erupt into a spasmodic kundalini jitterbug and knock a bunch of us down. Anderson himself would smack people on the head or across the face. He'd pull hair, yanking heads up and down with some vague allusion to releasing the innermost spirit heavenwards. Occasionally I saw him grab the breasts of the women, and some onlookers would cackle with laughter as though he'd broken some repressive taboo for the sake of us all. While striking a person, he would often verbally abuse them as well, yelling about their spiritual ignorance, complaining about the exertions he had to endure in order to wake them up. At the time, I bought into the rationalization—to the extent I was thinking at all—that he was stimulating some kind of embodied "release" of energy, that he was "converting" our "dark forms", and exposing us to "the light". I bought into the argument that he was abusing our egos in order to save our souls.

Today I understand all of the physical, sexual, and emotional assault as manipulative, hypnotic, controlling, and criminal. It put several hundred of us into an entranced, submissive, and vacant space for hours at a time. Not only did Anderson and the Academy's leaders demand that we turn off our rational, verbal, "ego" minds, the daily Session virtually guaranteed that would happen. This made us very compliant throughout the rest of the day. We worked in the Academy's front businesses for less than minimum wage. We took out credit card advances to pay for Anderson's grandiose plans. Some went personally bankrupt and became totally indentured to the group, and then were derided for complaining.*[196] Many of us drove in

* In *Wild Wild Country*, the Netflix 2018 docu-series about Rajneeshpuram, there are brutal hidden-camera sequences of group rituals that were similar in form to what I experienced at Endeavor, but apparently far more violent. (In fact, a core group of Endeavor members were former Rajneeshis, who had moved on, as many do, to the next cult.) What the filmmakers missed, aside from real input from Rajneeshpuram's actual victims, was any understanding of what the daily impacts of those group ritual assaults would have been. When outsiders are puzzled by the question of how 10,000 people could have wanted to work for free for 18 hours per day in the remote reaches of Oregon, they don't understand that the daily group ritual instilled such a deeply disorganized confusion of love and fear that most of the remainder of the day was spent in foggy dissociation that may have actually been relieved by mundane work.

a convoy from Wisconsin to Manhattan just weeks after 9/11 to proselytize. Every New Yorker we met told us to fuck off.

The story of how I slowly regained myself and reestablished contact with reality after my years at Endeavor is long and complex. For now, I'll sum up the basic connection between Stein's analysis and my own experience, with reference to the interview accounts I've gathered from Ashtanga practitioners.

On the surface, the rhythms, aesthetics, and worldviews of Endeavor and Jois's shala seem quite different, but they share an underlying structure. As I write this, it feels like Karen Rain is sitting beside me. It has taken us both close to 20 years to be able to articulate experiences that, in effect, robbed us of our powers of articulation. There's something moving about how when ex-cult members meet each other: they can help each other let it all pour out.

Anderson and Jois shared many of the same outward characteristics. Born just a few years apart, both were rotund, jocular grandfathers who could flip instantly in the eyes of their disciples between seeming to provide loving care, to selfish manipulation, or wrath. To follow Anderson was to know that humiliation was always near, but that the reconnection could be so sweet you'd go through anything to get it. I remember the inner circle of Anderson's followers literally running up the stairs, chasing him into his staging room after Session ended. When I joined them, I saw that they were running into a physical and emotional ambush in which they'd be smacked or verbally abused for hours. In the smaller quarters of his room, there was no buffer against his cruelty. To be in the inner circle was to submit to a full contact relationship to the leader.

When Karen spoke about the hypervigilance she felt upon waking up every morning in Mysore, I remembered the panic I felt as I approached morning Session. A cortisol buzz wicked up the back of my stiffening neck as I approached the building. Other followers would refer to this as rising "energy". I managed the terror by sinking into a kind of tunnel vision.

Sensations of inevitability coursed through me—an exhausting combination of tightness and weakness. I was equally split between wanting to enter and wanting to run away. The tension was intoxicating, it held me in a grip. There seemed to be only one possible pathway to relief: to walk straight into the thing that terrified me. This wasn't a new feeling, but something I'd gotten used to. In fact, I'd had it the first moment I walked up the steps of the building, before I knew anything about the group, or Anderson, or what the next three years of my life were to be like. Lightning jolted my nervous system. I paused on the threshold, stunned. Then I quickly interpreted the fear as a sign that I was embarking on positive and necessary growth. I had been exposed to a lot of propaganda leading up to the moment. My best friend had sworn by the place. I had been told that my ego was standing in the way of my happiness, and that it would have to die. *Of course I should be scared,* I thought. *Fear was a good sign.*

On those mornings, and in that feeling, I was isolated. I couldn't make eye contact with any of the hundreds of people who were there, waiting. Session itself was like some kind of anonymous group orgy in which everyone wore masks of ecstasy. Afterwards, what happened in Session stayed in Session. Not only because you couldn't remember it clearly, but also because it was so non-verbal and weird, it would have been impossible and shameful to share. The group's indoctrination enforced this. If you even tried to talk about Session, you'd be derided as "conceptual" or "stuck in your concepts", which meant "overthinking" things. (Recall Hassan's axiom that "thought" is one of the four key faculties a cult will try to control.) In the other high-demand group I was involved in, the leader used to emphasize the traditional Buddhist monastic vow against gossiping. He'd say that talking about your practice sapped it of its power. And Jois would say: "Yoga is 99% practice, 1% theory."

Stein's findings on these isolation tactics—deployed in the context of forming dysfunctional relationships—were revelatory. "Contrary to the stereotype of cult life," she writes, "followers are isolated not only from the outside world, but in this airless pressing together they are also isolated from each other within the group."[197]

The "airless pressing together" isn't a metaphor. At Endeavor, it was literal. At Jois's shala, likewise, students have historically been shoehorned into cramped, sweaty quarters. Several recent visitors to KPJAYI described to me near-stampede conditions as the hundreds of practitioners surge through the gates every morning after waiting in the dark. Wherever there is claustrophobia, Stein suggests, members "cannot share doubts, complaints about the group or any attempt to attribute their distress to the actions of the group."[198]

Why did I seek Endeavor Academy out? What was wrong with me? Why did Anderson's inner circle literally chase him down the hall so that he could abuse them? What were their issues? Why didn't they have enough sense to go to therapy before joining a cult?

Stein is adamant that the application of attachment theory to cult dynamics is not about analyzing *who cult members were before they joined,* but rather *how the cult dynamic transformed their attachment patterning from organized to disorganized.* "When I talk about attachment theory in this context," Stein writes,

> people are often prone to jump to the conclusion that I mean the follower has some type of attachment disorder that led them to seeking out a cultic or extremist group. "Aha," says the listener, "As I suspected, such followers are needy seekers, looking for some authority figure to tell them what to do." Let me make clear, at the outset, that this is not at all the direction of this explanation. In fact, it is my belief that followers start out with a similar variety of attachment-related dispositions as we find in the general population: some are well adjusted (securely attached) while others may be more or less so, and some, perhaps not well adjusted at all.
>
> My contention is that the system itself acts upon followers and, regardless of their original attachment status, attempts to change that status, to what is known as disorganized attachment. Further, the system aims to remove the follower's prior attachment figures and replace them with the leader or group as the new—and disorganized—attachment relationship. The people you love are pushed out and replaced by the leader or group as the new and sole focus of your emotional commitment.[199]

The high-demand version of Ashtanga culture that Karen Rain, T.M., and others encountered was able to foster many of the elements of disorganized attachment leading to dissociation, which prevented resistance to abuse, *while making it look like it was merely preserving a venerable, disciplined, modest, pragmatic, ancient spiritual practice.* The interviews with Jois's victims in this book show a pattern of being physically pushed and pulled by fear and attraction into states that tripped over into freeze responses, leaving many in chronic pain, and some with lasting trauma and PTSD symptoms. They felt isolated from the outside world, from each other, from their bodily autonomy, and from their own inner voices. And they were doing it all within the context of a seemingly humble, workaday practice community dedicated to introspection and growth. The Mysore environment presented a more hidden or digestible version of the physical, sexual, and emotional dominance that was overtly celebrated at Endeavor Academy. Charles Anderson made a virtue out of his chaotic personality, while Pattabhi Jois nurtured the affect of a simple, provincial, Brahmin priest. The latter proved to be a more commodifiable image. Anderson died of stroke in 2008, and the Academy has virtually ceased operations.

FAMILIAL PROJECTIONS

There are many other reasons why Stein's application of attachment theory to cult dynamics are particularly illuminating of the Jois event. Two of these reasons are related to the intimacy of an analysis that evolves from the close study of families.

First, many of the students of Pattabhi Jois not only venerated him as a yoga teacher, but also quite explicitly as a father figure.

Secondly, the setup of most yoga classes derives significant power through its capacity to suggest a regression into childhood and its dynamics. If a unison group class doesn't remind you of grade school, maybe lying down on a mat a little larger than a crib while an adult soothes you towards sleep will ring an earlier bell.

Over the years, I've come to understand asana education as a guided continuance of the individuation and growth we feel in our bodies through time. It is not separate from the intimate and relational stories—laced with the familiar tangle of tenderness and frustration—of how we come to know these bodies as dependent, independent, and finally interdependent. The environment of asana practice can recall the pre-verbal spaces of early childhood, in which foundational movements, breathing patterns, and sensual relationships are being learned through a blend of mimicry, touch, guidance, error, pain, and correction. I used to believe the colloquial individualist wisdom—that asana was about "meeting yourself on the mat." More than a decade on, this sounds oversimplified. The truth is that we meet many of our selves on the mat. These selves date from many different ages, and each of them was and is still formed by the physical relationships that governed those times.

It would be a mistake for yoga studies to continue to be silent on issues of family dynamics. After all, Modern Postural Yoga has globalized through family dynasties, with Krishnamacharya serving as great-uncle, adoptive grandfather, and actual father for Iyengar, Jois, and T.K.V. Desikachar, respectively, each of whom became clan patriarchs in their own right. Our childhood bodies are continually remembered and triggered by every physical activity we take up in later years, whether it's Zumba™, Crossfit™, or pickup basketball. Add to this the fact that everyone who enters a yoga studio even peripherally associated with these father figures is additionally entering a space in which both cultural and intimate inheritances inform many aspects of instruction. The modern yoga studio is a site where physical intimacies purportedly leading to symmetry, balance, openness, and strength are charged and motivated by the light and gravity of the family constellation.

As the schools descended from Krishnamacharya extend beyond their family shrines to cross cultures, languages, technologies, and eras, their genetic current must be converted into something more widely heritable. So far, mechanisms of succession have attempted to blend, in varying degrees, the power of bloodline, older ideals of parampara, and more contemporary models of matriculation. The most senior students of Jois and Iyengar distinguish themselves through personal anecdotes that prove familial contact with their teachers. The content of their instruction is strengthened by claims about where it comes from. Beneath the litmus-test-question of "Who's your teacher?"—commonly asked to verify whether a yogic instruction or the instructor has merit—a more important question might lie hidden: "What is your family like?"

This system is now strained. The Iyengar dynasty has attempted to decentralize the familial influence through a university-style syllabus of attainments that theoretically can be learned from anyone who has graduated from the late master's system. In actuality, however, few have attained high levels of certification without yearly practice-pilgrimages to Pune whilst Iyengar was alive (he died in 2014). Whether this requirement will continue in deference to his son Prashant and his granddaughter Abhijeet—who now carry on the family's teaching—is yet to be sorted out. At KPJAYI, as we've seen, the genetic process is more explicit.

If one is not the actual child or grandchild of the master in modern yoga, it seems that one must either be figuratively adopted in order to rise to the highest ranks, or work very hard to attain familial status in relation to the master and those who surround him. A cascade of reinforcing examples pour from the pages of *Guruji.*

JOIS AS "FATHER"

Over 430 pages, the word "father" appears over 100 times in Donahaye and Stern's book. Many of those instances come in interviews with students who are not his actual children. Students Mark Darby[200] and John Scott[201] quite frankly describe Jois as a father figure. Dena Kingsburg shares that she met Jois soon after her own father's death.[202] Peter Greve tenderly describes Jois's relationship to his wife, Amma, while remembering their familial hospitality, offering students food, love, and support. "She was doing the work in the background that gave him the opportunity to unfold as a father. He was like a father and grandfather to me at the same time."[203] Brigitte Deroses says:

> There is not one day when I do not think about him. His pictures are everywhere in my shala, he is like my father, somebody very important who transformed my life, who truly helped me a lot. And I experience always the same emotion when I see him.... I always have a lot of emotion.[204]

Sharath Rangaswamy says "the longer you spend with your guru, the more you understand him and his knowledge and his teaching. So it becomes like a father-and-son relationship."[205] The reflections of Nick Evans hint at the potential for disorganized attachment.

> There is no denying he means business, but with the people who are vulnerable and have a difficult time, he is the gentlest creature, the gentlest father figure. So he goes from having this terrible, intense authority to commanding your attention and your respect with very few words, just with presence, to being very, very supportive and kind, and he encompasses the whole lot in between.[206]

Another rich source of father-imagery in Ashtanga literature can be found in the two chapbooks of Jois devotee Ruth Lauer-Manenti: *An Offering of Leaves*[207] and *Sweeping the Dust*.[208] These are collections of talks given before or after yoga classes Lauer-Manenti taught in New York and beyond. A student followed her around faithfully for years to record them. Both books are dedicated to Pattabhi Jois, and to Lauer-Manenti's other teachers, Sharon Gannon and David Life, who are also Jois followers.

Lauer-Manenti first met Jois in 1991, and traveled regularly to study with him until the year of his death in 2009. The bio page on her website features a photograph of Jois holding her, pelvis to pelvis, in an extreme backbend, in the old Lakshmipuram shala.[209] Echoing the photograph, Jois provides the center of gravity for both books. The talks return to small moments with him again and again, but almost never related to yoga practice. Each story is conversational, familial. Amma is making coffee, Jois is musing about food or jewelry. "His kindness came through in the small talk," she writes, "and there wasn't any need for a teaching. It was just about being together. That was the teaching. Just being together. Not separate. Together."[210]

Shadowing Jois throughout both books is Lauer-Manenti's own father, Lothar, a Austrian-Jewish refugee who'd arrived in Manhattan at the age of 18 with ten dollars in his pocket. Lauer-Manenti doesn't give many details about her father's life, but she doesn't need to. You can feel the war-time hunger and trauma in his silences and tentative gestures towards connection. By contrast, Jois is large, jolly, magnanimous, endlessly giving. He is the opposite of a refugee: as a Brahmin, he actually broke religious taboos to travel abroad. His wife had to pack suitcases full of food for their journeys so that he would never taste anything that wasn't from home.

"Until he was ninety," Lauer-Manenti writes of Jois,

> he was physically robust and powerful; whereas my father, with his bad circulation, his Ace bandages around his ankles, his pale skin, slow walk, and slumped-over posture, always was an old man to me.[211]

The frontispiece of *An Offering of Leaves* features a photograph of the two men together that emphasizes the contrast. Jois beams for the camera; Lothar looks frail.

The photograph dates from 2005, when Lauer-Manenti brought her father to meet Jois in Encinitas, where he was being hosted by Tim Miller. Lothar was touched that Jois immediately offered him a chair. Later, Lauer-Manenti says, her father described Jois as "enlightened".[212] "One of the last things my father said to me before he died was how much he enjoyed meeting Guruji," she writes.[213]

But Lauer-Manenti also describes complexities. "All my teachers have yelled at me, often," Lauer-Manenti reports.

> Guruji yelled at me so much that I developed a reputation for being yelled at by him. I loved having this reputation, and I loved being yelled at by him. It was what I missed most when I returned to India in the summer after he died. Most people would agree that life seems overwhelming. We have to make decisions all the

> time, hoping those choices will be right, and wondering whether we have the tools to create the life we want. Life is coming at us and may make us feel confused and anxious and a little bit worried about everything all the time. Guruji thought his students were like that, worried all the time. Even in our better moments, that worry would still be there. If you are a little worried all the time, and then the teacher yells at you, fiercely enough to nail your attention but with the love of a mother, the yelling cuts through the worry and lifts you out of it. It gives you the feeling that someone whom you esteem is going to guide you, show you, teach you, actually give you instructions, and it comes as a great relief. That's the experience of being yelled at by the great and holy teacher.[214]

Lothar died before Jois did. The subtext of the narrative feels as though the biological father is blessing her adoption into a happier, warmer, more intimate house.

It was a house laden with confusions. Many years later, when Lauer-Manenti was sued for allegedly sexually assaulting one of her female students, she appealed to these intimate, familial feelings to provide context for her defense. When her accuser questioned her about her consistent boundary-crossing, Lauer-Manenti explained that she'd "cuddled with Guruji" and "sat on his lap and kissed him everyday that I had class."[215]

THE PATERNAL OR INITIATORY GAZE

The broad feelings of paternal transference onto Jois are obvious in these sources, but it's the micro-moments that really drive the intimate familial context home. Nowhere is this more primal than in how Jois's students describe his gaze.

It is now widely assumed that infants only hours old are capable of facial recognition, perhaps by virtue of a special "face-specific learning mechanism".[216] Some researchers claim that babies can respond to and even mimic happy, frightful, and neutral faces within hours of birth. But those of us who are parents don't need research. We've felt the power of these first face-to-face encounters.

In my own case, circumstances conspired to hand me my son while my wife Alix's postpartum surgery concluded. He and I were ushered to a recovery room and left alone for 30 minutes. I held him swaddled in my lap and gazed down at his face. He gazed back with his unfocused eyes. We breathed together in the same uncertain and exploratory rhythm, and the rest of the world disappeared. Later, after I'd handed him to Alix, I needed to leave the room to move the car to another parking spot. I could hardly see where I was going, and it felt dangerous to drive. My entire visual field was imprinted with his face, as though I'd been staring at the sun. He had branded me, hardwired me into his sphere of possession. How would I ever leave him?

Of course, I imprinted on him as well. Deep in the circuitry that secretes his attachment to me, an image of my face must dimly float, as large as the sky above him. It may at times be a fearful sight. But I hope against hope that it communicates love, patience, support, a home to which he can return in need, but more importantly, leave with confidence.

Given such primal beginnings, it seems like no coincidence that the "second birth" of spiritual initiation in many streams of Tantric yoga involves the penetration of the student's body by the guru's gaze. The *Kularnava Tantra*, for example, lists initiation by the guru's sight or gaze as a potent conduit of energetic awakening.[217] Here, culture meets biology, as "father" elides into "guru" through the eyes of reassurance and control.

Guruji is steeped with accounts of Jois's intense gaze. The surface explanation involves his instructions around *drishti*, or the gaze of concentration. But there are also strong themes of intimate surveillance. In the introduction, Guy Donahaye writes: "Guruji's eyes were always on us."[218] In an interview given alongside her husband Mark, Joanne Darby says: "You knew that his eyes were on you whenever you did something."[219] Graeme Northfield: "He was very strong and his eye was always on you."[220] Joseph Dunham: "My experience with Guruji has very much been… 1 percent talking… and 99 percent experiential. We look at each other. It's a lot of eye communication…."[221] John Scott takes it further, describing how eye contact can be a gateway for the negotiation of complex power exchanges.

> On many occasions, I had tried to resist his adjustment and just felt his adjustment intensify, and over the years I've learned you have to look him in the eye, which isn't the correct drishti… and submit and have the faith that he isn't going to put you into something further than you can go.[222]

In a blog post following her #MeToo disclosure, Karen Rain suggested that out of respect for Jois's victims, Ashtanga teachers remove Jois's portrait from the public altars of their yoga shalas.[223] It's not surprising that many disciples struggled with that suggestion. For some who had felt his gaze in person, it was like being asked to erase a primal imprint of safety and familiarity—something that gave them a bodily jolt of contact, however anxious or even disorganized, each time they looked at it. What seems like an obviously ethical decision—*don't display the image of a sexual predator if you want to create a safe space*—could feel like a psychic amputation.

KEEPING EYES WIDE OPEN

A father-figure gazes at a student who lies on a small bed-sized mat. He takes authority over the student's body, guides them, molds them, puts them into position. Maybe he touches them with boundaried ethics and care. But perhaps he touches them in confusing and intimate ways the student is supposed to learn from, but that don't feel right. He chants names and numbers that pulse the student towards sleep. When they wake, they feel emptied out, thoughtless, and wordless. They feel that their body and mind have been remade.

Do we really think that the history of postures and their relationships to medieval or older texts is an adequate framework for understanding the complexity of what's going on in such classes? Will we get closer to what transpired between Jois, Iyengar, Choudhury, or Yogi Bhajan and all of their respective students by studying what they said about triangle posture, meditation, or yoga philosophy? Will we get closer to the heart of what modern yoga—or the yoga of any period—actually is or was only by mining cultural data or tracking the influences of technology and globalization?

These are all worthy topics of material consequence. But not one of them will adequately speak to what happened to the interviewees in this book. If such topics are not studied in tandem with the patterns of interpersonal relationship through which yoga is always communicated, regardless of time and place, they risk remaining surface issues. At worst, they will obscure psychosocial drivers beneath veils of "objectivity" and shame. Yoga scholarship should be willing to consider a very yogic possibility: that texts, artifacts, and the discourses that surround them live parallel to another reality: that among the many things yoga practice is, it is also a delivery device for relational patterns.

NIZED ATTACHMENT: FROM ASHTANGA MATERIALS

ng background in attachment theory will help to make the following quotes from Jois students comprehensible at a deeper level than the propaganda framework through which they were originally presented. Stein's work, along with a close attention to embodied sensation can help us drop the confrontational, dead-end question of "Is Ashtanga yoga a cult?" and consider much better questions, with much broader applications for the yoga world and beyond.

1. What kind of relationships do I see in my community?
2. How are those relationships performed, questioned, or reinforced by the physical practices?
3. How am I interpreting discomfort and pain as I practice?
4. When I'm touched by my teacher, have I given full consent?
5. Do I feel like I have agency? Can I talk with my teacher about what is happening?
6. If an adjustment hurts me, is my instinct to wonder what I have done wrong?
7. Do I have friends within this community to whom I can say anything?
8. Are the relationships in this group controlling? Does it feel hard to leave?

The following passages are taken from Ashtanga media sources, including *Guruji*. They are quotes and not transcripts from therapy sessions. They are presented here not to diagnose the attachment patterns of the individual speakers. Rather, they are presented as evidence of disorganized attachment patterns functioning at a *community* level, communicated through speech and writing.

They propagandize by presenting the relationships they describe in positive, desirable terms. They communicate sentiments that reinforce positive group narratives, and possibly attract new students. Remember as you read them: the speakers are reminiscing about emotional connections that also happen to support business concerns.

If you read something here that simply does not make sense on a cognitive level, bear in mind that the output of disorganized attachment patterning can itself be disorganized. In particular, be alert for grammatical oddities, and words that seem to shift definition in mid-stream. If dissociation relieves the tension of the conflict, it would follow to see it as a feature of how that resolution is later told in story form.

Here, a new and chilling aspect of propaganda shimmers into view. In some cases, it seems that propaganda is not an intentional, top-down doling out of manipulative views and statements about the organization or its leader. It may in some cases represent the sanctification of what members say in the throes of dissociation.

It would be incomplete to pigeonhole *Guruji* as a mere hagiography. It may also record moments of dissociation that are reframed, performed, and published as praise.

"MIXTURE OF LOVE AND FEAR"

> **[Tim Miller]** He's probably the last of a vanishing breed of teachers of traditional yoga. He really seems to carry the energy of Shiva, that energy of both annihilation and creation. There's this mixture of love and fear that I've always connected to him.[224]

Quoted earlier, this statement highlights Miller's divinization of Jois as Shiva. His perhaps hyperbolic intent here is to praise, but is that the impact? Gods have often been used to integrate the conflicting forces of experience, but is it healthy to use this ideal to understand the volatility of a person? What part of "annihilation" and "fear" merit praise? The message here is that this mixed quality of loving and wrathful—the object of a disorganized attachment—is positive in nature, and desirable.

Miller also positively frames the peak experiences and loss of self provoked in relation to that mixed quality. The feelings he describes, though unnamed, are presented as necessary and helpful.

> On my first trip to India, in particular, oftentimes after practice, lying

> in *shavasana*, I would feel certain emotions surfacing. Sometimes I would just sit there and weep, not in a dramatic way, tears would just be running down my face and it was incredibly purifying and powerful. I would get up after and go out in the streets and feel almost as if I was transparent or something. Things were just moving through me, and somehow a great sense of spaciousness had been created inside me.[225]

It's important to note that Miller enjoys almost unanimous positive regard within the broader Ashtanga world. "He is amongst the greatest teachers on the planet, a true servant,"wrote one Ashtanga teacher.[226] In this light, Miller's reflections here would generally be quoted as proof of spiritual attainment in relation to Jois's teaching, rather than evidence for how a person managed a relationship complicated by fear.

"GOOD POP. NO PROBLEM."

The following comes from a video interview with Ashtanga-authorized teacher Gretchen Suarez, uploaded to YouTube in 2014.[227]

> I really felt that he was tuned in. He was tuned in to so many people, just energetically. He knows when to give the next pose, knew when to adjust. That fine level of attunement is mastery.
>
> I remember one day in Mysore, I was practicing, it was probably one of my first few years there. And there was a woman next to me who was doing deep backbends, and Guruji was backbending her. He's infamously known for having people grab their ankles. You know, bendy people, etc.
>
> So I'm there, doing my practice, and he's standing in front of me, and I'm pretending not to look, but you can't help but feel that energy. And Guruji starts backbending this woman, and I hear this loud POP!
>
> And I was in whatever pose, and I look up, really scared, because it was a really loud pop, and I thought "This woman, this poor woman, her back is broken, O my God."
>
> And I look up, he immediately [snaps fingers] looks at me and says [mimes Jois's Indian head-bobble]: "Good pop. No problem!" [laughs.]

> And that was the thing about Guruji. He had this energy that was so fierce, yet in the same, the very next breath, it was so loving. It was a really beautiful combination to have that experience as a teacher. To have that level of strictness, yet the love was there, and you felt it.

The video ends there, offering no further reference to what happened to the woman.

This was a common theme in the interviews I conducted with other Jois students. There would be references to other, unnamed practitioners who seemed to be in pain or distress. Not a single interviewee was able to report on what happened following the crack or pop or public weeping. The stories are not being told to report on an event. Rather, they seem to describe a moment in which the narrator produced an interpretation of the teacher that both reveals and resolves the mixture of love and fear they feel for him.

A similar scene plays out in the story senior certified Iyengar teacher Manouso Manos tells about his first meeting with Iyengar in the mid-1970s.[228] Manos went on to become one of Iyengar's top representatives globally, despite unresolved allegations of sexual misconduct brought against him by students that span from the late 1980s to 2015.

Manos couldn't get a spot in the class itself, so he sat on the dais with Iyengar, observing. A woman in the center of the room couldn't raise one of her arms in a standing pose. Iyengar questioned her, and she said her shoulder was frozen. The master stomped down from the stage and wrenched her arm up into place. Manos describes the woman's scream as "blood-curdling". Her knees buckled; Iyengar hoisted her upright, and commanded her to continue. He repeated the shoulder wrenching several times. The woman kept screaming. By the end of the class, according to Manos, she was raising her arms fully overhead like a football referee signaling a touchdown.

"I watched him cure a frozen shoulder that had been there for two years in a few hours," Manos reports, decades later. "It wasn't charisma. That's the easy word that we spit at each other. It was his command of the subject, his belief in the subject. His ability to inspire others into this was breathtaking."

Manos offers no notes about how the unknown woman fared the next day, or a year later. No consideration of whether she instantly regained her range of motion through a trauma response—because her body had no choice. Manos is not telling a story about the woman, but about his own conversion, using the alleged "opening" of the woman to illustrate his own moment of "opening" to an interpretation of Iyengar's violent act as a miracle. Her story has become his, and his story merges with the group narrative.

In Suarez's account, Jois's energy is totalizing, always palpable. He can look at Suarez, but Suarez is supposed to keep her eyes on her *drishti*. When she transgresses to peek, she sees him do something to someone like her. Initially, she thinks it's catastrophic. But this thought is quickly displaced by an interpretation that aligns with the general group narrative: Jois is providing a therapeutic balance of wrath and love. Jois looks down at Suarez and arrests her trespassing gaze with his own. The likelihood that he has injured the student disappears in the reward of this contact. The woman is forgotten in the relief of agreeing with the group's interpretation of Jois's action.

"Giving in," writes Alexandra Stein as she remembers switching off her critical mind under the pressure of a high-demand group,

> — dissociating and ceasing to think—is experienced as relief.... [O]verwhelmed with confusion and exhaustion, the thoughts that were trying to enter the cognitive part of my brain just could not make it there and they fell back out of consciousness. Simultaneously I stopped struggling and decided to commit myself more fully to the group *even though I disagreed with it*. That too felt like relief—I didn't have to fight anymore. key regions of the brain that connect emotional (largely right brain) and cognitive processing (largely left brain) are shut down in the disorganized and dissociated state.[229]

The reports of Suarez and Manos describe moments in which potential harm inflicted on a fellow student is instantly reframed as care, as if a cognitive switch has been thrown. This switch resonates with the simultaneous and contradictory impulses to withdraw from and approach the master.

Does this parallel the experience of the *students* Suarez and Manos are talking about? It's a hard question to answer with direct evidence, because it's difficult for any person in a high-demand context to develop a metaview of such critical, confusing moments. Stein's recollection of how and why she experienced relief through a trauma bond with the group comes after years of therapy and research. In my own case, it took similar years of work to understand why one of the first responses I had to a famous Iyengar yoga teacher who injured my spine in a non-consensual assist was to feel overwhelmed by feelings of love for him.

Tracy Hodgeman tells a story about a fellow student who protested and cried as Jois backbended her. She told him that she was in pain and asked him to stop, but he persisted. Tracy couldn't bear it, but felt powerless to intervene. She saw the woman the a few days later, beaming. "He healed my spine," she told Tracy. "My pain is gone." Tracy didn't question it at the time, and quickly lost track of the woman.

"STARING DOWN INTO THE ABYSS"

In his Preface to *Guruji*, Guy Donahaye writes the following.

> When being adjusted in a challenging asana by Guruji, I sometimes felt on a precipice staring down into the abyss at the prospect of death or debilitating pain, but also feeling that maybe salvation somehow was at hand. Then I was met in the present moment, because nothing will distract you from the moment when you face imminent death, by Guruji's smile: "Why fearing?"[230]

These two sentences deserve to be read over and over to be fully absorbed. First, we should note that Donahaye is describing a repeated experience. He feels that the outcome could be catastrophic, but that catastrophe is proximal to a benefit. It seems a familiar conflict.

The second sentence describes how the gaze and voice of Jois shuts down his defenses. But the second and third clauses of that sentence are grammatically incoherent. At first reading, it might seem that Donahaye is suggesting that the smile and question relieve his fear. But, read closely, Jois's smile and question *is equated with* the prospect of imminent death. Donahaye is not only the writer here, but also an editor. It seems as though the incorrect grammar and its implication was invisible.

> And then suddenly, before you know it, he has put you in the posture! The state of heightened awareness may persist for the duration of the adjustment, and during this time nothing else whatsoever troubles the mind. Afterward, there is a moment of suspension of belief, bliss, euphoria, openheartedness, ecstasy.[231]

Notice how the narrative does not veer into the other option—debilitating pain—which Donahaye admits to being a possibility in the first sentence. What the hagiographic structure must keep is the apparent miracle, the moment in which the person was filled with wonder, the moment the promise was kept. The "heightened awareness" can include a destruction of thinking, a loss of critical perspective, and a dissociation from emotion. Donahaye goes on to describe euphoria. Again, we have to ask whether such feelings of relief—which come to be associated with spiritual transformation—are coming from the adjustment, the posture, or the momentary relaxation of a conflict between the desire for care and the premonition of danger.

"BEFORE THE MIND CAN BECOME INVOLVED"

> **[Nancy Gilgoff]** I often tell people that [Jois is] the most compassionate person I've ever met because he'll take us into our fear and beyond it. When I'm teaching, if I read fear in someone, it's very hard to take them through it. So someone who can do that with you is the teacher for you because it's about fear, moving through it on all levels.
>
> **[Guy Donahaye]** *He says something similar about pain, doesn't he?*
>
> **[NG]** The pain element, there's good and there's bad pain. In terms of good pain, a lot of times you'll feel pain because you need to soften the muscle. A lot of times you'll see that the mind is actually creating the pain. Again, because pain is contraction, when the mind shuts down so does the body. Once you can open the mind you can release a lot of the pain and contraction. He definitely takes you into that realm where you have to let go of the mind in order to do something. He generally is taking you quickly into the pose. There's a moment when the mind is not present and he will take you through that time. It's very quick, you go right into it, and that's the trick of teaching asanas well. If you are doing hands-on adjustments, it has to be fast before the mind can become involved in it.
>
> **[GD]** *Probably, first-time Baddha Konasana, no problem.*

> **[NG]** First time is much easier than the second because the mind is present, it expects it. So each time, as the mind shuts down and the body shuts down with it, you have to trick a little bit differently and go in there and work just a little bit quicker or wait until the person's mind steps out of the way again. [232]

Gilgoff, like Miller, enjoys legendary status amongst the Ashtanga rank and file. In her review of *Guruji*, the aforementioned Ashtanga blogger praises this same interview for revealing Gilgoff's "humility and profundity and self-responsibility."[233] But from the outset of this passage, the potential for disorganized attachment is evident, with Gilgoff conflating compassion with the process of leading a student into fear and beyond. Then she reveals an assumption that the distinction between "bad" and "good" pain is universally accepted or even understandable. The end of the passage devolves into *an argument in favor of non-consensual adjustments.*

Within all of that, Gilgoff makes one substantiated point about pain, if we substitute "brain" for "mind". It's true that pain circuitry can fire inappropriately. The brain that produces unprovoked pain responses is the definition of pain as a stand-alone pathology. It's also true that mental techniques can help to disrupt pathological pain. Gilgoff is talking about using mental techniques, or abandoning the mind altogether, to resolve pain. But what if Jois is causing the pain directly?

Though the passage is mostly about being adjusted by Jois, Gilgoff starts with a generalized description of pain as often being self-inflicted, caused by the "mind" in "contraction". What is the difference, we should wonder, between "contraction" and the withdrawal of a fear response? At first, the reader might think she was describing practicing alone, as Jois isn't mentioned. But suddenly, Jois is there, taking the student to a place where you "have to" let go of the mind.

On one hand, Gilgoff is describing the brain or mind as an organ that contracts, that withdraws from something. On the other hand, she is also using the word "mind" to describe agency, the capacity to question, choose, and resist. She describes Jois as knowing when those functions are not on line—knowing, in effect, when the student is vulnerable:

There's a moment when the mind is not present and he will take you through that time.

The mind is pre-empted by the surprise of the adjustment. The power to choose, to say no, to ask for something different—all overwhelmed. The assumption is that this is good, because Jois knows what the student needs before they can articulate a request. Gilgoff actually reinforces this perspective by noting that the student's natural resistance to the intrusion will rise up after the first occurrence, and must be "tricked".

Gilgoff describes an ethos of not only implied consent, but *justified manipulation*. Gilgoff is literally saying here that being proficient at teaching asana requires that you manipulate students when they are undefended, *and* that you should contrive new ways of doing so when their defenses emerge.

Finally, notice how Gilgoff's usage of the word "mind" changes meaning in the last sentence. The mind that is "shut down" in a defensive response to fear and pain is presented as an obstacle to surrender. But then she describes the mind as something that must "step out of the way", be let go of, or as she suggests earlier, be nullified by Jois. What's the difference between a mind that is shut down and a mind that has vacated? It sounds like the shut-down mind is laying there, like the body, as an obstruction to the will of the teacher. The mind that shuts itself down is a bad thing, but somehow mind that is cleared out of the way by the teacher is a good thing.

The inconsistency of Gilgoff's language around the mind "shutting down" versus "getting out of the way" is complicated by a further anecdote. Earlier in the interview, she describes literally losing consciousness in some of the postures. "I even lost consciousness sometimes," she says. "When my mind was absent, my body did what he wanted it to do because I wasn't resisting and reacting at that moment."[234]

She's not the only one to lose consciousness in Jois's care. Another senior Jois student who wished to remain anonymous said that he regularly blacked out while performing the advanced postures.

This value of cognitive silence is by no means old-fashioned in the Ashtanga world, but rather an explicit and continuing value. In August 2018, under the shadow of the Jois abuse revelations, Mary Taylor co-taught a workshop with her senior student, Ashtanga-authorized teacher Ty Landrum, who has taken over the directorship of Freeman's and Taylor's Ashtanga Yoga Workshop in Boulder, Colorado. The advertising for the workshop, called "Teaching with the Hands", explains that

> Ashtanga Vinyasa is often taught in silence. In place of words, Ashtanga teachers use their hands. They use their hands to adjust, support and guide the breathing body deeper into the experience

> of the forms, *without breaking the silence and engaging the thinking mind*. This method of teaching is potent [intuitive] and highly suitable for the introspective and tactile nature of the practice. *Ashtanga Vinyasa is not an endeavor of the intellect*, but an exploration of embodied experience. It is through touch, *above all*, that this exploration comes alive.
>
> In this 5-day intensive, we explore the art of teaching with our hands. We consider how and when to use our hands, and when to use other means. We discuss the issues of intimacy, privacy and vulnerability that come along with using our hands to assist. *And we consider the crucial skill of making space for power dynamics to dissolve.*[235]

Nowhere in the copy for this event does the word "consent" appear. This is even more notable, given that beyond the value they place upon cognitive silence, Landrum and Taylor also suggest that the adjustment process can result in a "dissolution" of power dynamics—initiated, however, by the *teacher*. They seem to be suggesting that through an adjustment, teacher and student can come into a singular, boundaryless union. But have these teachers shown that such a state is both well understood and safe for vulnerable students?

"IT'S NORMAL: NO PAIN, NO GAIN."

> **[Mark Darby]** I had started on a Thursday but Guruji wanted me to do three days in a row, so he asked me on Friday, "You come in tomorrow, do Saturday"—traditionally the day off. So I came in the afternoon and he gave me a little class and I came back the next day. I did those three days plus the next week. By the next Saturday I was so thankful—I was so sore, so beaten up—to get a day off after a week and a half of practice.
>
> Then it continued basically for the next three months, continuous pain in different parts of my body. And Old Cliff Barber, he was a mentor. I could ask about practice and tell how my body was feeling, and [he would] tell me, "It's normal: no pain, no gain." Joanne came one week after I started. After three months, I'd had it. I needed to get out of there. I took a month off. Coming back, I had no pain and I'm all ready to go again and three days later my shoulder popped and here we go again.

> **[Guy Donahaye]** *Why do you think one keeps going in spite of the pain?*
>
> **[MD]** I guess it's belief in Pattabhi Jois. In this period I read *Autobiography of a Yogi* and also the atmosphere in India was starting to fuel an understanding about the teacher/disciple relationship. So Guruji is going to be my teacher, he is my guru, whatever he says to do I'll do, I have complete faith in what he teaches and wants me to do. And that was it, I just went with that belief. And it worked. I went away and after a month everything healed, the whole body healed by not being pushed. Where he had pushed me, I could now go to—I just needed to relax afterward. When I came back it was a different pain, more from getting stretched out, it wasn't that intense breaking down, so it did change.[236]

In Mysore, Mark Darby met his future wife Joanne—the woman whose rib Jois cracked while she was pregnant, according to her report.[237] They went on to become key Jois-certified teachers in the Montreal yoga world, where they continue to teach. In this passage, Mark describes *going back* to the person that hurt him by reframing the pain he expected to experience again—and did—as positive and progressive. He introduces this process by referring to the power of faith in Jois, and citing an indoctrinating comment from a mentor.

"GETTING ME TROUBLED"

> **[Annie Pace]** Medicine for me might be beating me up and hollering at me and getting me troubled and working me until I was a noodle, and medicine for the next person just might be a smile and a pat on the shoulder.[238]

Here, Jois certified teacher Annie Pace presents the premise that Jois is treating different people in different ways. She separates his wrath from his care to suggest that Jois had a keen sense of individual therapeutic need.

In so doing, Pace also describes a basic quality of the object of disorganized attachment—in this case, Jois. *You cannot be certain of what you are going to get from him. It is now widely understood within the neuroscience community that this uncertainty can be highly addictive.*

The inconstancy of Jois can in fact be viewed as a triple uncertainty.

1. The student is unsure if he will pay attention to them at all.

2. They are unsure which face Jois will show them.

3. They are unsure of the results of any given interaction.

The power of these multiple uncertainties might actually stimulate the biological root of devotion. Endocrinologists are discovering that when a person forms a desire, intuits the work needed to accomplish it, and then anticipates the reward of fulfillment, the neurotransmitter dopamine is released as a euphoric spark to facilitate goal-oriented action. Dopamine levels rise at the anticipation stage of the sequence, are maintained through the work-stage, and finally dissipate at the point of reward.

Oddly, in controlled experiments in which monkeys are made *uncertain* about the availability of the reward, something strange happens. They are first trained to perform a sequence of actions that lead to a treat. Over time, researchers can watch the dopamine levels of the monkeys surge as soon as they turn on a little green light to signal that the work-reward sequence is starting. But if the researchers cut the chances of the monkey being rewarded by half, dopamine levels spike sharply, forcing them to work much harder and much longer towards their goal than otherwise.

Some Mysore narratives resemble this pattern. Many interviewees refer to the special thrill of being adjusted by either Jois or Rangaswamy, and the strange depression that comes from being passed over. Drilling down to the moment of actual interaction, the oscillation is repeated: the adjustment might be terrifying or liberating. In the lab-shala, where we might imagine the chanting invocation that starts every class as the little green light that initiates the dopamine surge, the uncertainty of what Jois will do and how it will feel combines with yoga's uncertain promise of salvation.

Neuro-endocrinologist Robert Sapolsky, described aptly in the *New York Times* as a cross between Jane Goodall and a borscht-belt comedian,[239] explains that the dopaminergic systems of monkeys and humans are identical, and gives this wry analysis that carries both relational and existential implications.

> It's because you've introduced the word "maybe" into the equation. And "maybe" is addictive like nothing else out there.... Dopamine comes pouring out like mad. It's the uncertainty of the reward....

> Humans are profoundly manipulable in this realm.... What winds up being unique about us, with humans it's the time dimension. You get the signal, you do the work, you get the reward. And the question becomes: How much ... lag-time can there be between the work and the reward to still elicit the behavior...? We have just entered uniquely human terrain there....
>
> What we see is this astonishing ability of humans to keep those dopamine levels up for decades and decades, waiting for the reward. And in the most bizarre, unique realm of this in humans, sometimes we can maintain it with a belief system where the reward doesn't come in our lifetime. The reward comes after our death. The reward comes in our afterlife. The reward comes unto the next generations. And there's no monkey out there who's willing to lever-press all the time because of what Saint Peter's gonna think somewhere down the line.[240]

Perhaps the mechanisms of uncertainty that govern parental inconstancy, yoga pedagogy, and yogic aspirations can be fully synthesized into a potent motive for delayed gratification. You don't know if Jois will regard you, and if he does, whether he will hurt you or caress you. Devotees group these multiple possibilities under the banner of "love". Dopamine is high. You don't know whether the postures will harm or liberate. Devotees digest both possibilities through the name of "practice." Dopamine is sustained. Devotion entails tolerating an uncertain reward in both interpersonal and intrapersonal realms.

It is likely that each of us know people, perhaps very close to home, who are forever waiting to receive a certain love from authority figures. If we practice yoga with ideals of discipline, there might also be at least some part of us forever waiting to see the reward of what we ourselves will become. Such desires, bred of indeterminacy, can even survive the death of both parents and teachers, as we glean from the multiple portraits of Jois in the shala of Brigitte Deroses and how she refers to him in the present tense. What the neuroscience seems to be saying is that this layered uncertainty may provoke an ever-deepening secretion of ardor.

"LOOK HIM IN THE EYE AND SUBMIT"

> **[John Scott]** On many occasions, I had tried to resist his adjust-

> ment and just felt his adjustment intensify, and over the years I've learned you have to look him in the eye, which isn't the correct drishti, look him in the eye and submit and have the faith that he isn't going to put you into something further than you can go. In the submitting or even just the yielding to his pressure, my body has changed over the years. In fact, now when he adjusts me I feel so secure.[241]

John Scott is originally from New Zealand, and is beloved throughout the European Ashtanga community for his gentle passion and pirate-fairy eccentricity. Here he introduces the experience of being adjusted by Jois as governed by non-consent. As he resists, Jois overpowers him. He does this not only through muscle, but through his arresting gaze. Like Mark Darby, Scott also invokes faith, and describes how he has been changed through submission. Ostensibly, that change is good.

But Jois's gaze was no guarantee of safety. Kim Haegele Labidi, a student of Richard Freeman, went to Mysore in 1991 at the age of 30. On the first day, Jois lay on top of her in same way he lay upon Karen Rain, T.M., and who knows how many other women, while she was in a supine split position. A ligament in her hip ruptured. She describes it sounding like a gunshot. She also describes gazing into his eyes while he was above her. She started to weep. She remembers that he didn't look the least bit troubled. She has a vague memory of a flicker of amusement in his eyes, but can't be sure, she said.

"IF YOU TRIED TO RESIST YOU WERE IN SERIOUS TROUBLE"

> **[Peter Sanson]** You had to surrender to his adjustments, and then you would be safe. If you tried to resist anything you were in serious trouble. Many times I could hear things tearing in my body—like the sound of sheets ripping—I thought I was going to be finished. But in the end I would just let go, and surrender up to him, and allow him to take me into the different asanas, and then I was safe.[242]

Sanson, originally from New Zealand, is transforming an experience of harm into an experience of safety. It appears as though this was effected by a collapse of resistance. Again we have to ask whether the "safety" described here was actual safety from Jois, or the safety that comes when the crisis of a disorganized attachment event has tripped over into the false relaxation of dissociation.

"IT'S A BIRTH PROCESS"

As of this writing, a haunting photograph of Jois assaulting a women sits on the website of Gary Lopedota, who along with his friend Brad Ramsey opened the first Jois-dedicated practice space in the world outside of Mysore, in Encinitas, California, in the mid-1970s.[243] They had both studied with Jois during his early trips to the United States. They rented a vacated church building at the corner of La Veta and Marcheta that had once housed St. Andrew's Episcopal. Inspired by the radical 19th-century German "cleansing" diets, they planted a garden of wheatgrass and herbs in the front yard.

Classes at Ashtanga Yoga Nilayam (the "Abode of Ashtanga Yoga") were Mondays, Wednesdays, and Fridays at 5pm, and taught with Jois's signature individual attention and intense adjustments. Lopedota and Ramsey led newbies slowly but firmly through the postures, up to the point of exhaustion. The buzz amongst the in-crowd was that the practice provided ecstatic sensations, and relief from depression and addiction.

It also drove people to extremes. Stan Hafner, a student at the time, said that many of the women students got hooked on laxatives to lose weight and be able to go into the deep twists more easily.

The colors in the photograph are as Polaroid-intense as the postures. In the background of the photo you can see a CD in a jewel case on the table in the background, which means the year must be 1980 or later.[*244]

The scene shows a woman in her mid-to-late 20s, supine on the carpeted floor in hand-to-foot pose (*Supta Padangusthasana*: *see* Figure 1, p.28). Her right leg is extended out and her straightened left leg is up and out to the side. Pattabhi Jois has draped himself over her body, his left leg on her right, his right hand pinning down her left ankle up and out to the side. His left hand is openly fondling her right breast. He's looking at her face with an enigmatic side-eye—half beatific gaze, half smirk.

Her face is averted and her eyes are closed, as if she's dissociating from what is happening to her.

Jois is doing exactly what Karen Rain and T.M. described him doing on a daily basis, in the same posture or versions thereof, more than a decade later.

* In his record of Jois's visits to Encinitas, Tim Miller writes that Jois was there in 1975, 1978, 1980, 1982, 1985, 1987, 1989, 1993, and 2000.

Lopedota didn't respond to a request for comment about the photograph.

Other students from that community and era noted many things about the photo. They talked about how young Jois was in it. They noted that he still had his hair. They identified Brad Ramsey adjusting another student in the background. They described the kinds of fabric mats they were using at the time. But nobody knew the woman's name.

The photograph caught Ramsey in the moment before applying the final twist to the student. The student's back glistens with sweat. Ramsey, sprung and wiry, gazes into the distance.

If you were to crop out Jois and the nameless woman, the remainder would leave a poignant composition of the key elements of Jois's legacy: intensity, focus, stoic application of adjustment to the body. What the photograph doesn't record is the rhythm of slow and heavy breathing, which gives every Jois-inspired room an intimate, humid pulse. There can be something both primal and disciplined about it, like some ritual group orgy in which no one touches each other, except for the teacher touching the students. The intensity of the postures drives focus inward.

Understanding this picture involves understanding how many of Jois's early students, especially the men, were potentially high on a cocktail of physical intensity, pain, and spiritual devotion. This blinded them further than any garden-variety misogyny could to what Jois was doing to the women they practiced with. Many of these men may have spent intense amounts of moral energy building metaphysical explanations for what that pain meant and how they had to deal with it. Their gaze was on the perfection of the postures towards the transformation of their inner selves. They organized every bit of their attention around that goal. No testimony shows this more clearly than Ramsey's.

> **[Brad Ramsey]** It was extremely painful. I don't think there's one part of me that wasn't sore. He wasn't as restrained on his home turf as he was in the U.S., so it was transformative. That's where I really got my leg to stay behind my head, and that took a lot of torque, a whole lot. I felt like I was being dismembered. My body was changed.
>
> **[Guy Donahaye]** *Why do you think we allow ourselves to go through so much pain?*
>
> **[BR]** The benefits, I guess. You can feel it working, you can feel the

quietness after. And I don't think it's the endorphins; it's because the system really works. You can almost hear your mind shutting down. Even the pain, if you give that up to God, I think that's part of the practice, really. I don't know. Manju always says, no pain, no gain. [Manju Jois is the son of Pattabhi.] And there is a great amount of truth there, I think. The pain is almost necessary. The pain is a teacher also.

[GD] *Usually you take that as a message to stop what you are doing because you are about to do some damage.*

[BR] Yes, that's the American way, probably the rest of the world, too, but Americans especially. In a lot of schools of yoga, if it hurts you are doing something wrong. And if you were a perfect physical and mental specimen already, then I can see how that might be true. If you are altering the status quo in an unpleasant way, you might want to stop if you were already perfect. But if you feel growth coming from it, and see things changing that need to be changed… the series is just a mold toward a body that meets the requirements for spiritual advancement, I believe. I don't think you can get there without pain. I never met anybody who did. For me, it hurt from the first day to the last, at least something. There's always something.

[GD] *I think for everyone there comes a point where the pain gets moderated, you learn how to practice in an intelligent way and sustain yourself, rather than trying to break through.*

[BR] That's true, it does get better.

[GD] *It's a hard lesson to learn, and a difficult one.*

[BR] Sometimes even to make the effort is painful.

[GD] *Why do you think that is?*

[BR] It's the nature of the beast. It's a birth process really.[245]

***

The first thing to note here is the dissociative isolation of the entire quote. Ramsey begins with a single reference to the fact that he's talking about being adjusted. But in the following sentence, he erases Jois from the scenario, as if the "torque" was something that he was applying to himself. As in Gilgoff's account, Jois is both there and not-there. His presence seems internalized.

Ramsey knows enough about the neurochemical possibilities involved in the post-adjustment cognitive shut-down to dismiss them. But he offers nothing but faith in place of the dismissal.

He goes on to say, as Kino MacGregor will later repeat to a million followers, that "pain is a teacher." But not in the "American way" of indicating approaching harm. Change will be painful, he asserts, and necessary, and constant.

Ramsey doesn't quantify how much of the pain he endured came from the fact that Jois was brutalizing his body. There's a series of 1986 videos of Ramsey practicing under Jois with a small group of devotees doing the Third (Advanced A) Series in what looks like someone's garage in Kealakekua, Hawaii.[246] Jois circles the room for two hours, calling out the poses and the breath count. He wrenches feet behind heads, steps on thighs, leans his full bodyweight into the tangle of surrendering flesh. He's harder on the men. The cohort is both obedient and impassive towards him. For the most part, their eyes stare forward, limiting eye contact with Jois, even when he peers into their faces to murmur or bark an instruction.

Jois pays special attention to Ramsey, who is less flexible than the rest of the cohort. As they enter the full forward-splitting posture of *Hanumanasana*, Jois applies the adjustment of stepping down with weight onto the top of each practitioner's back thigh. His toes extend up the buttock as he lifts their arms aloft. When he gets to Ramsey he applies the same technique, even though Ramsey's pelvis is a full foot off the ground before Jois adds any pressure. Under the weight of Jois's foot, to which he jerkily transfers his entire body weight, Ramsey's pelvis lowers, marginally. He's shaking. Jois disengages, and the camera lingers to show Ramsey slumping forward, his hard-sprung body dripping with sweat, bowing his head in weary acceptance.

"Really it's all preparation for your death moment," Ramsey goes on to tell Donahaye,

> that's the whole idea behind it. Because if you can put your mind on God while you are hopping around on the floor doing mildly painful things, that's practicing for the last moment of greatest extremity. And if in your death moment you can put your mind on God, the theory is, you save yourself a whole lot of births, you save yourself many travails.[247]

Brad Ramsey died of suicide in 2012.

A LETTER TO HER TEACHERS

On July 17, 2007, Tracy Hodgeman wrote the following letter to her teachers David Garrigues and Catherine Tisseront. It shows how the push and pull of disorganized attachment trickles down through time and spreads outwards from Mysore.

> dearest david and satya,[248]
>
> i found out yesterday that i have a torn rotary cuff. i got some unanticipated financial encouragement a couple of weeks ago to get an mri, and so i went to the shoulder specialist at the university of washington sports medicine clinic, dr. green. he explained it all to me. the only way to stabilize my shoulder is to reattach the missing ligaments surgically. he says he could put anchors in my bone, two or three, and sew the missing muscle back on to those arthroscopically. he also says my shoulder is way more worn out than most people my age. he occasionally sees this sort of wear and tear in professional weight lifters and old people. he says i have worn down the cartilage that cushions the joint. he says we are built to stand upright. he told me that human arms aren't built to be weight bearing, and he says i have arthritis in mine. he suggested that i look for a different kind of yoga, one that is easier on the arms.
>
> he also says the surgery is $9000, and takes 9 months of physical therapy to recover from... with a 90% success rate. 100% chance of being painful. many nerve endings in the bone... ouch.
>
> i can remember the day i tore it, if i remember correctly, i was coming up from *ashtavakrasana* (or trying to change sides), trying not to touch my feet. and boing!!! my collar bone moved under

my skin, i heard it. my ribs felt strange, my shoulder hurt. the end of my collar bone stuck up funny and was really sore. when was that? can you remember? it was before david went to india last winter. can you remember david, when i first started complaining? was it november??? before???

the surgeon was really surprised that i had done so much damage by myself. before the mri, i was trying to explain what happened, and he formed an idea of what he thought was wrong, based on xrays and a physical exam and my explanation (i took in pictures of iyengar in the poses to show what i meant). but when he saw the mri he was surprised that i could pull myself apart so thoroughly with yoga. usually takes an impact. i told him i must have impacted myself.

i stubbornly pulled myself apart. i so very badly wanted to be able to do those poses and even more frustrating, the vinyasas in between.... i wanted to "progress." to keep up w/the program, keep getting new poses, keep moving ahead. to perform well. to be a good student. to be a good teacher by example. all that stuff i was telling you before that my self worth was and still is caught up in...

i ignored the tiredness. i ignored the soreness. i ignored the tightness. i did not listen to my pain. i told myself i was getting stronger and more flexible and more open. i thought i was noble. i thought i was brave. i thought i was a good worker. i thought i was doing the right thing. instead i was beating myself up. over and over, day after day, year after year. and calling it yoga. i am starting to think i had a yoga disorder. like an eating disorder. i couldn't see what was right in front of my face until i finally came apart and i had no choice but to look reality in the face.

now i don't know what to think. i am discouraged and sick and sad and angry and confused and scared. and at the same time, i am hopeful and excited to have some clarity on what has been so puzzling and "limiting" in my body.... i think i am going to get the surgery. god knows i have tried every other possible thing out there. if there was no surgery, no way to fix it, i would survive, i could manage. but it pulls funny on my ribcage, my shoulder blade can't move properly, i feel like i'm constantly under this weird stress.

my shoulder clunks every time i try to use any muscular force, to lift the tea pot, to use the clippers to cut branches, to pick up a heavy object, to do a pushup. all day long i am reminded that things aren't where they belong. and it is somewhat painful, at times. but not debilitating. as long as i don't use it much, it's not too bad...

and of course my faith in ashtanga is sorely tested. is this the right thing for the average human being to be doing w/their body? or even the above average??? what is the purpose of the really difficult and tricky poses??? are the benefits heavy enough to balance the cost? for me, no. i don't think so.

the main reason i am telling you all this is because i think you need to know. i think there is not enough honest discourse about the dangers of yoga between yogis. between ashtangis in particular. i hear myself and other people talking about their pains as if they are awards of honor, badges of courage, something to be proud of, to brag about. it's just common chatter after and before practice. the yoga blogs are full of it. macho talk about what hurts today. and how far we are along in our practices, as if the further along the better a person you are. the more spiritually advanced!!!!! i think the linear style of ashtanga is really dangerous for many people. the perfect self destructive weapon for the over achiever. push more, go further, always further. i think it's almost a sickness. a cultural sickness...

and you are both a part of it too. david, you are so good at pushing people to go further, you are like a coach: "come on!" you say. and man, we want to do what you say. you are so compelling. you are powerful. you are more powerful than my own delicate common sense, my own unsteady and underused intuition. i like giving up my power to the guru. it is comfortable and i feel good doing it. listening to my own voice is foreign and difficult. i'm not very good at it. and it's fun to go further, to do better than you thought you could. it's intoxicating, and it makes you want more. like a runaway cart w/o brakes. until you hit a tree. bam!!! you both have that "work harder" ethic. which is good right? up to a point. but where is that place where good work turns bad???? obviously i don't know. and if i don't know, i would suspect that there are a lot of others like me.

i feel like i am waking up from a drug, recovering from a cult. what was i thinking????? my poor shoulder. i am so sorry. i didn't know what i was doing. i was under a spell. i thought i was doing a good thing. i didn't know enough. now it's too late for me. but it's not too late to try to help other people see the potential dangers waiting there on their mats.

i hope you can understand me. i love yoga so much. i love my practice so much. i love you both so much. i love the poses that were my undoing. i was so very happy struggling w/those third series poses. i wanted to be able to fly. i miss it and i am lost in the world w/o that to define me now. i don't regret what i did, exactly, because that is not very useful, but i would like to imagine a world where these poses are only done w/the utmost ahimsa. i thought i was doing that already, but obviously i wasn't. this is almost impossible to do. very advanced. the most advanced. i can't even imagine how to do it yet. i am going to be looking for that place.

my surgery is scheduled for august 29th. the first 4 weeks i will be in a sling. then slowly rehab starts, little by little, for the next 8 months after that. i have not figured out how i will pay for this, and i do not know how i will work—i suspect i can tell people w/o showing... i'm also not sure where i stand as a teacher, i don't know what to think. i would really like to take a break from all of it, do something completely different for a while so i can think... but what??? i don't know. we'll see...

i don't know if i will be very useful to you in the teacher training, but i would be happy to do what i can. as i mentioned, i will be gone from the 16th to the 23rd of aug...

satya, i will see you tomorrow at 3.

love, tracy

Neither Garrigues nor Tisseront answered the letter, Tracy says. But the day after Tracy sent it, she saw Garrigues at the studio, she says.

"We had a two-minute interaction where he told me that he didn't hurt me, Ashtanga yoga didn't hurt me, but that I had hurt myself."

I asked her how that made her feel.

"I don't want you to get the impression that I hate him," Tracy says.

> I actually love the man deeply. I got hurt under his care, and I am disappointed that he was not more willing, at the time, to question the "flawed" system and himself to see how he may have played a part in my injury because I am worried about other people also getting hurt. But I also forgive him. I chose to go there. I kept coming back, day after day, year after year. Until I couldn't any more...
>
> He is flawed just like his beautiful Ashtanga System. I think he was drawn to Jois in part because Jois was also famous for deflecting questions. *Because I said so*—was always the answer from Jois. *You listen. You do. Do the practice and all is coming. 99% practice, 1% theory.* All this talk is just avoiding the work at hand....

Tracy says that Garrigues did offer her some private classes, which she accepted. And when Tracy's friend wanted to raise the $9000 that the surgery would cost, Garrigues kindly offered to host the fundraiser, she says. "I was in this elite corps of yogi athletes," she told me.

> And now I've become a pedestrian, someone who does normal things in the morning. Water my plants. Pet the cat. For a while I thought I would get back to a regular practice that was more sustainable, but it seems I don't need it. There are other things I'd rather do.

Garrigues didn't respond to a request for comment on Tracy's story, about Catherine's experience of Jois, and about Nicola Tiburzi's account of being assaulted by Jois at the Seattle event that Garrigues hosted (p. 323). But in a statement posted to his Instagram account, he expressed sadness and remorse in response to the public disclosures of Jois's victims.

"I have been reflecting on the allegations of sexual abuse committed by Sri K Pattabhi Jois," he wrote.

> I'd like to say that my heart and prayers are with the victims. Many years back while studying in Mysore I didn't listen to my gut feeling and speak up when I felt something not right was taking place. I don't know if Pattabhi Jois had perverted thoughts in his mind when he was giving the adjustments but I know that the adjustments were inappropriate and that no yoga teacher should

> touch his or her students in these ways. I apologize for contributing to anyone's pain by my silence. I was afraid to speak up, to question authority. I was confused as to what was inappropriate or appropriate. I believe the fact that I was sexually abused as a boy contributed to my remaining silent. I hope that by me speaking up people who were hurt by Pattabhi Jois's inappropriate behaviors will feel that there are those of us who support them, want them to exercise their right to speak out, be heard, and take the steps they need to heal. I will continue to reflect, confide in those I trust, and to utilize the past and present as important sources of growth and healing for building a better, more loving, courageously honest, and spiritually alive future for me and all within our community. I remain committed to allowing truth to emerge even in the most difficult circumstances so that I continue to evolve as a student, teacher, and person.[249]

Soon after Tracy's surgery, Garrigues and Tisseront separated, and Garrigues moved across the country.

Sometime after her cancer diagnosis, Tisseront changed her name to Satya, which means "truth" in Sanskrit. She died in hospice in Seattle in 2010.

Part Five

A Long Shadow, Brightening

In 2001, Katie traveled to South India on a two month retreat to practice and study with a senior Ashtanga yoga teacher. Heartbroken and vulnerable after a breakup and redundancy, she traveled alone to immerse herself in the healing and safe environment of an ancient, spiritual practice in order to find a sense of clarity and calm.

Katie had heard amazing things about a European yoga teacher who ran retreats in South India and her hopes for learning more about the sacred teachings of yoga with him were high. What she didn't anticipate was a full-on and repeated sexual assault over the course of eight weeks.

— Genny Wilkinson Priest, reporting on allegation against a certified Ashtanga teacher. "Katie" is a pseudonym.[250]

Gurus demand total surrender from disciples. Disciples have an irrepressible need for the guru's approval. This is one subtle driving force of the relationship.[251]

—Sharon Gannon and David Life[251]

BARGAINING WITH HISTORY AND THE PRESENT

Elisabeth Kübler-Ross's five responses to grief—denial, anger, bargaining, depression, and acceptance—are typically used to understand personal responses to terminal illness, tragedy, or death.*[252] But they're also useful as a framework for exploring social responses to group trauma. After all, for many, revelations about Jois's assaults constitute a kind of death, of both idealization and community trust.

In this book, we've seen denial on full display in group responses to the Jois adjustment video. There were also cruel and discrediting comments that appeared in response to the disclosures of Karen Rain. Anger has also been palpable, but with a dual target. Some expressed outrage at Jois for having assaulted women and betrayed the community, and at his family and senior disciples. But others turned the tables to vent at both victims and whistleblowers.

Clinical psychologist Jennifer Freyd has named this table-turning **DARVO** ("**d**eny-**a**ttack-**r**everse-**v**ictim-and-**o**ppressor"). She writes that the

> perpetrator or offender may **Deny** the behavior, **Attack** the individual doing the confronting, and **Reverse** the roles of **Victim** and **Offender** such that the perpetrator assumes the victim role and turns the true victim—or the whistle blower—into an alleged offender. This occurs, for instance, when an actually guilty perpetrator assumes the role of "falsely accused" and attacks the accuser's credibility and blames the accuser of being the perpetrator of a false accusation. [253]

But it was Kübler-Ross's "bargaining" phase that was most evident in some of the first responses from leading Ashtanga figures to the revelations of Jois's abuse. These eventually gave way to the voices of Ashtanga leaders who expressed not only depression and acceptance in their range of response, but also found the capacity to speak for change.

There is a formula to the bargaining statement

- "Yes, that happened...", or
- "It *seems* to have happened...", or

* Kübler-Ross's term is "stages". I'm using "responses" here because the claim that grief follows a staged and orderly arc is contested in clinical psychology, and because the model of stages suggests that those who move through more of them are either more mature or more healed.

- "The victims *say* it has happened and we should honor their truth…",
- *But…* [insert mitigating statement that redirects away from the victim's point of view and reestablishes empathy with the accused]."
- Mitigating statements might sound like: "But he didn't mean it," "He's really not like that", "He's a family man", "Many people never had a problem with him,"* "So many people love him," "He does such good work in the world."

That didn't happen. But when it did, he was doing it on purpose.

In the months following Karen Rain's disclosure, crisis statements from leaders acknowledged her account, often without naming her. But many also spent more space on personal reminiscences about the wholesomeness of Jois, assertions that the issue had been addressed, and appeals to followers to focus on the benefits of his practice.

All such add-ons contribute to a key feature of the bargaining statement posing as an accountability statement: its *length*. Statements limited to apology and accountability are succinct. This has the advantage of giving space back to the victim. "That is horrible. I'm so sorry that happened to you. I'm going to examine the ways in which I might have contributed to this happening, and take steps to help make sure it never happens again."

On December 26, 2017, global Ashtanga celebrity and Jois disciple Kino MacGregor issued a 3800-word statement that established common cause with Jois's victims by disclosing that she too had been sexually assaulted by a yoga teacher. The post expressed empathy, offered some action items for reform, but was also heavy on bargaining while it subtly cast doubt on Jois's accusers.**[254] In a podcast with J. Brown four months later, the bargaining became literal. "I would be very happy to have an open dialogue and a discussion with them to discuss what atonement are they looking for," she said, referring to Jois's victims.

> Is it monetary? Because if they want a GoFundMe for monetary remuneration to make up for what they have experienced, I would

* While writing this chapter, political supporters of US Supreme Court nominee Brett Kavanaugh produced a letter from 65 women attesting to his good character and relations with women in high school. The letter was in response to Christine Blasey Ford, who accused Kavanaugh of sexual assault and battery when she was 15 and he was 17. In deciding to confirm Kavanaugh, the Republican Majority Senate Judiciary Committee highlighted the letter along with other character witness statements, while minimizing Blasey Ford's corroborating evidence for the assault.

** At the bottom of this lengthy article, MacGregor forbids anyone from quoting from it, except in full, with her permission. This might be understood within the context of the high-demand drives to manage image and control information (cf Mann, Hassan).

> be more than happy to facilitate that. What do they want? Do they want a formal apology?[255]

In her written statement, MacGregor explained to her million-plus social media followers that while she believed Rain and others, she herself had not seen Jois giving any student anything but love and care. She spent a number of paragraphs subtly casting doubt on Rain's claims by showing how, in her own teaching, she offers students some of the same adjustments that Rain and others identified as assaultive when performed by Jois. She worried that observers could misinterpret *her* actions—implying that it was still possible that Jois's actions were being misinterpreted—if they saw nothing but a photograph. She lamented that Jois was dead and couldn't be asked about his intentions.

MacGregor confessed that the daylight between her perceptions of Jois and the reports of his victims brought up strong cognitive dissonance personally. But she also passionately argued that the Ashtanga movement had overcome Jois's "mistakes".

"It would be a grievous misunderstanding of the yoga tradition," she wrote, "to throw out the entire lineage of Ashtanga yoga because of the mistakes of one man (whose actions have been largely accounted for and removed from the system of Ashtanga yoga)."[256]

MacGregor's claim is unsupported. At the time of her blog and through to the time of this writing, there has been no third-party investigation and no Ashtanga-wide policy initiatives undertaken to protect students or establish grievance procedures. There's been no offer of restorative justice to Jois's victims. There have been no substantive changes to the code of ethics that authorized and certified Ashtanga teachers must follow, and no official statement from KPJAYI or members of the Jois family.

Before a brief review of other statements like MacGregor's and comparing them to more substantive accountability statements, we'll look at three stories that unfortunately show, contrary to MacGregor's view, that some disciples of Jois have followed him into what is now a cycle of abuse. In this sense, a bargaining statement might be difficult to separate from a denial statement. The stories feature unresolved allegations against a Jois-certified teacher, a teacher authorized by Rangaswamy, and a Jois disciple who has a leadership position within the Jois-inspired Jivamukti Yoga School. We'll also examine how a risk factor for yoga-related abuse—the premise of implied consent given to the yoga teacher to manipulate the bodies of students—has been normalized, popularized, and even sexualized.

These stories are presented to heighten the urgency of the action items presented in **Part Six**. Abuse in the Ashtanga world did not magically die with Pattabhi Jois. Facing it squarely calls for tools that will be of use to every community of wellness or spiritual practitioners.

ALLEGED ASSAULTS, FOLLOWING A PATTERN

Eight days before MacGregor posted her blog, Genny Wilkinson Priest, an authorized Ashtanga teacher, seasoned journalist, and yoga manager of Europe's largest yoga company, published an article that highlighted the problems with the suggestion that the Ashtanga community is self-correcting.[257]

Wilkinson Priest opened by reporting on the experience of a practitioner who traveled to South India in 2001 to study with a senior student of Jois. The article did not name the teacher.

"Katie" (not her real name) "had heard amazing things" about this popular Ashtanga teacher, "and her hopes for learning more about the sacred teachings of yoga with him were high. What she didn't anticipate was a full-on and repeated sexual assault over the course of eight weeks."

The article then describes an abuse scenario that corresponds with reports about assaults committed by Jois. Jois's student would "grab, squeeze and move Katie's breasts as she folded forward." The teacher went further than Jois, using "his intimidating personality and position of authority to try to persuade her to 'finish' her practice in his bedroom down the hall."

The correspondence to Jois's classroom assaults is made more explicit when Katie tells Wilkinson Priest that Jois's student assaulted Katie in a supine splits posture—as Jois did with Karen Rain, T.M., Kim Haegele Labidi, and an undetermined number of other women.

"He placed his thumb between my legs on my clitoris and made circular movements," Katie tells Wilkinson Priest. "I thought maybe his hand had slipped. But he did it again on my last day there, and I knew there was absolutely no way it was a mistake."

ALLEGED RAPE IN MYSORE

In her post, MacGregor insisted that there is a "new culture" in Mysore guided by Sharath's "impeccable" ethical behavior. Her claim was echoed in comment threads around the world.

But the report of an Ashtanga practitioner from Australia who traveled to Mysore to study at KPJAYI suggests otherwise.

The practitioner, who wishes to remain anonymous, alleged on social media and via email that on the night of October 31, 2014, she was raped in Mysore by a Level 2 authorized Ashtanga teacher from the United States. Because the alleged incident happened in India and involved foreign nationals—and therefore jurisdiction complexities—it was very difficult for the practitioner to pursue criminal charges.

She later learned that the assailant was a registered sex offender in Venice, California. The registration came from a 1999 conviction in Isabella County, Michigan, for "sexual assault with intent to penetrate". He was sentenced to 104 days in jail, to be served on his winter, spring, and summer breaks from college.[258]

She alleges the rape occurred after she had gone to a party with the accused. "Because I was scheduled to fly out the next day," she writes, "I did not have time to process the situation nor report to Sharath or the authorities."

She told no-one about the incident until she returned to Mysore in February 2016 and informed Rangaswamy.

In a private meeting, Rangaswamy reportedly told the practitioner that the alleged attacker had been de-authorized, and that she "shouldn't worry anymore". He did not offer an explanation for the de-authorization.

But in June of that year, the practitioner saw photos of her alleged attacker on social media, attending classes with Rangaswamy in a gymnasium at UCLA. One photo shows him in the front row as Rangaswamy walks by, instructing. Another shows him smiling, with his arm around a young woman.

"This is what pushed me to go public and assert for an explanation from Sharath," the practitioner writes. "Imagine how I would feel?"

She made her grievance with KPJAYI public in a Facebook comment.

"From where I stand, the bubble is looking all too fake and plastic," she wrote.

> What happened to having a voice? Where have all the feminists gone? Why is it so hard to stand up to him? To question him? Since when were we so meek? How different is it from having your own child harassed by his/her teacher and the school principal saying, "Well, that's why boys shouldn't be hanging out with girls." Will you tell your kid, "Well, you should've gone to the police!" or maybe, "Well, that's "school" (India)—deal with it."[259]

Rangaswamy did not respond to a request for comment on the practitioner's statements.

"I SAT ON GURUJI'S LAP ALL THE TIME"

More evidence of a pattern of sexual misconduct amongst some Jois disciples is revealed in the documents of New York County Supreme Court Case 150790, filed in Lower Manhattan on February 1, 2016.[260] Holly Faurot, a teacher for the Jivamukti Yoga School, alleged that her mentor Ruth Lauer-Manenti, a senior Jivamukti teacher and Jois disciple, sexually harassed and assaulted her as many as 25 times between 2011 and 2013. When the suit was made public, Jivamukti released a statement decrying the complaints as part of a "negative campaign."[261] The allegations were never tried, and the case was settled out of court.

Lauer-Manenti's co-defendants in the lawsuit were Jivamukti founders Sharon Gannon and David Life, and Carlos Menjivar, their long-time business manager. The suit alleged that Gannon, Life, and Menjivar covered up the abuse, in contravention of Jivamukti's ethics policies.

The court documents report that Faurot had been Lauer-Manenti's teaching apprentice at the Jivamukti Yoga School during 2009–10, and had graduated to assisting and occasionally subbing for her classes as a favored student. In Exhibit A, the "Report of Sexual Harassment by Complainant",[262] Faurot writes:

> I heard countless stories from Ruth throughout my study with her about the transformative and enlightening nature of her relationship with her guru, Shri K. Pattabhi Jois. She repeatedly emphasized the importance of her devotion, dedication, and obedience to him as his student. Devotion, particularly guru devotion, is a dominating theme found throughout the teachings imparted by the Jivamukti yoga method. Chapter 5 of the *Jivamukti Yoga* book entitled, "Guru: The Teacher You Can See and Feel" states, "You must also be willing to let trust develop between you and a teacher."

That chapter also says, "Gurus demand total surrender from disciples. Disciples have an irrepressible need for the guru's approval. This is one subtle driving force of the relationship."[263]

In 2011, Lauer-Manenti asked to stay at Faurot's downtown apartment on nights before having to teach early morning classes. "I was so excited at the opportunity to be of service to my teacher," Faurot writes in the Report. Faurot says she intended for Lauer-Manenti to sleep in the guest bed, but the teacher said she wanted to sleep in Faurot's bed. When Faurot agreed, Lauer-Manenti initiated spooning and cuddling. So began two years of increasingly intimate intrusions, including Lauer-Manenti making sexual comments about Faurot's body in the apartment and also at the studio, and asking to take erotic photographs of Faurot. "As Ruth initiated more and more intimate and sexually charged contact and encounters in private," Faurot writes, "in public my position as her student became increasingly more privileged."

According to Faurot, Lauer-Manenti asked to speak with her in February 2014. They met at a tea shop in lower Manhattan, a few minutes' walk south of the Jivamukti Yoga Center.

Faurot includes excerpts of their conversation in the Report. In them, Lauer-Manenti says that she was showing innocent affection, and that Faurot misinterpreted her.

"It was inappropriate as a teacher," says Faurot in the transcript. "To cuddle in bed with your students."

"Alright!" says Lauer-Manenti. "I cuddled with guruji, okay!"

"In your bed?"

"No, but I sat on his lap and I kissed him everyday that I had class."

Later in the conversation, Lauer-Manenti reaffirms, "I sat on guruji's lap all the time."

No one but Faurot and Lauer-Manenti will ever know for sure what happened between them. If Faurot's allegations against her former teacher are true, an argument could be made that Lauer-Manenti was acting out behaviors learned in part through her relationship with Jois.

Eddie Stern dismissed the link. "The Jivamukti problem has nothing to do with Pattabhi Jois," he wrote by email.

> If it had to do with Pattabhi Jois, then ALL of his students would be engaging in sexually abusive or invasive acts, but they are not. The problem is with individuals, the problem is not with some Guru somewhere.[264]

JOIS'S ECHO IN THE CULTURE OF IMPLIED CONSENT: EXAMPLE FROM A POPULAR BOOK

In an article published before her suit was settled, Faurot suggested that the alleged sexual harassment by her mentor that took place outside of class was continuous with Jivamukti's in-class culture of constant intimate physical adjustments. When Lauer-Manenti helped her with dropbacks—an adjustment appropriated from the Jois method—Lauer-Manenti would "thrust her thigh into my crotch," Faurot said. "She'd drop me back and then pull me back up on her thigh. Things were way more intimate then they would be with a stranger."[265]

The Jivamukti Yoga School has been a key influence in the spread of Ashtanga values in digestible and popular form. Sharon Gannon and David Life founded the school in New York in 1984. Initially, their teaching drew on the simpler sequences of Sivananda yoga, but after traveling to Mysore to practice with Jois in 1989, they began to cite him as their primary asana influence.

"We loved him from the start," they write in their flagship 2002 book, *Jivamukti Yoga: Practices for Liberating Body and Soul.* (A careful read of the following quotes renders signs of the disorganized attachment dynamics discussed in **Part Four**.)

> He was demanding but gentle, as he drove us through the strenuous Primary Series of asana postures of Ashtanga yoga. He laughed at our awkwardness one moment, then shouted admonishments the next.[266]

> Pattabhi Jois has tremendous charisma and pulsates with the aura of a true *siddha*, one who has acquired the unusual powers earned through dedication to yoga practice and teaching for over six decades. Injuries that refuse to respond to any kind of therapy or bodywork disappear under his touch.[268]

> Pattabhi Jois knows where all your buttons are located. With a few words he can make a devotee feel like a maharaja or a bad child. The work is subtle and psychological when one commits to a master. The asana practice becomes mere structure for the real work, which is transformation.[267]

A class in the Jois-inspired Jivamukti technique was grounded in devotion to the teacher—whether it was the person standing at the front of the room, or the Teacher-as-Archetype, represented on the altar photos. It began with chanting and sun salutations, moved towards a posture of peak difficulty that resonated with the crescendo of the music playlist. Most importantly—especially for its influence on some of mainstream yoga culture—the class was measured out with a rhythm of constant physical adjustments, which were presented as spiritually helpful.

In the manual for the Jivamukti teaching apprenticeship program, trainees are told that when adjusting their colleagues, "Your hands should almost never leave them."[269] Teacher trainees at Jivamukti were encouraged to adjust as many students in the room as possible. As with Jois, Jivamukti adjustments were believed to transmit healing energy. But, as with Jois, they carried the possibility of violation. And if things went wrong, the injury suffered in relation to the adjustment could be attributed to the student's "resistance", or seen as a necessary by-product of "opening". Finally: as with Jois, the Jivamukti adjustment protocol operated under the premise of implied consent, and through a belief that a yoga posture lays bare a person's soul before the intuition of the teacher.

"I certainly feel that we were being trained to be abusive, bullying teachers following in the tradition of ... Jois," says a former Jivamukti teacher, who co-founded a Facebook page called "From Darkness to Light" that focuses on revealing abuse in the yoga world.[270] The page was created after Faurot brought her suit.

> There is such an emphasis in all these traditions of just mimicking your teacher and kind of 'faking it till you make it', that it's like we were being taught how to be abusers and fakes. We were being groomed to be abusers or abused, or both.[271]

In 2014, Gannon and Life published a book entitled *Yoga Assists: A Complete Visual and Inspirational Guide to Yoga Asana Assists.* [272]Not once amidst the detailed psychosomatic instructions does the word "consent" appear in the text. Nor "permission". This makes sense, given that the book reads like the distillation of typical Jois-informed Ashtanga rationalizations for adjustments.

In the introduction to the book, they write that Jois "taught us the healing touch of hands-on assists."[273] Later, they write,"Sri K. Pattabhi Jois said, 'Without touch, progress is very slow.'" They elaborate:

> There is a magic to touch that is the very thing that draws many people to a yoga class in the first place. Through hands-on assists we have the potential to convey information clearly, directly, without words.
>
> Touch can accelerate progress. Touch can provide directional cues, help identify and release unconscious resistance or tightness,

> increase awareness and help diminish pain. Gentle, medium and strong touches all have their unique applications.
>
> Gentle touch moves the skin and provides clear and precise directional cues that indirectly guide the underlying tissue and muscles. The quality of touch must be direct, purposeful and clear, not distracting, confusing, annoying, or susceptible of [sic] misinterpretation as an uninvited caress. Gentle assists can give information, focus awareness, release skin tightness and impart confidence without intimidation.
>
> Medium touch moves not only skin, but also directly moves underlying muscle and tissues. Medium assists can provide a sense of support and thereby relax psychological and physical resistance.
>
> Strong touch moves skin, fascia, muscle, bone, organs and perceived limitations. Strong assists can guide skeletal alignment, inspire, create space and open up new physical and psychological range.[274]

Gannon and Life make brief reference here to the potential for the space of implied consent they are creating to produce "misinterpretation" in the arena of touch versus sexual assault. Later, they do acknowledge that adjustments could cause or contribute to injury. This particular discussion begins with the assumption that the teacher should be able to gauge a student's readiness to be manipulated by monitoring their breathing patterns.

"The quality of the breath reveals directly the experience that the student is having," Gannon and Life write.

> When there is hesitation or stuttering in the breath, doubt and anxiety are present. If you hear shallow breathing, that could indicate fear, or lack of trust or confidence. Heavy breathing can reveal aggression. If the student is not breathing in a strong, calm, clear, rhythmic way, that is an indication to the teacher not to push them into an assist. To push in this circumstance is to assert your dominance and force the student to yield to your will, which among other things can lead to injury. This is not a proper assist! The first rule for avoiding this kind of interaction is to only assist a student to move deeper into an asana to the extent that you can hear the student's breath remaining strong, calm, clear and rhythmic. An essential step in giving a good assist is to tune in to

> the student's breathing. Begin to make the sound of your breath audible, strong, calm, clear and rhythmic … and the student will often naturally modify their breath to follow yours. *Ujjayi* breath can be very helpful here.[275]

As we've seen, however, rhythmic breathing can be used to dissociate from both pain and whatever else is happening in the room, or even happening to you. "If you focus really closely on your breath," Karen Rain said, "you're not going to be paying attention to anything else."

Additionally, the notion that a teacher should influence the student's breath in relation to their own has to be handled with care. While encouraging a student to mirror a slowed breathing rate might have supportive effects in many cases, the teacher has to remain aware of problematic power dynamics that might unfold during the exchange. How would a teacher know that their student wasn't matching their breath in order to please them? A student is not necessarily indicating consent by mirroring their teacher; they may be indicating a surrender of agency.

Yoga Assists offers no guidelines for training or competency in touch, nor does it articulate a scope of practice. Like Jois's (or Iyengar's, or Choudhury's, or many others of that generation) physical adjustments, the Jivamukti scope is seemingly unlimited. Through good intentions and the power of yoga alone, Jivamukti teachers are empowered to look deeply into their students' bodies and subtle energies, discern what ails them, and offer healing.

"Before you assist anyone," Gannon and Life write,

> observe carefully, not just with the physical eyes but also with your feeling self, increasing compassion. Your subtle sight will reveal resonance or dissonance with the energetic form of the asana. You will be able to spot some things very easily, like dissymmetry [sic] or unequal weight distribution. But some things are difficult to perceive, especially physical, emotional or psychological trauma suffered in the past. Using the chakra system as a model can help you to understand deeper causes for misalignment that are apparent in the physical body. For example, alignment problems in standing asanas, especially in how the feet and legs connect to the Earth, may speak of misalignment with nature and/or unresolved issues with money, home or parents. Moving upward from the

> feet into the various body parts and the associated chakras can provide valuable insight into causes for the physical misalignment and energetic blockages that the teacher can see.[276]

Yoga Assists was written for public consumption, and conveys a basic plausibility. The postures are common enough, and the manipulations are easy to understand. If you overlook vagaries like "skin tightness" and "skeletal alignment" and feel intrigued by the mixture of premodern body poetry with scientific terms like "fascia", it's a functional book. But passages like the above endow the teacher with special charismatic powers that can become dangerous objects of belief.

ADJUSTMENTS AND SEXUALIZATION OF PRACTICE

In the section on how Jois's assaults were sometimes rationalized as "*mula-bandha* assists", we explored how this deception both recalled and manipulated information about medieval yoga practices, taught by and for men, that employed sexual techniques towards sublime goals. We've now looked at two stories that correlate with this deception in Ashtanga sphere beyond Jois: the sexual assault of "Katie" under the guise of adjustment, and the fuzzy boundary between Lauer-Manenti's assists and her "cuddling".

However, just as a reminder: this book examines the Jois event to shed light on issues that are in no way limited to Ashtanga culture. In 1991, the *San Jose Mercury News* published an investigation of B.K.S. Iyengar's most senior disciple, Manouso Manos. Journalist Bob Frost wrote that

> Manos allegedly rubbed his pelvis against women students in a sexually provocative way as the women were doing yoga poses, touched them in private places during classes under the guise of pose adjustments, and asked certain women students individually into an institute classroom after group classes, where, behind closed doors, he performed sexually charged physical manipulations, and had intercourse.[277]

Manos reportedly made a public apology, and was removed from his position at the San Francisco Iyengar Institute. Several months later, he was reinstated by Iyengar himself. But according to an investigation by the radio station KQED, Manos allegedly re-offended in 2015.[278] The Ethics Committee of the Iyengar Yoga National Association of the United States ruled it had received insufficient evidence to sanction Manos. Though the complainant brought corroborating witnesses who she told about the incident when it happened, the Committee said it needed eyewitnesses, despite the fact that the incident occurred during a posture in which the students would not have been looking at the teacher.[279]

In December 2017, yoga activist Rachel Brathen released excerpts from over 300 #MeToo yoga stories she received in response to a social media call-out. She has reportedly received many more since. The allegations included rape, groping, assault and harassment.[280]

Such stories are among the worst outcomes of a broader trend, where physical adjustments in global yoga culture play out against the unexamined sexualization of practice. The subject is receiving increasing attention, with feminist scholars leading the way in mining the gender politics involved. The work of Melanie Klein and colleagues in the yoga and Body Image Coalition[281] as well as in academic anthologies[282] give sharp insight into the complex intersections and disagreements between yogic ideals, disciplines, and performances and feminist notions of reclaiming agency and self-acceptance. At the heart of these discussions is the problem of the objectification of women's bodies—even within a practice that often promises access to female empowerment. The arguments are informed by an awareness of the objectifying "male gaze" on both cultural and internalized levels.[283]

Remembering the power of Jois's own gaze can open a window onto how the objectification of women's bodies in yoga relates to the elevation of male teachers as subjects with special knowledge of and power over women's bodies. In keeping with the framework of this case study, two examples from the current Ashtanga world will help to show that the objectification of (silent) women's bodies through gaze and touch has become intergenerational in spaces that continue to foster the notion of *implied*, as opposed to *explicit*—or even better, *affirmative* —consent. Both show the eroticized social power this can give a charismatic male teacher.

EXAMPLE ONE: A VIDEO

"Mysore Style with Tim Miller" is a 2016 promotional video shot and edited by Agathe Padovani.[284] Miller is certified as one of Jois's oldest American students, having started practicing with him in 1977. Padovani has produced video content for both Fox and the Disney Channel and now creates polished promotions for international Ashtanga stars like Kino MacGregor.

Padovani is also Miller's student. Her Instagram feed features a video clip of Miller assisting her in a version of the backbend that comes at the end of the Primary Series. Miller holds her lower back/upper buttocks as she goes down. He then drapes his chest over her abdomen so he can help her catch the back of her upper calves with her hands. Once she's in the posture, he straightens up and lays his hands on her bare abdomen. After a moment, he makes a drumming motion with his fingers to alert her that she should come up. She comes back up with closed eyes and, smiling serenely, kisses him on the cheek.[285]

Padovani's four-minute film focuses entirely on Miller adjusting students during a Mysore-style practice session at Miller's Ashtanga Yoga Center in Carlsbad, California. As of this writing, the AYC has no formal consent policy for physical assists in its classes. Like a great many Ashtanga teachers, Miller does not hold licenses in any manual therapy regulated by a state authority.

Miller is famous in Ashtanga circles for the intensity of his physical adjustments. Chad Herst, an old friend of Karen Rain and a student of Miller, said that colleagues used to call Miller "the human can opener". Padovani's video, however, foregrounds the intimacy instead of the intensity of Miller's touch.

It's highly charged. In the 16 interactions between Miller and individual students in the montage, 13 are with women. Like the majority of Ashtanga practitioners, they are younger than Miller, who is in his mid-sixties, and framed by Padovani's lens as silver-fox-handsome. The camera catches his hands lingering on the students' bodies, and the loving gazes that pass between them. One women hugs and kisses the beaming Miller on the cheek after coming up from an assisted standing pose. Another hugs him after his backbending assist. He also holds a male student close after supporting him up from a backbend.

The film's soundtrack is Krishna Das singing "Good Old Chalisa", a hymn to Hanuman, the virile-but-celibate Hindu deity featured in the shala's logo. Das's rich, singular baritone voice backed by a female chorus provides an auditory echo of the gender dynamic playing out visually. Through Padovani's lens, Ashtanga practice in Carlsbad is a delivery device for bodily and emotional access to the master, wordlessly eroticized by his community.

EXAMPLE TWO: AN ESSAY

Ty Landrum is the Ashtanga-authorized teacher who co-presented with his own teacher Mary Taylor the "Teaching With the Hands" workshop referenced earlier. One of the workshop's stated goals was to encourage students to *consider the crucial skill of making space for power dynamics to dissolve.*[286] An essay on Landrum's site called "Yoga and Sexual Fantasy"[287] offers insight into Landrum's gendered understanding of those power dynamics.

The essay, which ostensibly offers ethical guidance for teachers and students in the #MeToo age, presents the student–teacher relationship as a kind of spiritual romance. The student is depicted as not only female, but as the archetypal "feminine", whom the male teacher, symbolizing guidance and awareness, longs to love, selflessly. This "feminine" energy, however, is also synonymous with the teacher's own breath. Whether as an essentialized archetype or as a part of the teacher's body, the silent female student in Landrum's essay is not a person with a voice, not a citizen with rights with whom the teacher discusses their needs or establishes consent.

"Yoga and Sexual Fantasy" seems to be intended to add to the conversation around safety and touch emerging in the wake of the Jois revelations and the excerpts from 300 yoga abuse stories published by Rachel Brathen three weeks earlier. Throughout, Landrum presents a consensus position towards the sexuality of *hathayoga*: the practice makes use of erotic energies, he explains, but the point is to use them to dissolve ego-centrism. Indulging them selfishly is a grave error. This is dangerous stuff, he explains, because few people have the psychic training that would allow them to sublimate the drive for gratification. The evidence for this, Landrum says, is clear from the "troubling profusion of recent allegations of sexual violation made against prominent yoga teachers by their students."

Landrum argues for psychological maturity in yoga culture, but, in the process, assigns equal responsibility for sexual abuse to both teacher and student.

> [W]e have not, as a community, braced ourselves adequately against the psychological perils of the practice. Too many of our teachers, *not to mention our students*, have failed to handle those dangers gracefully. They have allowed their sexual impulses to overcome them at crucial moments, causing others irreparable psychological harm. [Emphasis added.]

The essay edges Landrum close to the orbit attributed to Jois: that of a yoga master both knowledgeable about sex, and beyond it. "The intimacy of Hatha yoga," he asserts, "can involve the reciprocal exploration of human sexuality, but even then, it must be devoid of fantasy, objectification, and power imbalances of any kind." With references to extrasensory perception, no mention of consent, and wordless assumptions about what the female student is feeling, the writing attains full first-person male omniscience—or, as the title has it, fantasy.

> The touch of a teacher who is grounded in the present moment is very different from one who is silently indulging sexual fantasies. When a teacher imagines his student as an instrument of pleasure, *she can feel the shift immediately.* This shift is something that untold numbers of yoga students must have experienced, but it is rarely if ever mentioned. For it amounts to a violation which, though deplorable, is nearly impossible to prove. It involves no overt indiscretion, and registers only as a sudden feeling of vulnerability and estrangement.
>
> Or perhaps there is a shared sense of arousal, and a quiet reciprocation. The teacher indulges a fantasy, and the other is excited in turn. She starts to indulge some fantasy of her own, however tenuous it might be. Either way, the conditions of yoga, as mutual presence with the reality of the other, have just been undermined. [Emphasis added.]

Landrum's presentation makes use of the aforementioned erroneous centering of intention as the defining aspect of sexual assault. This model depends on the student feeling the teacher's intention shift. Further, it depends on the teacher having a *sexual* intention, whereas the motivation to sexually assault might simply be to wield power. Using this reasoning, Landrum implies that the student must be able to discern a sexual "intention", and will know something is wrong. But this shames the victim if she doesn't speak up immediately. As Karen Rain points out, "Why *should* a sexual assault necessarily feel sexual to a victim? It might feel confusing. It might feel painful. It might feel like nothing."

Landrum takes care to assert that yoga teachers who indulge sexual fantasies cannot model selfless love. He also says that "openness is not possible when fantasies and power dynamics are in play. Since the student-teacher relationship is structured by certain power dynamics, it is simply not fit for sexual intimacy."

But the message is garbled. "Nor can any yoga teacher use sex as an instrument for teaching," Landrum writes. "And if he pretends otherwise, he only shows the depth of his confusion about the possibility of sexual exploration as a vehicle for yoga." As with the rationalizations that surrounded Jois, a double possibility is left open: the teacher does not use sex, but his yoga must not exclude sex. Because he doesn't indulge in mundane sex, his sexual mastery can give spiritual insight.

How can such doubletalk provide clarity to a community with a rape culture problem? Are speculations on the sexualized spirituality of medieval misogynists really useful at this point?[288] Especially when they've been used to deflect, minimize, and obfuscate assault? At a time in which both the Ashtanga community and the wider global yoga world is trying to understand and recover from sexual abuse and institutional betrayal, clearer conversations might be in order: about consent, gender equality, trauma awareness, and evidence-based approaches to mitigate structural power imbalances.

Ty Landrum did not respond to a request for comment.

BARGAINING AT AN ASHTANGA CONFERENCE

Loaded language and self-sealing reasoning might make it hard for Jois disciples to have clear conversations about accountability. At the same time, the diffusion and diversity of the global Ashtanga community would make any policy initiative challenging to organize.

But Jois's senior students do occasionally gather for joint teaching conferences. They did so in March 2018 in San Diego, under the cloud of a growing uproar over the revelations of Jois's abuse. The schedule included a public panel entitled "Do Your Practice and All Is Coming—Sri K. Pattabhi Jois".[289] The panelists were prepared for questions about the abuse allegations. The non-profit yoga credentialing body Yoga Alliance provided funding for a representative from Rape, Abuse & Incest National Network (RAINN) to be in attendance and answer questions that attendees might have about sexual assault. The organizers did not invite any of the women who had disclosed having been assaulted by Jois. Still, this would have been a good opportunity for strong collective action.

The discussion exposed concerns and regrets, but also in-group jargon, emotional bargaining, a lack of resources for dealing with the impacts of sexual assault, and no clear pathway towards organizational accountability. Mary Taylor described what a confusing time it was for everyone who loved Pattabhi Jois. She spoke of the value of listening to victims, but then suggested that community healing would come through the development of mutual understanding between Jois's victims and his disciples. If Jois's victims were listened to, Taylor implied, they in turn would start listening to Jois's disciples.

Certified Ashtanga teacher Dena Kingsberg echoed Taylor, reinforcing the importance of listening to both the victims and the concerns of the community as a whole. She contrasted her perception of Jois as a transformative figure with his victim's experience of him as an abuser.

"Is it possible," she asked, "that we can embrace both ends of this spectrum with respect for one another?"

There was no one there to respond on behalf of Jois's victims.

David Swenson, who first studied with Jois in 1977, said he hadn't been aware of the accusations against Jois until a month before the panel. He spoke about the need for ethics in teaching and adjusting, and emphasized that students need to be empowered to say no. At some points, however, he employed the same loaded language that was used to subtly (and perhaps unconsciously) shift responsibility from Jois to his victims, suggesting that students are at fault for giving too much power to the teacher. "The Guru is not a person," he said. "It's the practice." Mary Taylor shared this sentiment, cautioning students to not put teachers on pedestals, and that Ashtanga practice itself would provide the main support the community would need to transcend the crisis.

Manju Jois, Pattabhi's middle son and also a revered Ashtanga teacher, pled ignorance. "I didn't know anything about it," he said, explaining that he had left both India and his family's influence, in 1975. "I was shocked when I heard the allegations." Manju repeated this when an audience member stated that he'd heard that the Jois family had been alerted to the allegations many times.

The panel event ended on a dissonant note. Tim Feldman, authorized Ashtanga teacher and husband to Kino MacGregor, read from a "scribble" he'd posted online, in which he regretted having been in denial about the stories he'd heard and the pictures he'd seen.[290] Feldman said that as a result of reflection and talking to colleagues who verified the assaults, he concluded that Jois had definitely touched students "inappropriately". Then, turning to the question of Jois's intention, he found an opportunity to break the tension.

"My next question was why did he do that?" Feldman continued.

> Because I have never received an adjustment from Guruji that was anything else than bringing me closer to myself, and under-

> standing what he wanted. I don't have an answer. I do not know why he touched some women in this particular way. I just don't know and I'm still trying to figure out. So I'm actually speaking to friends that have received adjustments that they found were inappropriate and I'm trying them out at home in a safe space with my wife.

The audience burst into laughter.

STRUGGLING TO LISTEN

That uncomfortable panel rounded up a winter of online responses that struggled to metabolize the revelations. On December 8, 2017, Mary Taylor was the first prominent Ashtanga figure to publish a statement, in which she acknowledged the "sexually invasive and inappropriate" adjustments administered by Jois, and expressed regrets about not speaking out sooner. She wrote that his "behavior was wrong." But she also chalked this "flaw" up to "cultural differences".

"I can say that my experience," she wrote,

> was that he began doing these adjustments after foreign female students came to practice with him wearing very revealing Western-style clothing. To a provincial, orthodox Brahman [sic] from a tiny village, who knows what these women looked like? Certainly they probably didn't appear to be chaste or well bred.[291]

On December 17, 2017, London-based Jois-certified teacher Hamish Hendry gave a talk on the issue. It was recorded and transcribed, and then posted by his long-term student Genny Wilkinson Priest.[292] The post and recording were loudly criticized for what many heard as notes of deflection and minimization. It was quickly deleted.

***

In February 2018, Wilkinson Priest launched a petition on *change.org* for Sharath Rangaswamy to acknowledge the abuse.[293] Wilkinson Priest is the yoga manager of Triyoga, Europe's largest yoga corporation. Five of their six London locations open their doors at 6am for Mysore-style Ashtanga classes.

"With great respect for the Ashtanga Yoga system," Wilkinson Priest wrote,

> we ask KPJAYI Director Sharath Jois to issue an official statement that acknowledges Pattabhi Jois gave inappropriate adjustments to some of his students over the course of many years.
>
> We believe a KPJAYI apology on behalf of Pattabhi Jois is the first step toward healing old as well as new wounds in the global Ashtanga community. We have a great love for this practice and would like KPJAYI to publicly champion an ethical teacher-student relationship. Together as a community we can lay the foundation that spurs action around the world to protect students as we find a safe, supportive environment in which to teach and practice yoga.*[294]

In a podcast several months later, Wilkinson Priest explained that her petition was:

> benignly written, because what I was trying to do was to plead with him to take some kind of action here. The vocabulary and the language that I used was quite soft. Basically, it just said we need you to come out and acknowledge that this happened in order for us to move forward. Please, can you do something about this? This is about the practice, really. We need to preserve this… Sharath, we need you to lead us out of this, because we're in really dangerous territory right now, and my concern is for the longevity of this practice.[295]

As of this writing, the petition has gathered 588 signatures. "Every time somebody signed that petition," said Wilkinson Priest, "Sharath would receive an email." Perhaps there weren't enough emails to be worth addressing. The global Ashtanga practice population, after all, numbers in the tens of thousands.

Ashtanga archivist Anthony Hall reported that Sharath Rangaswamy had briefly addressed the issue of his grandfather's behavior at a closed "conference" meeting in early January 2018, but noted that there was no official statement.[296] Later that same month, Sharath posted a new "Authorization/Certification Code of Conduct", the title of which might have led some to believe that he was taking concrete steps towards community reform. The

* In addition to this public letter, Rangaswamy also received an unknown number of private letters, asking him to acknowledge his grandfather's victims. One was sent by Chad Herst in June 2018. Rangaswamy did not respond, and Herst shared the letter on Facebook in September 2018. See **Appendix 3** for the full letter.

14-point document, however, which all Ashtanga teachers are now required to sign, includes only one bullet-point forbidding teachers from sexually harassing students (without defining it), and demands teachers be held accountable for their "actions, behavior and speech, including anything which might be defined or perceived as abuse, harassment or otherwise immoral, unethical, or illegal conduct". The *sharathjois.com* website, however, lists no grievance procedure for how that accountability might be enforced. Eleven of the 14 commitments in the new code are pledges of brand and financial loyalty to the Jois family. The move appeared to be more about group cohesion than apology, accountability, or ethical reform.

So was Sharath's next move, which was to seemingly randomly remove teachers that Jois had certified or authorized, some decades before, from the official online list of those permitted to teach the method. This initiated another wave of instability and consternation throughout sections of the global community, with many wondering whether he was purging those who had begun to denounce Jois's behavior. Within a month, however, some of the teachers were reinstated.[297]

For London-based Ashtanga teacher Sarai Harvey-Smith, the unceremonious list-slashing followed a recognizable pattern of control. "I think one of the biggest problems is it's arbitrary," she told a podcaster, referring to the authorization process. She suggested that authorization didn't depend on passing distinct learning thresholds, but rather simply continuing to make pilgrimages to Mysore.

> I think that's about power and control. It creates a culture of fear. This striking people off the list creates that fear, that if I teach differently or the way that I believe, or if I speak my mind, if I talk about ideas that are different from Sharath's ideas, then I can lose my authorization. I think that's very dangerous. I think that's what brings it into this cult-like culture, where if you step out of line, you're out. That's not to mention the money that one has to invest going to Mysore. It's very expensive to get those qualifications. Going to Mysore, but also paying for the certificate.[298]

Sharath Rangaswamy and his mother Saraswati Rangaswamy did not respond to requests for comment.

LISTENING

On a podcast in February 2018, Richard Freeman referred to the reporting on Jois as "yellow journalism" and complained that critics had not had the courtesy of reaching out to him and his partner Mary Taylor before speaking out.*[299] But in July, Taylor walked back some of her husband's defensiveness by posting a lucid and wide-ranging acknowledgment and action plan on behalf of them both.[300] The post was mainly inspired, she explained, by their conversations with Jois's victims. It acknowledged the intersection of physical, emotional, sexual, and spiritual injury caused by Pattabhi Jois. "Even since his death and to this day in some Ashtanga communities," she added, contradicting MacGregor, "sexual abuse and injury from adjustments continue."

Taylor criticized the hierarchical nature of the culture. It is, she wrote,

> fertile ground for disaster; establishing a power dynamic between teacher and student that can sour into an abuse of power. Abuse of power may manifest for students as consciously or unconsciously giving your power away to the teacher. For teachers, who have the upper hand in this power dynamic, it can manifest as fanaticism, narcissism, demands for obedience and loyalty—the stripping of another's intelligence.

The post also specifically addressed the reception of Freeman's podcast statements.

> I also know that some of his statements on podcasts came across as if he doesn't care and is in denial. Unfortunately, the statements hurt, rather than helped victims.
>
> Richard moves at his own pace and in his own time—as do we all. I live and work with him and see him every day gradually coming to grips with the situation. We talk about it a lot. From the beginning he has been deeply troubled by it. He has expressed to me and some others that he has been struggling to find the most truthful, authentic and supportive ways to express his sadness, dis-

* I began emailing with Mary Taylor in April 2015 to request an interview with Freeman. We exchanged emails in which I was transparent about the subject of my study: about wanting to ask about Jois's behavior and how Freeman understood it and felt about it. At one point, we confirmed an in-person appointment time at their home in Boulder. Via Taylor, Freeman canceled at the last minute, citing a scheduling conflict.

> appointment and disgust at the needless harm and suffering that has occurred due to Pattabhi Jois's behavior, while the true insight and depth of the yoga tradition was being ignored. He also deeply regrets any role he played in the perpetuation of the problems.
>
> Richard and I both apologize to those who have been hurt by us, Pattabhi Jois, or within the ashtanga practice. We also apologize for the roles we played in allowing the problems within ashtanga—in particular Pattabhi Jois's sexually abusive behavior—to be glossed over or go unchecked for years.

***

While older or more visible Jois devotees bargained with the tragedy—and perhaps struggled to separate community accountability from brand protection—a parallel stream of younger Ashtanga teachers were already risking a different message.

On December 18, 2017, the same day as Hendry's statement was posted, Greg Nardi published a lucid reflection on the community's crisis.[301] It was the first highly visible statement from an Ashtanga-authorized teacher to name Karen Rain. Nardi co-owns an Ashtanga Yoga Shala in Fort Lauderdale with his husband, Juan Carlos.

Nardi, who practiced with Jois from 1999 to 2009, acknowledged the assaults and expressed confusion about his own blindness to them. "Many well-intentioned and good people were complicit in upholding a harmful power structure," he wrote.

> Any attempt to defend Pattabhi Jois invalidates the experience of the victims. At this time, it is incredibly important to stand with women who are speaking out to shift power structures that enable sexual assault. The silencing of victims is part of the power structure that we have all been indoctrinated into and when we participate in it, we are its unwitting agents. When we shift the focus away from the victims, this amounts to silencing.

***

"I feel ashamed to have been part of a community where this happened, and to have not been fully aware of it."

March 2018 saw the publication of the first clear and *actionable* statement of accountability from an authorized Ashtanga teacher.[302] Originally from

New Zealand, Sarai Harvey-Smith had studied the method with several London teachers for many years. She also made eight trips to Mysore to study with Sharath Rangaswamy, and a ninth to attend Jois's funeral in 2009.

Writing about the Jois abuse revelations, Harvey-Smith criticizes Sharath Rangaswamy for his silence, and calls for transparency, a "reparative message for all women who wish to practice", and "a more professional structure with official channels of feedback, complaints, communication, accountability."

> In the absence of Sharath Jois taking responsibility, perhaps ... we should boycott Mysore, and challenge the cult-like tradition of Guru worship and Mysore pilgrimage, and separate *yoga teaching as a profession* from spiritual seeking.

Harvey-Smith goes on to commit to five restorative actions, several of which directly address concerns raised by Karen Rain.

1. I have taken all pictures of Pattabhi Jois down from my studio altar, website and social media and will no longer use his image in relation to my teaching.

2. I have stopped using the term "Guruji" I will now refer to my one time teacher as Pattabhi Jois. Elevating someone to Guru status creates a culture of idealisation and unquestioning acquiescence and deference. This contributed to the power this man had and abused, as well as the culture of silence around it.

3. In my Mysore classes I have drastically reduced my use of physical adjustments. I now ask whether students want to be assisted by me before commencing. In my led classes I now limit my approach to corrections and verbal guidance only.

4. I will share the stories of the victims and those teachers in the community who have made statements, and direct anyone who enquires to their blogs and testimonies.

5. I apologise to the victims for being part of a culture that enabled

this to happen, having studied with Pattabhi Jois in Mysore annually from 2003 until his death in 2009. I am accountable by:

A. Not being aware of the extent of the abuse. I had heard jokes about historical finger up the bottom mula bandha adjustments, but nothing else or current – only one friend during a Mysore trip, saying she was uncomfortable with certain adjustments made by Pattabhi Jois day after day. When I questioned what she meant she said "it's just too intense"—now I still don't know what she meant by that, but I regret not thinking about it and the rumours in a serious way. I think this suggests a culture of covering up, and a wish to turn a blind eye towards something that if seen and challenged could threaten my position within a cult like community where there is the fear that speaking out against the Guru would mean being ousted from the community and possible loss of livelihood.

B. Venerating the teacher and therefore contributing to his position of power, where boundaries could be transgressed.

C. By encouraging my own students to go to Mysore.

D. By desiring the qualification and therefore being part of a culture that grants Authorization like an arbitrary anointment from the 'Guru', rather than an achievement of clear-cut goals and pedagogical achievements.

***

"During my last stay in Mysore in 1999," wrote Gregor Maehle in a post to his blog on May 17, 2018,

> I shared all of my doubts with a friend. I talked to her about the process of projection, about idealizing a person, about giving up one's power, hypnotizing oneself into beliefs and finally about taking self-responsibility. She said to me, "What you say sounds much too difficult and tiring. I just want to totally surrender to a

> person that fixes all my problems in return." I think [this] really sums up the crux of the matter nicely. I realized then that I was a member of a cult.[303]

Maehle had had prior experience with high-demand groups. German by birth, he began his travels to Pune, India, in the mid-1980s as a devotee of Bhagavan Rajneesh, later known as Osho. Craving a more disciplined physical practice, he began to split his days between the ashram and Iyengar's Institute, six kilometers away. He hid his participation in each group from the other.

Maehle met his partner Monica Gauci, now a Doctor of Chiropractic, in Mysore. Jois certified her to teach Ashtanga in 1996, and Maehle received his certificate the following year. By the early 2000s, they had both been removed from the official list of certified teachers. Undaunted, Maehle went on to become a popular writer and commentator in the Ashtanga world, and together with Gauci travels from their home close to Byron Bay, Australia, to teach internationally.

In her own post from the same day, Gauci lists the reasons she left the Jois community in 1999.[304] She couldn't accept the ableism that required students to advance through harrowingly challenging physical postures before receiving instruction in breathwork or meditation. She noted the absence of pedagogical training, and that authorization was doled out on the basis of little more than attendance and payment of fees. While the sexual assaults weren't apparent to her at the time, she did "witness and personally experience the dangerous adjustments given by K. Pattabhi and Sharath Jois at that time."

> I would cringe watching others being adjusted and avoiding doing certain postures when they were watching. To the loud "pop" of ligaments being torn Pattabhi Jois would comment "Mmmm, good. Opening." Mysore became known for My sore knee, My sore back, etc. This damage was not only done in the practice room in Mysore but is perpetuated by many teachers who have simply copied the same adjustments their teacher gave them.

Gauci writes that she often treats injured yoga practitioners in her clinic. Maehle echoed these same criticisms in a follow-up post. Together, their comments have further challenged a community shaken by controversy.

"There were no spiritual teachings or guidance," Gauci writes, remembering Mysore.

> In the eight months that I spent studying with Pattabhi Jois in Mysuru, I attended every "Conference" held. This time was spent discussing all sorts of things from rasam recipes (a South Indian soup) to the price of gold, but never spirituality. I never heard Pattabhi Jois say anything profound.

A week after her first post, Gauci published a follow up to address the victim blaming questions and assumptions thrown at Karen Rain —Why did she let it happen? Why did it take her so long to disclose? —through the lens of her own memory of being sexually assaulted by the late Iyengar teacher Martyn Jackson.[305] Gauci was 19 at the time. Jackson was in his mid-fifties, and made his living on the Australian workshop circuit. Disclosing took all that time, Gauci explains, because of the shame and guilt, and fear of DARVO-type responses.

Maehle's direct appeal to Karen Rain, enriched by his personal memory, modeled what Gauci would have needed from a colleague all those years before.

"I want to thank you for coming out with your story", Maehle writes, addressing Rain.

> I was trying through the night to remember how close your mat must have been to mine. The old shala held 12 mats and my spot was front row, left corner in the 4:30am time slot. Sharath's spot was front right and I think you practised next to him. This would have placed your mat about 3 metres maximum from mine. I am completely shocked that you had to go through all of this a few metres away from me and I was ignorant of it. I am deeply sorry.
>
> I am asking myself how I could not notice the extent to which these things were going on. I didn't initially. We all focused on our *drishti* and practiced as if the devil was breathing down our necks, literally. But I remember at some point I performed a twist, while KP Jois adjusted the girl next to me in drop backs. When I spun around I saw what looked to me like him grabbing her buttocks and rubbing himself against her while he stood between her legs and she was back arching. I was totally shocked. After

> practice I approached her, told her that I saw what happened and that I was happy to accompany and support her if she wanted to take it up with him. I remember to this day her clarity and steely determination in her eyes when she looked straight at me and said with a smile, 'Forget about it. That did not happen. You are making it up.'[306]

***

Also in May 2018, Jessica Blanchard posted an article entitled "Why We Need To Talk About The Sexual Abuse Committed By Pattabhi Jois" to the website of the yoga studio she runs in New Orleans.[307] An Ashtanga practitioner for 18 years and authorized by Jois in 2006, Blanchard asserted that Jois's actions were "abusive on several levels".

Following the lead of Sarai Harvey-Smith, Blanchard used her post to commit to removing all photos from her studios—not only of Jois, but of all teachers. She committed to offering consent cards that will allow students to indicate whether they would like to receive physical assists. Her teachers would "look beyond the physical manifestation of yoga postures." She would "encourage ongoing dialogue between teachers and students."

"We continue to listen to the women who were abused by Jois," writes Blanchard under the heading "What's Next?"

"We continue to practice all the limbs of yoga. We continue to heal."

***

As this book goes to press, a small collective of next-generation Ashtanga teachers has banded together under the name "Amayu", a Sanskritic term for "boundlessness" that they say implies "together we are a global family/lineage." Greg Nardi and Scott Johnson are the co-founders, and have attracted a number of partners from across the United States and Europe.

Their mission statement opens with the promise of providing "excellence in Ashtanga yoga training, mentoring and development driven by consent and student empowerment." The statement goes on to highlight the value of universal accessibility, of mitigating power imbalances between teachers and students, and of platforming the "disadvantaged, disenfranchised, and disempowered." They hope that Ashtanga yoga can become "a global force for social change."

By email, Johnson noted that Amayu is currently drafting a Scope of Practice, a Code of Conduct, and an accountability protocol for its teachers.

When asked if the expectation was to displace the KPJAYI as the center of the Ashtanga world, Johnson was modest, and diplomatic.

> There are currently many teachers and schools offering Ashtanga teacher training across the world. From our perspective becoming part of Amayu does not preclude teachers, studios and students also being part of other schools, training programs or yoga communities. We feel Amayu will be adding value to the process of people becoming highly skilled Ashtanga yoga practitioners and teachers.[308]

PART SIX

Better Practices and Safer Spaces: Conclusion and Workbook

There's a deeply troubling pattern of sexual misconduct within our community, a pattern that touches almost every tradition in modern yoga.

Every human being deserves to practice yoga free from abuse, harassment and manipulation.

In honor of those who have spoken up, and in honor of those who have been too hurt to speak, we have to start somewhere, and we have to start now.

—Shannon Roche, Chief Operating Officer, Yoga Alliance, January 5, 2018[309]

But what is at stake here is that we show how much we care about the victims. That's at stake. And if you look back from history at this moment, the question won't be: "Has Ashtanga yoga been discredited, etc., etc." What is at stake is our humanity. Did we live up to the challenge? Getting off our high horses as yogis and actually helping those people who basically have been bucked off to that extent that, you know, they got abused.

So we need to support the victims. We need to support the victims. This is not about being right and wrong, this is about doing the right thing by them, doing the right thing that they are acknowledged. And I've stood up before in writing, you know, I will do that again: "I apologize for what I have done there. It happened under my nose, under my watch. Karen Rain was basically more or less next to me. I've seen those things. I didn't act as I should, I'm sorry about that. You know, there is no making it better. There's no excuse. There is no justification. I should've acted better."

—Gregor Maehle, interview[310]

It was left to us to put ourselves back together again in such a way that the cracks would surely show.

— Interview with filmmaker Mike Hoolboom, remembering his studies with the late Michael Stone

TOWARDS "NETWORKS OF EMPOWERMENT"

In 2018, Professors Peggy Cunningham and Bill Foster at Dalhousie University's Faculty of Management teamed up with Professor Minette Drumwright, who teaches Advertising and Public Relations at the University of Texas, to work on a multi-year research project called "Networks of Complicity and Empowerment".[311] They are studying more than a dozen instances of organizational and institutional abuse in business, academia, media, the military, and the entertainment sectors. These abuses, they hypothesize, emerge not only from the unethical or criminal behavior of leaders, but also from what they call "networks of complicity" that enable those behaviors.

One thing they want to understand is how some victims are able to breach these networks by speaking out, naming what is happening to them, and gathering allies who help them petition for justice and reform. How do they form "networks of empowerment"? What conditions and supports coalesce for them, but not for other victims? These fascinating questions provide an inspiring framework for the conclusions of this book.

While the project's data is not yet fully collated and analyzed, Professor Cunningham has been able to offer a few reflections via email. Preliminary findings suggest that the victim-ally network of empowerment forms bonds that are in some sense symmetrical with the abuser-enabler network of complicity. Empowered victims can themselves become movement leaders to whom allies—who may find common cause with the victims through a shared trauma—show deep loyalty and contribute moral, therapeutic, journalistic, legal, or financial resources. Allies will help to create effective communications campaigns, and offer resources and advice from beyond the bounded reality of the group.

The origin story of this book exemplifies this process. My initial resistance to Diane Bruni's story was eventually overcome not only through positive shame, but also because we both had a history of participating in abusive spiritual groups. Across age, gender, and experiences, we shared a common cause. Then, reaching out to Anneke Lucas after reading her blog seemed to electrify a hidden network of connections waiting to glow. Contacts multiplied. People who would become interviewees for this work and other articles started talking to each other. Social media accelerated everything. Connections between members of yoga and Buddhist groups dealing with abuse histories were forged through Facebook groups. An emergent ally network shared resources and emotional support. People who knew lawyers asked for and got pro bono advice on the liabilities of publishing about their experience.

By the time Karen Rain had disclosed, Anneke Lucas had reissued her 2010 blog piece, and Jubilee Cooke had published her Mysore story, there was still a network of complicity there to resist them, but there was also a network of encouragement and empowerment, ready to amplify their voices. My editor at *The Walrus*, Lauren McKeon, a prominent feminist cultural critic who's written powerfully about her own experience of sexual violence, accepted the pitch of the story only minutes after I sent it. One network of empowerment began to intersect with another.

Overall, the process has been characterized by a kind of breathless speed. Though often guarded to begin, and at times anxious, there was something instantly receptive and expansive about the communications. Trauma happens quickly, is profoundly isolating, and healing takes such a long time if it happens at all. But in some cases, it seems like the social bonds that help with that healing can form instantly through a shared knowing that can no longer be restrained.

The values expressed in an empowerment network directly oppose those in the abuse-enabling network, because the goal of victims and their allies is to deconstruct and redistribute power, rather than to capture and hoard it. Where secrecy silenced harm, there will now be transparent speech. Where deception confounded critical thinking, there will now be evidence and research. Where power had crystallized vertically, there will now be a horizontal sharing of space and dignity.

The symmetry is elegant, and palpable. Over the course of researching and writing this book, the concentrations of power in the Ashtanga yoga world have visibly shifted. The posthumous influence of Pattabhi Jois over the community's discourse has slowly but steadily been pushed to the margins, as the voices of his victims and their allies have been pulled towards the center. If somehow the totality of that discourse was accessible to comprehensive real-time analysis, it might reveal a strange tipping point—the moment when more people in the Ashtanga world are talking about what people like Karen Rain thinks and needs than they are talking about what Pattabhi Jois taught them.

The symmetry also epitomizes what might be the mantra for this book: *Harm is not inflicted in a vacuum, and healing is not accomplished alone.*

When it is complete, the data compiled by Cunningham and her colleagues might help yoga and other spirituality community members and leaders to better understand how and why a network of empowerment was able to constellate around women like Karen Rain and Anneke Lucas, or at Kripalu after the crisis over Amrit Desai's abuses, or in relation to the Satyananda yoga organization. (This last case was exposed and addressed through governmental intervention.) It may also help us to understand why such networks have *not* emerged in numerous other communities known to harbor abuse histories. But whatever the specific answers are—assuming they're out there—the general contours of collective resistance to and resilience in relation to abuse will involve an intersection of personal and structural strengths and skills that may never be enforceable or guaranteed to work, but can certainly be learned and researched further.

It's to these strengths and skills we'll now turn, distilling the voices and analysis of this book. First we'll look at personal better practices for resistance and resilience, including enhancing critical thinking and psychological awareness in relation to palpable group dynamics. While these will be useful for every reader, they won't be enough on their own, given the mantra of this book. Structural supports for safer practice spaces are also necessary for systemic change to take root. These are presented with teachers, trainers, and organizational leaders in mind. The discussion will explore the powers and limitations of codes of conduct in industries like yoga, which have historically resisted regulation in the US-dominated market. The value of achieving a culturally accepted scope of practice for yoga teaching will also be explored.

The **PRISM** model (p. 267) forms a bridge between personal and structural tools. It is, essentially, a process for transforming personal listening and research into the basis for community action. It asks us to listen on two mutually supporting levels. The private story is rarely speaking explicitly to structural issues, while the structural narrative can never fully grasp the mystery of the private.

Each section of this conclusion ends with workbook-style essay questions that students, teachers, trainers, and administrators can use individually and in groups to reflect on the themes, and ways they might apply to their own lives and communities. *These questions are not diagnostic or therapeutic, but exploratory and educational.* They are offered to summarize and activate the findings of this particular case study. They are informed by my personal experience with recovery from high-demand groups, as well as years of speaking with other survivors. If they bring up points of personal concern, it may be appropriate to seek qualified therapeutic or in some cases legal help.

BETTER PRACTICES: PERSONAL SKILLS

While most cult analysis literature emphasizes that individuals can do little to defend themselves in the vulnerable moments before, during, and after they are deceived by and recruited into a high-demand group, it also uniformly suggests that education about how high-demand groups work is key to weakening their power and reach. Education is emphasized over policy or legal initiatives. This is because the bounded reality of the group, which may support criminal activity and its concealment, is not in itself illegal.

If we want to take the matter of toxic group dynamics seriously—researchers estimate that there are 5000 high-demand groups in the United States alone, engaging between 10 and 20 million people—it is perhaps best faced as a public health issue.[312] Anti-smoking campaigns, for example, which focus on health literacy and better personal choices, have helped lower smoking rates by as much as 50% in Canada.[313] What would public education about high-demand groups look like? What would it ask people to consider?

I believe the following eight areas should be at the top of the list:

1. Assessing situational vulnerability.
2. Feeling and understanding transference and idealization.
3. Feeling and understanding disorganized attachment sensations.
4. Assessing the value and effects of trance states.
5. Listening for loaded language.
6. Assessing the honesty and transparency of the group or its leader.
7. Rejecting the "Bad Apple" argument: thinking structurally instead of individually.
8. Rejecting "I've-Got-Mine-ism".

1. ASSESSING SITUATIONAL VULNERABILITY

While many people live with the chronic effects of trauma, illness, or marginalization, everyone goes through periods of situational vulnerability. A death in the family, estrangement or divorce, an illness, a depressive period, an accident, losing a job, not being able to find a job, losing a strong home base—these are regular life events. They are also isolating junctures at which researchers suggest vulnerability to the promises and attachments offered by a high-demand group is heightened.

It's good to clarify that these are also the points at which many people turn to yoga, Buddhist, and other spiritual communities for answers and support, and have generally beneficial experiences. Many Ashtanga practitioners were drawn to their local shala while navigating situational vulnerability and didn't wind up on a "transmission belt" towards the hotspots of indoctrination we've explored. Then there are those like T.M., for whom "thin social ties" increased her vulnerability to group pressures.

Keeping all this in mind, you can use the following questions to reflect on the relationship between your own "low points" and the groups you've found yourself close to or in. Perhaps you will learn a little more about how those groups either served or exploited your vulnerability.

You can also use these questions to reflect on what you know about the circumstances of a family member or friend you know well. Though speculative, reflecting on what you've observed in others might shed light on your own story.

QUESTIONS FOR REFLECTION: SITUATIONAL VULNERABILITY

1.1 Consider a point (or several) of situational vulnerability in your personal history. Did you find yourself strongly attracted to an authority figure or group?

1.2 Did the authority figure or group help you to find your own power and resources to navigate situational vulnerability?

1.3 Did the authority figure or group offer solutions contingent on spending time with the leader, in the group, or in performing activities on behalf of the group or the group's ideals?

1.4 Did the "completeness" of the answers offered by the authority figure or group seem to contrast favorably with your own "incompleteness" at the time?

1.5 If the group made increasing demands upon your time, attention, and loyalty, did this mend the feeling of vulnerability, or replace it with a feeling of dependence?

1.6 Have you had a truly *empowering* experience of becoming involved with a group during a period of situational vulnerability? What elements do you believe were involved in making it work?

2. FEELING AND UNDERSTANDING TRANSFERENCE AND IDEALIZATION

This book has only glanced at the psychological notion of "transference", mainly in relation to how some of Jois's disciples felt and saw him as a father figure. Strictly speaking, however, transference is *unconscious*. Disciples who literally call Jois a "father figure" show that they understand at least some, if not all of what that relationship meant to them.

Transference in its fullest sense is said to be at play when any powerful influence from a person's past is unconsciously impacting the way in which they are relating to a person in the present. Often the transference—which *transfers* the meanings and dynamics of a past relationship onto a current one—flows towards a person of authority.

In the world of psychotherapy, transference is not understood as either a positive or negative phenomenon in itself, but rather something that simply happens between people as they negotiate present relationships through the lens of their relational history. In fact, the therapeutic process can make healing use of it. Accordingly, psychotherapy training pays a lot of attention to helping the therapist learn how to detect the transference of the client—onto them, especially—so that it can gradually be recognized and brought to consciousness, and its tensions worked through.

Therapists are also trained to recognize the same phenomenon when it flows the other way. Through "counter-transference", they may begin to unconsciously treat the client not as a separate person in the present moment, but through the lens of past relationships. When unrecognized, this tendency can obstruct the therapeutic process. If, for instance, the counter-transference means the therapist is responding unconsciously to the client as someone who seems to have less power than them, they might wind up using the encounters as an opportunity to gratify their need to be seen as an authority.

If Pattabhi Jois had been trained in psychotherapy, he would have recognized that some of his students were transferring onto him, or more simply projecting idealized values upon him. That recognition would have been a cue for an *increase* of care, boundaries, and ethics. He also would have examined himself to see whether he was counter-transferring, or using students to gratify his own needs, and taken steps to manage this. He would have learned the basic ethics of therapeutic relationship. Obviously, this didn't happen.

The only field in which therapeutic relationship is a subject of serious study in the yoga world is in the emergent global discipline of Yoga Therapy. Organizations like the Interational Association of Yoga Therapists (IAYT) have made mighty efforts to establish consensus around things like the nature of evidence, scope of practice, codes of conduct, and informed consent.[314] IAYT and its member schools face the necessary and daunting task of bridging the aforementioned transcendent and therapeutic modes. To be clear, none of this is meant to suggest that South Asian *paramparas* or initiated learning relationships do not have their own understandings of and safeguards against things like transference and counter-transference.

The most important variety of transference to consider in relation to one's vulnerability to an abusive leader or high-demand group is the *idealizing* type, or "idealization". Unless people are forced, after all, they won't hang around a person or group they instinctively don't like. It's when you think you've found your ideal teacher or communal heaven that the red flags should go up.

That warm feeling of pleasure and connection that comes with the immediate engagement with the leader or group, promising good things to come, is compelling, and not necessarily a sign that you are heading towards a high-demand situation. It is merely worth paying attention to. Most ex-members of high-demand groups report an initial falling-in-love or honeymoon period. This might be provoked or intensified by the group itself if it engages in techniques like "love-bombing", by which the potential recruit is showered with attention and fondness that makes them feel loved at first, but then indebted.

An initial flush of idealization can be overpowering. You can't believe you've found the answer you've always been looking for, or that the leader who will care for you in ways you've been deprived of is miraculously paying you attention. You may feel high, sublimely energized, perhaps to the point of hyperactivity or insomnia. You may feel released from all tension and concern. It can be an addictive feeling, and the group will be set up in certain ways to keep you well-supplied. Your friends and family may notice changes in your daily habits, facial expressions, bodily posture, and language. If you've emerged from a depressive episode, they might feel relieved along with you that you've found something that finally feels good. But eventually, they'll start looking at you sideways, and wondering what exactly is going on. They'll recognize that whole parts of you have gone offline. These would be the same parts that might buffer you from total commitment to the group.

The idealization of Jois as a spiritual teacher and healer was part of a machine that led women to Mysore, where he assaulted some of them. From his side, it seems, idealization is about the last thing he needed. He needed to understand his boundaries and act within them. Failing that, his freedom to teach should have been rescinded. In addition, as with any assaulter, there should have been police intervention, jail time, sexual assault education, and perhaps other social services. Yoga wasn't enough.

When you enter the sphere of someone you or others assume has a special glow and who is meeting unmet needs, and you feel a surge of love and longing rise up, let it ring an alarm bell. What will you do to keep that feeling alive? What will you give away? What does that feeling exclude or cover over? The following study questions can help mine some of these potential danger zones.

As you answer them, keep in mind, that an idealizing transference is not a mistake or sign of immaturity. It's not a *causative* factor in recruitment into a high-demand group or victimization. *Women idealizing Jois did not make him assault them.* What we can say is that:

- The idealization of Jois by the group gave him more access to women, and then later,
- Inhibited some of those he assaulted from resisting and speaking out.

Again, these are questions you can consider in relation to your own experience, or use to privately contemplate stories you've heard from people you are close to.

Finally, I highly recommend reading Donna Farhi's *Teaching Yoga: Exploring the Teacher–Student Relationship.*[315] This groundbreaking resource examines in detail the many types of projection, transference, and idealization that crop up in yoga learning environments.

QUESTIONS FOR REFLECTION: IDEALIZATION

2.1 Have you ever felt a compelling charge or sense of enthrallment in relation to an authority figure or group you've just encountered and know little about? How did that feeling influence your behavior?

2.2 Can you remember a period of time when the compelling figure or group seemed to be all-good? What did it feel like when a more complex picture emerged?

2.3 How did you begin to articulate that more complex picture? Who were you allowed to share it with?

2.4 When engaging with a compelling figure or group, did you ever have a sense of repetition or familiarity? What do you think it reminded you of?

2.5 [For teachers and trainers:] Have you felt students or trainees idealize you? Is it gratifying? What does it gratify? What do you do when this happens?

[Note: Contemplating these questions will *not* provide the tools needed to understand and manage any counter-transference responsibly. But it can provide insight into whether it happens often in your work. If this is the case, it might be appropriate to study the subject formally and under supervision.]

3. FEELING AND UNDERSTANDING DISORGANIZED ATTACHMENT SENSATIONS

As we saw in **Part Four**, the paradox of wanting to both *approach* and *withdraw* from a person or group you *explicitly* associate with care, but *implicitly* associate with harm, can feel electrifying, on-edge, pressured, or paralyzing. The sensations are at high pitch, conveying a continual conflict of hope and trepidation. It can feel claustrophobic or "airless" (to use Alexandra Stein's term), in the sense that it seems like there is nowhere to go, no space to maneuver, and that you're running out of time. The constant pitch of high arousal intimates that something important is happening, or about to happen. Uncertainty is the key note. The resulting panic can be strangely magnetizing, or even addictive.

If you are being harmed by the person or group, but can't articulate that harm to yourself or others because the harm has been conflated with care, and this magnetic quality keeps you close for repeated and intensifying encounters, you may be feeling the chains of a trauma bond. At unpredictable points of exhaustion, these chains might seem to dissolve entirely, leaving you with a sense of profound relief. This can reinforce the sense that the caregiver really is taking care of you. This, in turn, can rekindle the approaching behavior. It can feel like a vicious cycle.

The above paragraph is an attempt to describe some of the sensations of disorganized attachment behavior at its most acute, as well as the periodic "relief" that comes from dissociating from intolerable pressure. If you are currently experiencing these sensations in relation to a group, it might be appropriate to seek out therapeutic help or counseling from outside of the group.

Therapy might be helpful in learning to pre-emptively identify when you are close to disorganized sensations or spaces. It's one thing to study yoga (or any spiritual practice) from books, and another to feel it work in practice. Attachment theory is no different. If you're keen to learn more about how it works in general and has informed your relationships thus far, and whether it has anything to tell you about the dynamics of a group you're currently in, you might benefit from seeing a psychotherapist who is well-versed in attachment theory. Some therapists do educational counseling, which would allow you to learn more about the ideas in the context of your particular circumstance.

Deeper levels of therapy over longer time periods use the therapeutic relationship itself as a touchstone for exploring attachment styles. The idea is that if relationship tensions are at the heart of our strife, they will be at be at the heart of our integration.

The good news is that you don't have to become a whistleblower or expert in high-demand group functions to figure this all out and make a difference for those around you. You may just need to experience, if you haven't already, what it feels like to be secure in a relationship. Once you feel that, and know something of what it takes to offer that to others, you may not want anything else.

The following questions, while not diagnostic, can help illuminate acute symptoms of toxic or disorganized attachment, but also milder sensations worth noticing and contemplating. Disorganized attachment behavior doesn't have to start at peak levels, and you don't have to be fully expressing it in order to participate in and support an environment that harms others with its full impact.

QUESTIONS FOR REFLECTION: DISORGANIZED ATTACHMENT SENSATIONS

3.1 Have you ever experienced a confusing, "double" feeling in relation to a teacher, group leader, or group? This might feel like both *wanting* and *not wanting* some kind of attention or contact at the same time. How did you handle that feeling? Did you do anything that surprised you in response to it?

3.2 Have you had a similar double feeling towards a practice space? This might feel like a moment of high arousal when on the threshold of the room in which you seem frozen between entering and leaving.

3.3 Did the leader or group have explicit instructions deployed to help you navigate double feelings, override doubts, and continue on with the group activities and commitments?

3.4 Have you been in group environments that seemed to run at a continual high pitch of excitement and pressure? If so, did you notice that at times this intensity seemed to stop and leave you floating and thought-free? Did you associate those moments with progress?

3.5 Have you been in group environments in which members speak about the leader or leadership in contradictory terms meant to convey intense value? For example, "He is wrathful, but loving," or "When he acts like [euphemism for abuse], he's trying to tear down everything within you that is not love."

3.6 Do you remember a moment in which the actions of a group leader or group harmed you in some way, but you felt yourself accepting that harm as if it were care?

4. ASSESSING THE VALUE AND EFFECTS OF TRANCE STATES

A certain portion of many spiritual cultures is dedicated to the pursuit of altered states of consciousness. Through disciplined prayer, meditation, and trance techniques, practitioners reach for tastes of ultimate or transcendent reality, often thought to be above, beyond, beneath, or within the "disguise" of the conventional world of things, thoughts, and worries. Yoga practitioners of various eras have used meditation, chanting, breathing, and posture work to refine or alter their experience of the "normal" world, and break free of it. When they do break free, they often describe their experiences in other-worldly terms: *luminous, expansive, empty, silent, motionless, timeless.*

These peak experiences are intrinsic to many practitioners' sense of dedication. They can provide feelings of emotional renewal and renovate self-perception. But these same sensations, especially when provoked by contact with a high-demand leader or group, can (but not necessarily) have a hidden edge. Not only might they wear down resistance to undue influence; they can also overlap with responses like dissociation that act as safety valves against intolerable stress or pain. As noted in **Part Four**,

> How these sensations might emerge in relation to abuse in a yoga or spiritual setting are crucial to understand, because each and every one of them can be reframed by the priest, teacher, or even the indoctrinated person themselves as a sign of spiritual attainment. The person's thoughts have stopped, and they may have

> disidentified from their body and emotions. This can feel euphoric. According to a manipulative reading of several yoga philosophies, it could be said that they've attained a kind of liberation.

How do we tell the difference between the sensations of peace or true resolution and the sensations of dissociation, especially when it's unclear whether they have emerged through personal effort or interpersonal stress? It is a difficult question. One possibility, inspired by the work of Stein, might be to see whether the trance states facilitated by group experiences increase or decrease the sense of isolation she describes as central to the cultic dynamic. Put simply: do the high points of practice actually enhance your sense of secure relationship and interdependence, as often promised? Or do they leave you feeling alone and uncertain?

Also worth noting here is the prevalence of dissociative sensations *after* one disengages with a high-demand group.

> Former members of groups that use a lot of chanting, speaking in tongues, intense group criticism, hypnotic and guided-imagery sessions, and meditation or other trance techniques frequently experience floating episodes. Floating occurs because the mind has been trained and conditioned to dissociate during those practices, and so under certain conditions, a person so trained may involuntarily slip into a dissociated state.[316]

If this is resonant for you, it might cast new light on previous group experiences.

Recognizing the negative trance state is one thing. Truly assessing and recovering from its impacts are another, especially if it has been experienced in conjunction with a decline in personal agency, a loss or abandonment of familiar activities, and tangled up in "loaded language", covered in the next section. A personal anecdote here can illustrate this point.

I was a lifelong writer before entering high-demand groups in my late twenties. I was bookish, introverted, and didn't come from a therapy culture. Writing for me was compulsive—it still is, which brings its own problems—but the dialogue it provided was also a touchstone for self-regulation. I wrote to focus upon, understand, manage, rage at, and sometimes even forgive both myself and the world. Writing was not just an activity I did, but a place I went to, where I was safe and independent. Where I could afford to feel my own feelings, and to express love.

Both high-demand groups that recruited me featured lengthy, intense daily practice rituals with singing, chanting, thought-suppressing meditations, and relentless self-questioning. I stopped writing for six years. This is unimaginable to me today, and one of the greatest indicators for me now of how unduly influenced I was. I rationalized it at the time: my interest in writing had simply evaporated, I thought. What would I write about, now that trance or altered states of consciousness had shown me the "truth" about myself? *I found my own thoughts—whether they were about the banalities of breakfast, or doubts about what I was doing with my life—uninteresting to me.*

The practices I was given moved into my body and asserted themselves as more important than my familiar internal life. There were some benefits to this, but the process also muted the singular voice that carried my history, meaning, and uniqueness. Many cult researchers describe this in terms of "doubling": that as the group member takes on required ideology and behaviors, they develop a second, group-related identity. Their pre-cult identity recedes into the backdrop, living on in painful silence.

Hassan expands on this:

> One can almost observe the process in some young people who undergo a dramatic change in their prior identity, whatever it was, to an intense embrace of a cult's belief system and group structure. I consider this a form of doubling: a second self is formed that lives side by side with the prior self, somewhat autonomously from it. Obviously there must be some connecting element to integrate oneself with the other—otherwise, the overall person could not function; but the autonomy of each is impressive. When the milieu control is lifted by removing, by whatever means, the recruit from the totalistic environment, something of the earlier self reasserts itself. This leave-taking may occur voluntarily or through force (or simply, as in one court case, by the cult member moving across to the other side of the table, away from other members). The two selves can exist simultaneously and confusedly for a considerable time, and it may be that the transition periods are the most intense and psychologically painful, as well as the most potentially harmful.[317]

I also developed definite cognitive and attentional problems as a side effect of dedicated practice. When I sat down to write, I felt empty and blank, as though the inner voice I'd known since childhood had gone into hiding. The repetitious nature of the practices had rewired something to make the voice unavailable. Moreover, the *content* of the practices effectively shamed that inner voice, if it were ever to emerge. If I did have a strong internal thought that began to rise up, my reflex was to question, discredit, or otherwise disarm it. In the Buddhist group, this was actually spiritualized. Higher awareness, it was claimed, would be attained by distancing oneself from thoughts tainted by "me" and "mine", which we were taught were cognitive errors. That group went further by weaponizing private writing against us. The leader prescribed journal-writing six times per day, but not to strengthen the internal voice. We were meant to journal all of our micro-infractions of the various vows we had sworn to keep.

The double bind was hard to see. "Me" and "mine" were illegal concepts if they expressed agency, but then actively used to identify with and take ownership over transgressions. The "I" that wanted food or recognition or to express anger was an illusion, whereas the "I" that broke a vow against letting a Buddhist scripture touch the floor, for example, was very real, and had to make amends.

When I left high-demand groups, it took more than a year to be able to write again, to feel centered, curious, and unashamed. I'd sit down and be torn between needing to write something, anything, and the reflex to completely blank out. I had to start from the beginning, slowly, with pen and paper. I couldn't deal with screens. Connecting thoughts over the span of a paragraph seemed almost impossible.

Somehow I stumbled upon a trick. If I wrote in cursive (joined-up) writing and didn't let my pen leave the page, not breaking between words or even pages, the continuity of my internal voice seemed to strengthen. I also committed to not making any corrections at all. This helped too. The unbroken line of my internal voice, unapologetic and uncorrected, tied together hundreds of pages of a journal that felt as continuous as a body.

It's also significant, I believe, that my post-cult practice has been to write mainly in the early morning. This would be during the same time that I'd spent six years meditating and "emptying" myself out.

Lalich and Tobias write that difficulty in concentrating is common for ex-group members.

Many former members report that immediately after leaving their group, they were unable to read more than a page or two of a book in one sitting, incapable of reading a newspaper straight through, or forgot things a minute after reading or hearing them. This is due in part to the loss of critical thinking abilities caused by the cult's thought-reform program and controlled environment, and in part to the loss of familiarity with their native language. Although it can be overwhelming at times, this inability to concentrate is generally temporary.[318]

The following questions can help you to explore whether the intense rituals or peak experiences of yoga or spiritual practice in relation to a leader or group feel developmentally healthy or not. Are they temporary respites from tensions the leader or group are escalating or even creating? Do they enhance or degrade your capacity for concentration? If applicable, these questions can also help to assess whether trance or other altered states you have experienced in relation to a leader or group have increased or decreased your sense of empowerment and agency, and the strength of your internal voice.

QUESTIONS FOR REFLECTION: VALUE AND EFFECTS OF TRANCE STATES

4.1 If you have had peak experiences in relation to a leader or group, how do you believe they were triggered? Were they preceded by periods of stress or periods of openness and calm?

4.2 Have you ever found yourself wanting to repeat peak experiences in relation to a leader or group?

4.3 Does the trance or altered state leave you feeling more or less connected with your co-workers, friends, or family?

4.4 Does the trance or altered state leave you feeling more or less cognitively active and critically aware, especially in relation to the leader or group that facilitated it?

4.5 Have you ever had trouble focusing, thinking, reading, writing, or speaking after being in an intense group ritual environment? Were you encouraged to view these effects as signs of progress?

4.6 Were you ever associated with a group that engaged in intense rituals or practices that in hindsight you realize altered some fundamental sense of internal stability?

4.7 Were you ever associated with a group that diminished or negated your relationship to an activity or skill that was, up until that point, very meaningful for you? This might include writing, reading, drawing, dance, music...

5. LISTENING FOR LOADED LANGUAGE

In **Part Three,** we looked at ways in which the "loaded language" evident in parts of Ashtanga literature can deceive the public and group members, and foreclose discussion on complex topics. The very title of this book presents a key example of loaded language, albeit turned against itself.

It's worth quoting Robert Jay Lifton, who coined the term, more extensively:

> The language of the totalist environment is characterized by the thought-terminating cliché. The most far-reaching and complex of human problems are compressed into brief, highly reductive, definitive-sounding phrases, easily memorized and easily expressed.
>
> Totalist language then is repetitiously centered on all-encompassing jargon, prematurely abstract, highly categorical, relentlessly judging, and to anyone but its most devoted advocate, deadly dull.[319]

Lifton's guideposts of "repetitive" and "reductive" are apt. Loaded language sounds simple, and rolls off the tongue. But it also hides something. It points at information that seems so important, it must remain inaccessible, except through continued and deepened contact with the group. If you're not in the group that's using it, it might sound mysteriously attractive. But on closer inspection, it may also reveal itself as incoherent, undefined, and garbled. It is not designed to communicate information so much as to take up space and attention, and express the affect or performance of authority.

In its spoken form, the repetitious and vague quality of loaded language can contribute to group trance states. One good way of seeing whether this is happening is to use an inexpensive transcription robot like *temi.com* to record portions of talks or sermons by charismatic teachers or group leaders to see how they check out in written form. If the speech was delivered to a rapt audience but the transcribed text seems bland or littered with word-salad, this is a powerful clue. The speaker is not delivering information; they are performing power. They are not teaching, but casting a spell. The audience is there to feel the leader's presence in their act of speaking, but not necessarily to understand or care about what he's actually saying. This is different than rhetoric, which pairs content with powerful presentation.

A near-future technology may also be helpful for students wanting to investigate the words that are repeated so often and in so many contexts that they lose definition—a sign that a word is beginning to convey more power than meaning. If and when a platform like Google Books improves its search tools, a researcher might be able to create complete keyword indices and concordances for books like *Guruji*—or even better, a searchable collection of dozens of popular Ashtanga books—to find out which nouns and verbs have become central to the group's language. Looking at the top hits, the student might ask: "Is it clear from the literature what these words really mean?" If it's not, this may be a clue that the actual meaning of a given word for the group has been displaced by its capacity to deliver a sense of emotional gravity. If you were to transcribe such a word from the flow of a speech, you might feel like capitalizing it to capture that important-yet-vague quality.

Students and teachers of spiritual cultures rooted in languages they do not speak face a particular challenge here. Untranslatable terms from Sanskrit, Pali, Tibetan, or texts in other languages are often crucial for trying to understand the worldviews at play in practices like yoga and Buddhism. But because educated access to their actual meanings is often limited, these terms can easily be "loaded up" with group power and sentiment, and become central to a jargon that suppresses rather than enhances discussion. The way in which the Sanskrit term *parampara* has been used in some parts of Ashtanga culture is a rich example here.

Lalich and Tobias report that ex-members of high-demand groups can experience "extreme difficulty speaking so-called normal English" even it is their native language. "I spent time every day for the first few weeks out of the group relearning English," they report one ex-member saying, "until I had every cult word replaced with a known English word."

According to Lalich and Tobias, several seemingly simple activities can help with the re-languaging process.

"Television, magazines, crossword puzzles, and books of all kinds can re-acquaint you with language and help rebuild vocabulary," they write.

> Reading the newspaper and listening to the news are also highly recommended for retraining your mind, gaining vocabulary, and keeping up with world events. Another useful technique is to list all specific words and phrases to the cult, and then look them

up in the dictionary. Seeing the accepted definitions and usages can help reorient your thinking and reestablish your capacity for self-expression.[320]

The following questions will help to enrich critical listening and reading skills, and might point the way towards personal writing and other forms of language engagement as a way of reclaiming inner agency.

QUESTIONS FOR REFLECTION: LISTENING FOR LOADED LANGUAGE

5.1 Have you encountered an authority figure or group that seems to rely on key words and phrases repeated in its communications? Make a list of the terms you remember, and see if you can clearly define them.

5.2 Can you think of an interesting or charismatic teacher who has moved you emotionally with their speaking skill, but if you were asked to summarize or paraphrase their message, you'd be stumped?

5.3 What words in your community seem to carry great emotional weight? (The word "community" itself can carry a lot of freight and expectation.) How do you feel in your body when you hear them, or speak them?

5.4 Have you ever tried to ask a leader or fellow group member to clarify the meaning of a key term, and had your question deflected or ignored?

5.5 Have you ever found yourself shy to the point of not speaking when outside of a group that uses specialized language?

5.6 If you come across a lecture or speech by a leader that you suspect is packed with loaded language, try running a recording of it through *temi.com* or other automated transcription tool to see what it looks like in print. Is it as coherent as it sounds? If it sounds coherent but isn't upon reading it, what is the speaker doing (body language, posture, rhythm of speech, position in the room, pageantry, clothing) to convey the impression of authority?

5.7 Have you ever found it difficult to read or comprehend either mainstream media generally or media that conveyed new information about the group you were involved with?

6. ASSESSING THE HONESTY AND TRANSPARENCY OF THE GROUP OR ITS LEADER

Often, leaders and groups will make claims and offer information that a new member cannot possibly evaluate in detail. Or the new member may not want to evaluate the claims, if they temporarily seem to satisfy their desires and needs. The vast majority of travelers to Jois's Mysore shala, for example, had no tools to assess the integrity with which he and others were using Sanskrit terms and ideas from yoga philosophy. They would have had no way of knowing how unlikely it is that Jois's series of postures dated back many centuries.

A competent *performance* of knowledge might be all that is required to gain a member's implicit trust. Another anecdote may help.

In the first lecture I attended by the leader of the high-demand Buddhist group into which I was recruited, he apparently recited from memory several dozen verses from a medieval Tibetan philosophical treatise. I was enthralled by the chanting rhythm, the way in which he closed his eyes, the way the syllables seemed to tumble out of him. It never occurred to me that the leader's recitation could be garbled, his pronunciation might be terrible, or that—as became apparent later—he had a twisted and self-serving view of the subject matter. Within a few minutes, his credibility in my eyes was established.

He performed competence. He seemed to be doing what I wanted him to be able to do, something that signified value. For whatever reason, he presented what was for me at that time a seductive possibility: that someone like me, having grown up in suburban North America, could seemingly rewrite his entire internal landscape with the mysticism of an ancient culture. This is where, in my case, the reflex to idealize met an educational deficit.

I may have been more naïve than others in not asking some basic investigatory questions, but I'll note that the teacher attracted others who had actually studied enough Tibetan in college to get the sense that he really was accomplished. They seemed to trust him, and so I trusted them. We all came to trust the leader for different reasons, at different ratios of aspiration, need, and credulity. This all would have been harmless—except for the wasted time—had he not gone on to deceive and exploit people.

Magicians know that there's little defense against a good performance.

But there is at least one simply prophylactic against performances that deceive. Students of complex subjects like yoga and Buddhism, offered on the free market and outside of peer-review systems like academia, should always ask themselves three questions.

- Does the teacher seem to be fond of making strong claims about what an ancient philosophical system or text says?
- If they are, are they equally fond of citing sources that you can access on your own?
- Failing citations, is there anyone in the room who would be able to assess whether the teacher is bullshitting?*[321]

If you're not given citations and there isn't anyone around to provide quality control, it doesn't necessarily mean the teacher *is* bullshitting, but it does mean you don't know enough to be able to simply take their word on whatever they are telling you. They may be emotionally compelling, but they have not earned your intellectual trust. Recognizing that those are two different things might save a lot of trouble.

In the same vein, the analysis in this book shows that when you encounter writing that portrays a leader in an all-good light, such as *Guruji*, it may well be because important things have been left out.

It's hard to avoid being deceived, but *you can become aware of the contexts in which deception is more likely to occur or harder to detect.* These questions will help to sharpen your understanding of those contexts. They also begin to point to a structural aid proposed in the last section of this book: what it would mean for yoga teachers to commit to a *scope of practice*.

QUESTIONS FOR REFLECTION: HONESTY AND TRANSPARENCY OF THE GROUP OR ITS LEADER

6.1 Have you ever found yourself in a situation in which the proficiency that a leader or group shows in one area leads you to believe, without examination, that they are proficient in another?

6.2 When a teacher or group makes strong claims about human nature,

* "Bullshit" here is the technical term philosopher Harry Frankfurt uses to describe the speech acts of a person who doesn't care about the truth of something so much as he cares about persuading others.

why there are problems in the world, or any other highly complex problem, what forms of evidence do you expect them to provide?

6.3 If you come to believe that knowledge of Sanskrit, Pali, Tibetan, or any other language is important on your spiritual path, but you don't have time or access to study it yourself, how will you choose a translator or explicator you can trust?

6.4 If a teacher or group has published literature that makes strong statements that are not disclaimed as subjective opinions, what kind of review process did that literature go through?

6.5 [For teachers and trainers] Do you provide citations for every bit of data you teach? Do you make distinctions for your students between popular/aspirational literature and peer-reviewed scholarship?

7. REJECTING THE "BAD APPLE" ARGUMENT: THINKING STRUCTURALLY INSTEAD OF INDIVIDUALLY

As of November 2018, the English-speaking yoga world is responding to new allegations of sexual assault against senior certified Iyengar teacher Manouso Manos. The unfolding Manos story brings a common theme into sharp relief. As yoga communities grapple with abuse revelations, disciples and apologists tend to default to *individualistic* as opposed to *structural* analyses. On one side, they put blame on the victim for not having shown discernment, given boundaries, or speaking up. On the other side—if they are forced to discuss the abuse at all—they will describe it as the isolated and unfortunate damage caused by a single flawed teacher.

These are two sides of the "bad apple" argument. Naïve students and bad actors are said to be the core problem. If the former would only grow up and the latter were simply removed—so the theory goes—the structure can continue making apple pie. Recall the certified Ashtanga teacher writing that Jois's "actions have been largely accounted for and removed from the system of Ashtanga yoga,"[322] as if the "system" had not itself enabled those actions for decades.

If the bad apple theory is allowed to sacrifice victims and scapegoat individual abusers, the structural power dynamics of the community can avoid examination. This study section will help you to examine whether you use the bad apple argument in a way that unintentionally distracts you or others from the challenges of structural reform. A brief overview of the Manos situation, and one individual's paradoxical response to it against the backdrop of the Jois revelations, will provide helpful context.

In the spring of 2018, Iyengar teacher Ann West made a complaint against Manos to the Ethics Committee of the Iyengar Yoga National Association of the United States. West alleges that in 2015, Manos groomed her into somatic and emotional compliance with unwanted comments and attention over several years. Then, one day, she alleges that Manos caressed her breasts and nipples under the guise of adjusting her in a backbending posture.

A month before making the complaint to the Ethics Committee, West filed a report with the police in San Diego. The detective told her that since the caress happened over her clothes, the incident would be classified as a misdemeanor, and would at that point be outside of the two-year statute of limitations.

West's report to the committee echoes testimony from other Manos students published in 1991, private communications between members of the California Yoga Teacher's Association (CYTA) and its publishing arm *Yoga Journal*,[323] and an additional testimony from yoga teacher and author Charlotte Bell published in September 2018 of a similar assault by Manos in 1988.[324]

The committee dismissed West's complaint in September 2018, ignoring key aspects of her claim. They also cited a lack of eyewitnesses, despite West's description of the class as being "chaotic" and alleging that the assault occurred while everyone was upside down. West provided corroborating witnesses but this was not enough. The meeting notes also show that committee members first decided that West's allegation was unsupported, *then* reasoned that previous reports of Manos's misconduct were irrelevant.

"The past history," they wrote, "would have significantly impacted the nature of sanctions if there were a determination of an ethical violation beyond reasonable doubt in the present case."[325]

While the committee deliberated, Manos held a seat on the Senior Council of IYNAUS. At least one of the committee members was a long-term student of Manos, enrolled in his three-year Yoga Therapeutics course. The meeting notes cast additional doubt upon the committee's impartiality. Members questioned West's perceptions of the incident, but found Manos's explanation of his intentions "logical". Several mentioned that his "strong" or "offensive" teaching manner might "confuse" some students. One member, despairing of how "complex" the situation was, suggested the committee punt the file to the Iyengar family in Pune.[326]

The parallels to the Jois case are striking. Manos is a charismatic, world-traveling master-teacher said to have healing powers linked to a direct line of spiritual transmission. When accused of harm, all manner of excuses are deployed by him and in his defense: he's a family man; the victims "misinterpreted" the touching; the victims were sexually abused themselves and therefore confused; he had a problem but he stopped; American students are immature or have prurient imaginations; Manos touched men and women the same way; the Iyengar family should take care of it.

One Manos disciple went so far as to publicly post a long, DARVO-driven letter addressed to West, turning *Manos* into the victim of the allegation, and blaming *West* for jeopardizing the disciple's relationship to Manos, and therefore, she claimed, her very survival.

"I rely on Manouso for my life," the disciple wrote. "He is my most steadfast and worthy anchor in human form. He holds a powerful lineage of healing and he has served as an honest and clear conduit for that information for thousands of students." The disciple feared that Manos would no longer want to teach classes under a cloud of suspicion. "He may also decide the stress of teaching his American classes is more than he cares to handle."[327]

What is extraordinary about the Manos case is that, unlike with Pattabhi Jois, allegations about his sexual assault and misconduct were actually public knowledge, at least for a while. The fact-checked and legally vetted publication of the 1991 feature article had been a watershed moment in the American Iyengar community. Several prominent members of the Iyengar Institute of San Francisco, including the current world's expert in Restorative Yoga, Judith Hanson Lasater, resigned when Iyengar himself reinstated Manos after "pardoning" him. IYNAUS was formed in the following year, in part to increase accountability for Iyengar teachers.[328] Internationally renowned yoga teacher Donna Farhi was on the Board of Directors for *Yoga Journal* at the time and reports that the magazine voted to stop carrying advertisements for Manos's tour and workshops, along with other male yoga teachers who at the time were accused of sexual misconduct. And yet, despite all of this open coverage, Ann West, who started studying with Manos only a few years later, in the late 1990s, had heard nothing about it. Nor had many of her contemporaries. The community had effectively buried it.

When West's allegation disinterred that history, its parallels to the Jois revelations drew out a striking ramification of the bad apple theme. By scapegoating single abusers, bad apple-ism can also cling to the myth of perfect leaders.

In late September 2018, a male yoga practitioner posted a letter to the IYNAUS President to Facebook (not publicly available). He bore witness to multiple instances of watching Manos sexually assault women in yoga classes in the 1990s. The letter was significant because, as this book has shown, witness statements from men are hard to come by.

However, the letter was written by someone who that spring had spent a lot of time online defending Jois. When asked whether his views on Manos had coincided with a shift in perspective on Jois, he said they hadn't. He repeated all of the rationalizations for Jois's abuse from months and decades before. They were rationalizations he was willing to apply to Jois, but not to Manos. Paradoxically, the allegations against Manos seemed to provide further passion to his argument that Jois was stainless. *That guy is a criminal, but my guy would never do such things.*

The commitments of discipleship can be incredibly strong, and they operate in the sphere of individualistic logic. Psychologically, Manos might be scapegoated for behaviors a Jois disciple knows on some level Jois acted out as well. Most importantly, this capacity for splitting—Manos is a predator, while Jois is misunderstood—depends upon a near total absence of structural critique. It nurtures the opposite of the pattern-seeking thinking required for reform.

Making Jois into a perfect apple seems to reinforce the tendency to make someone else into the bad apple. But part of rape culture is the fact that men in leadership positions share a lot more than they differ. If you are arguing the bad apple theory in the face of an obvious structural pattern, you may also be suppressing other things.

To sum up, the bad apple argument does three things.

- It uses the same individualist logic that isolates and blames victims for the harm they suffer.
- It diverts attention away from the analysis of patterns and structures of power and harm.
- It furthers the potentially toxic glorification of the "good apple".

The following questions will help to focus on where you might unconsciously use elements of bad apple-ism, thereby missing opportunities for examining structural patterns and remedies.

QUESTIONS FOR REFLECTION: REJECTING THE "BAD APPLE" ARGUMENT: THINKING STRUCTURALLY INSTEAD OF INDIVIDUALLY

7.1 Can you think of an offender in yoga or spirituality community to whom you have applied the "bad apple" theory? As in thinking or saying: "If only he would just leave, everything would be fine."

7.2 If the bad apple was the leader of a community you weren't part of, did contemplating their actions contribute to a subtle assumption that your own community was too smart or ethical to suffer from the same harm?

7.3 Have you ever watched a community fire or excommunicate a long-term offender and then take no further steps at structural reform and harm prevention? (These might include adopting formal codes of conduct and accountability mechanisms.)

7.4 Is there any leader you think of as being a "perfect apple"? Do you know enough about them to say for sure?

7.5 Has the "perfect apple" feeling in relation to a leader ever given you a sense of security you later discovered was unwarranted?

8. REJECTING "I'VE-GOT-MINE-ISM"

"I've-Got-Mine-ism" (IGM) is a defensive strategy by which the member of a high-demand group who has not (or believes they have not) directly experienced abuse or institutional betrayal within the group deflects stories of abuse from within the group by immediately self-referring.

I've-Got-Miners will say things like: "I don't know about other's experience; I find/found the teacher/teachings/community to be profoundly helpful in my life." The statement is usually couched within an unwillingness to act on behalf on victims or mitigate future harm.[329] If the statement is transparent about the harm under discussion, it might engage in a form of "harm calculus" by which the benefits of the teacher/teachings/community are used to bargain down or dismiss the harm.

This book has recorded numerous statements in this vein by Jois disciples. The immediate effect of IGM is to change focus from the disclosure of harm to a promotion of good. This automatically begins to minimize, relativize, or even discredit the harm disclosure, as if a person's alleged activity is somehow balanced or cancelled out by the good experience some people have with him. It turns something obvious—that the same person can do both good and bad things—into a defense that can obstruct fully investigating the latter and the damage that's been caused.

When a leader in the yoga or other spirituality fields is accused of abuse, members of his or her group should think very carefully about the logic and ramifications of signing a character witness letter (or joining a social media campaign) that may then be used to discredit the accusers. You may have had a good experience with the person or group in question. Don't make that sour by asserting that that is equally or more important than the harm that person or group may have caused. If you had a good experience, you're in the position to use that privilege to help those who didn't. But you'll have to listen to them first.

There are two final aspects to consider. First, to what extent does the IGM response function to protect the disciple's own perception of the leader/group/community. If a disciple eases off on the IGM response, do they risk feeling like they must doubt their positive experience?

Secondly, when understood as a statement of privilege, IGM brings up the mystery of benefit attribution. How does one know for sure that the positive benefits one attributes to a leader, practice, or group are not rooted in other supports? What if the difference between the victim perspective and the IGM perspective is not only that the latter has not or does not believe they've suffered abuse, but that the latter had more supports to begin with? What if IGM is not only the expression of privilege within the particular group, but also of privilege *in general*?

The following questions will help identify and disarm the IGM impulse.

QUESTIONS FOR REFLECTION: REJECTING "I'VE GOT-MINE-ISM"

8.1 Can you think of an instance in which a report of harm associated with the group you were in provoked an immediately *defensive* response, in yourself or others? What did you do?

8.2 Can you think of an instance in which a report of harm associated with the group you were in provoked an immediately *apathetic* response, in yourself or others? What did you do?

8.3 Have you ever given an IGM response to someone who disclosed a story of harm about a group in which you were both members? Is it possible to reconnect with them, apologize, and—if they're open to it—ask them to share their story again?

8.4 When you think of the benefits you received from a given leader or group, are you able to confidently separate them out from other forms of privilege in your life? How are you sure, for example, that the emotional well-being you feel within a practice community is not supported or even made possible by secure attachments formed outside of it?

8.5 Have you ever found yourself engaging in "harm calculus", in which you try to balance the harm a group causes against its purported good? If so, why was this important for you to do? What might it dissuade you from doing?

THE PRISM MODEL

Personal best practices are good, but, like yoga and meditation, they cannot on their own lead to social justice. Sharpening your internal radar for situational vulnerability, idealization, the sensations of disorganized attachment, loaded language, bullshitting, bad apple-ism, and IGM can help you individually. But everyone in a high-demand group responds in different ways, and will have different levels of access to these skills. If you want to really help to create safer spaces for everyone, you'll also want to learn how toxic group dynamics and abuse affect people in ways you're not aware of. By listening carefully to victims, you can come to know more about systems in which you may be embedded. You can let them lead the discussion towards levels of justice and equality you've never pondered.

The **PRISM** model is a listening practice designed to bridge the gap between personal and collective approaches to harm reduction, and directly effect structural change. It is intended to foster transparency and care in spiritual communities. It is meant to help prevent retraumatization, to obviate the stress of disillusionment, and to help (yoga) teachers, trainers, and scholars avoid the psychological, institutional, and spiritual drag that accrues when abuse histories are hidden. Hopefully, it can also help to reduce the material and emotional labor of backtracking and mending necessitated when hidden histories explode.

Whatever yoga is—whatever a spiritual practice community is—we approach it like beams of light approach a prism. The cut glass, flashing, presents different angles and entry-points. When we enter in, our outwardly similar experiences are spliced into a spectrum from transcendent yellow to tranquil blue to blood-angry scarlet. There are unseen colors as well, experiences that have not been processed, or named.

Yoga teachers, scholars, and service providers who wish to "first do no harm" can no longer accept the uncritical, single-color narratives of modern yoga hagiography, evangelism, and marketing. If they do, they risk giving legitimacy to communities and leaders whose values, actions, and education will potentially not live up to their standards of care. Worse than that, they may unwittingly convey the impression of endorsing a group that has abused members. In some unfortunate cases, they may platform people who enabled or even participated in abuse. This can be hard to avoid, given how successful some organizations have been at hiding their abuse histories.

Elsewhere, I've covered two cases in which well-meaning yoga enthusiasts have legitimized yoga groups with abuse histories.[330] In the first, two feminist scholars lauded Eddie Stern for his work with his non-profit "Urban Yogis" program, which brings Ashtanga yoga to marginalized teens.

> Our engagement with the Urban Yogis program has inspired a confidence that a feminist-informed social justice orientation to community engagement emphasizing ethics of care, commitment, shared power, and mutual political vision is indeed possible.[331]

The scholars were unaware of the abuse history of Ashtanga yoga.

In the second case, trauma and addictions recovery specialist Gabor Maté works closely with a Canadian organization called Beyond Recovery, which offers a yoga-based training program "for individuals seeking to develop healthy habits and overcome addictive behavior, for health professionals and yoga teachers who work with addiction."

The yoga community providing content for the program is 3HO: the "Happy, Healthy, and Holy" organization founded by Yogi Bhajan in 1969. Recent scholarship has shown that Bhajan's postmodern "Kundalini" blend of Tantric yoga and Sikhism has few historical roots in any stream of Indian wisdom tradition, despite the community's lofty claims.[332]

PAUSE

Pause to reflect on the idea that each yoga or other spiritual method
and community carries both value, but also,
potentially, a history of abuse.
These can be disentangled.

The first step in the **PRISM** process is for the yoga enthusiast who is poised to become a yoga teacher, trainer, scholar, or advocate to **P**ause. In that pause, the teacher, trainer, scholar, or service provider can relax the understandable personal enthusiasm that is inspiring their desire to share yoga, and begin to ask: what exactly is this thing to me, and to other people?

So many people who wind up professionalizing in the yoga world (as with other spiritualities) started with a powerful moment of private transformation. They found something that seemed to change their lives in a profound way and in a very short period of time. Before long, they find themselves advocating for the practice they've found.

This understudied process has been a driving force in the steep global adoption curve of yoga. Practitioners have intensely transformative experiences. The available language for describing those experiences points to ideas of vastness, union, universality, love, and light. This in turn seems to encourage the practitioner to speak of the yoga they've found in broadly all-good terms. It's not a practice they stumbled upon that just happened to work for *them* uniquely in harmony with countless other factors. It is *the* way, and it is very good. The method spreads on the wings of enthusiasm.

We should be cautious when learning about love from honeymooners. There's no question that practitioners the world over have benefited from the basic practices and ideas of the yoga movement generally. But no yoga method is inherently safe for everyone, and no yoga community in the globalization period has created a uniformly safe space. This is no surprise, given that yoga communities are human communities. If we simply pause to allow for the fact that value and harm are tangled together in a knot of postures and breathing, we'll stop pretending that yoga communities are other-worldly.

Jules Mitchell, an exercise scientist who has done groundbreaking work in the science of stretching in relation to posture practice, told me about a great phrase she uses when teaching postures: "This may work for some of the people some of the time." Her circumspection expresses the value for a judicious pause that may lead to more realistic thinking.

QUESTIONS FOR REFLECTION: PAUSING

P.1 Are you familiar with the "honeymoon period" of involvement with a leader or group? What did it feel like?

P.2 Were you ever "love-bombed" in the initial period of joining a group? How long did that last?

P.3 Did you ever love-bomb someone during your own yoga honeymoon? Might that have been intrusive?

P.4 Is there a key moment you remember realizing that a particular practice or relationship that was effective or even life-changing for you may have had very different impacts on other people?

P.5 If you feel strongly inspired to share yoga, is there an element of this that's related to a need to validate your own experience? For example, might you think "If other people report similar benefits, I know I'm not fooling myself."

P.6 Can you think of spiritual marketing language that presents practices and groups of practitioners as universally helpful and all-good? Choose one such statement and rewrite it in more ambivalent language. Try using Mitchell's phrase.

RESEARCH

Research the literature on the method to find and understand that history.
It can educate everyone towards doing less harm.

The yoga worker will be better prepared for ethical service to the extent that they learn the specific ways in which a method or community has, in some instances, weaponized its spirituality against its members for the sake of accumulating power or money.

If a teacher, scholar, or service provider wants to engage the methods of the any yoga or spiritual community, they should prepare to **R**esearch the hidden literature on the method to find that history.

As this book shows, this can take a lot of work. The stories of harm are hidden, because abuse victims often ghost away, and the method's most prominent adherents do not want to remember them. It takes effort to discover hidden stories. And even more effort to really listen to them.

RESEARCH AS A LISTENING PRACTICE

Research is a listening practice, and listening is a real skill. People like Karen Rain teach us that trauma stories can rarely be remembered *and* told in a linear arc. The reason for this is that trauma disorganizes the continuity of the self. Details are broken, and their fragments are retrieved in an unpredictable order. Therapists have known this for a long time.

Imagine trying to pick up the pieces of a smashed mirror. You'll never be able to do it in the precise order or radius in which they scattered. You'll pick up what you can, according to the energy you have. You'll cut yourself in the process. It will take a long time, and what you put back together will never be complete.

The conventions of journalism and law often cooperate to enforce a general societal demand that cannot accommodate this reality of the trauma story. They ask the trauma survivor to present something like a news item or a legal writ, scrubbed of jagged emotions. The survivor is asked to present the mirror of their continuous self as though it had not been smashed.

This demand is so unreasonable, so tone-deaf, that the person trying to pick up those pieces can be easily discouraged, humiliated by the mess that somehow they must make whole again for it to be heard, let alone believed.

The common hope is that the trauma survivor is working this all out in therapy. But what's missed is that the way they are listened to in the public sphere may be playing a critical role in whether it can be worked out at all. The responses of listeners can have a direct impact on the accessibility of those memories. A denial or deflection from a listener can easily and shamefully reinforce the very repressions of denial and deflection that the speaker is trying to break through.

Everyone can be better listeners to trauma stories through this single practice: when the trauma story begins, don't interrupt. Not with questions, contexts, challenges, equivocations, or it-can't-be-that-bad-isms.

Try to imagine that you've started to watch someone picking up those shards. This may not look like a familiar action to you. This could be because you can't see the shards. You'd need professional training to come close to seeing them through the person's eyes. Without that training, the least you can do is stay out of their way and let them know you are listening. A further step might be to indicate you understand how much it costs them to speak at all. It may be hurting them to speak.

If all you can offer is a fraction of the time and space that was stolen away by the trauma, that's really something. It will help protect victims against the inevitable blowback enacted by a culture in crisis.

After Karen Rain disclosed Jois's assaults on her, she immediately encountered exactly what shed expected—a barrage of victim-blaming questions and defenses in hundreds of comment threads, many raging on Ashtanga group pages. Here's a partial list of the type of rationalizations and defenses thrown at her.

> *Jois didn't have an erection, so it wasn't about sex for him.*
>
> *I heard that Jois adjusted men and women in the same way. So it wasn't necessarily sexual.*
>
> *It wasn't so bad, because it was in public.*
>
> *You're saying "assault", but other people didn't feel it that way.*
>
> *It doesn't make sense that you kept coming back. Why didn't you resist or say something? You must have wanted that treatment on some level.*
>
> *But he was such a heart-exploding teacher for so many people. That must not be forgotten.*
>
> *He had a healing touch and hands.*
>
> *He had a problem, but he stopped when asked.*
>
> *He didn't know what he was doing.*
>
> *He was only human, not perfect. Everyone makes mistakes.*
>
> *He's not here to defend himself.*[333]

Given the stress and messiness of the listening process, yoga and other spiritual communities should take care to resist premature calls for unity or appeals to emotional compliance. These "showing" strategies come from mending instincts and require caregiving labor, which is disproportionately provided by women, who are also more likely to be victimized by institutional abuse. The strategies are also often distorted by a group's will to self-preservation, which can survive well into any period of reform.

Group members have to ask themselves: What's more important? Recovering the feeling of group unity (which might have been manufactured in the first place)? Or continuing to learn and grow by grappling with stories that don't fit the mold? Integrity teaches that the more we learn, the less we can assert that we share the same experiences or beliefs. If we assume we do, we continue to shut out the voices and stories that can help us grow. Listening to and absorbing the stories of Karen Rain, Tracy Hodgeman, T.M., and the rest is not an easy process. But it may lead to the capacity to recognize our interdependence—not through platitude alone, but by grappling with experiences that are not our own. This also teaches us about democracy, which is built on the friction of misunderstanding. If, like honest democrats, we expect to misunderstand each other or disagree, we become free to do so in good faith.

Finally, we learn that democracy does not guarantee equality. Our social positions are never equal in terms of power. The 16 voices in this book have been talked over and mansplained to by decades of bookwriting and lecturing. Listening to a victim of institutional abuse requires reversing the ratio of broadcast space typically given to each.

QUESTIONS FOR REFLECTION: RESEARCHING

R.1 Have you ever become involved with a yoga or spirituality group without researching their history? What did you later go on to learn?

R.2 Did you ever catch wind of a negative story about the leader or group you were involved in and simply didn't want to hear it? Do you know why?

R.3 Have you encountered instances of victim-blaming in a yoga or spirituality group?

R.4 Are there ways in which the teaching content of a yoga or spirituality group you've been involved with support victim-blaming? These might include the teachings on karma or the primacy of personal responsibility on a spiritual path.

INVESTIGATE

Investigate whether the harm has
been acknowledged and addressed.
If it has been silenced, it can also be given a voice.

It has taken three years to compile the testimonies on which this book is built. That alone is a powerful clue that some parts of the Ashtanga world—including those with administrative power in Mysore—may not have moved on to the acknowledgment stage. If they haven't, how exactly can the new practitioner or the service provider who wants to make use of a group's methods or materials be assured that they're receiving knowledge rather than propaganda?

If you wanted to investigate whether the harm of a group had been addressed, where would you start? You could start with your own teacher, or your local studio owner. Almost everyone who has professionalized in the yoga world has some connection at some point to a well-known method or community like Ashtanga. In many cases, that connection has evolved through generational change and rebranding. Jois's method, for example, has inspired Power Yoga, Rocket Yoga, Vinyasa Yoga, Vinyasa Flow, and several other offshoots. At this point, it is reasonable to expect a teacher of any one of these brands to know about the Jois issue.

You can ask:

> So I've heard this method is inspired by Pattabhi Jois. It's now widely known that he assaulted students under the guise of adjusting them. How has this impacted your own understanding of teacher–student dynamics and policy around touch in a yoga class?

In an unregulated industry, policies shift according to market demand. The simple act of asking questions like this may help catalyze the last two steps of the **PRISM** model: that teachers and service providers **Show** how they will honor the method they are using *without* passing along its trauma, and how they will **Model** transparent ethics for future generations.

Asking questions, however, may be uncomfortable, especially of elders one admires or has learned from, and who may have suppressed their own stories, disappointments, and wounds. On the bright side, such questions can also lean into the relationship in fruitful ways. They can reveal the depth of communication one has with that elder. They can show whether their understanding of yoga includes the ongoing practice of transparency.

One-to-one inquiry, however, might be as limited as any personal "better practice". We should also study, and where appropriate, support growing efforts in yoga and other spiritual communities attempting to acknowledge and rectify harm, and support third-party investigations. Current examples point to an array of possibilities and liabilities, such as that of Rigpa International[334] and Shambhala International,[335] both Buddhist communities.

Investigation is not easy. As the Manos case shows, even when it happens in a public manner, the results can disappear—although this may become less common in the internet age.[336] Exploring the personal and structural barriers to transparent investigation can only help make it easier.

QUESTIONS FOR REFLECTION: INVESTIGATION

- I.1 Have you ever asked a group leader or senior member a question about group history and had your question deflected?
- I.2 Are the financial records of the group in which you are or have been a member publicly available?
- I.3 If members or ex-members make ethics complaints against an organization, are they handled transparently?
- I.4 Have you ever seen a group attack a complainant?
- I.5 Under what conditions would a third-party investigation return a report with real integrity?
- I.6 What are some of the ways in which a yoga or spirituality group might address harm that has been discovered and substantiated?

SHOW

Show how you will embody the virtues
and not bypass the wounds of the community.
There is no bypass to healing.

Moving from personal to public integrity involves Showing how you will acknowledge and address a shadowy history. You can show how you will embody, for yourself and others, the virtues and not bypass the wounds of the method.

Showing, however, is not necessarily doing, as we see with the co-optation of trauma discourse by Kausthub Desikachar, only a year after being accused of sexual misconduct and without showing any evidence of training or therapy in the areas of gender inequality, assault, or trauma.[337] In another example, the director of Jivamukti's flagship studio in New York City claimed in a 2018 podcast that historically, the studio has been "a safe haven". Now that they are offering consent cards, he explained, Jivamukti was "at the forefront" of the conversation on consent in the yoga world.[338] This gloss on this important safety practice completely overlooks the women who have been doing this work for years.

It's crucial to remember that the industry is unregulated, and that a number of its most popular teachers have backgrounds in the performing arts.[339] The point is that statements are easy to make. PR firms can write them for hire. They can cover over the fact that the real work may not have been done on any deep level.

Beyond explicit showing, there are subtle ways in which a community can self-correct in relation to its history. For example: many second-generation Ashtanga practitioners describe having moved on from "traditional" adjusting techniques in favor of a softer and more attuned approach that attempts, above all else, to avoid injury. This may not have happened within an explicit framework of naming and rejecting the manipulations of Jois as assaultive, but it does seem to carry the in-group knowledge to its natural conclusion that something was wrong with some of those adjustments.

There's a difference between a practice gradually becoming socially unacceptable, and actual policy that names and sanctions that practice, and becomes part of an explicit curriculum. For the most part, the implicit changes in Ashtanga adjustment culture seem to rely on unstable things like intuition and good intention. Both are impossible to measure, and neither *explicitly* empowers the student. In fact, the teacher who has relied on intuition and good intentions to shift to a less-intrusive adjustment protocol may still be relying on, even unconsciously, some of the same processes of mystification through which Jois's own skill was idealized. Without the teacher explicitly seeking a student's consent to be adjusted, and discussing what adjustment means, why it is being applied, what their scope of practice is, and where on the student's body touch is never appropriate, the student is left to simply trust the good will and indefinable wisdom of the teacher. In the absence of open discussion, power structures can persist. In short, the **S**how step of **PRISM** really can't fully work without the background of **R**esearch and **I**nvestigation—as well as the proof-in-the-pudding stage of **M**odeling transparent ethics.

In this light, Karen Rain becomes a very important and realistic storyteller within Ashtanga culture. Through studying Rain, people will come to a more balanced understanding of what can actually happen in a yoga practice, and perhaps what yoga practice can really mean. That is, if yoga is about understanding your social conditioning, working to undo the bonds of trauma, and finding a pathway, by hook or by crook, towards integration.

QUESTIONS FOR REFLECTION: SHOWING

S.1 If you come from a yoga community with an abuse history, how do you show your students, trainees, and the public that you are not passing along that legacy?

S.2 What measures would you expect from a teacher or service provider to substantiate their claims that they have recognized and addressed the harm history?

S.3 How will you assess claims made by yoga or other spirituality teachers or group about their new awareness of issues like trauma in the yoga or spiritual space, or informed consent?

MODEL

Model transparent power sharing and
engaged ethics for future practitioners.
Cycles of abuse, silence, and neglect can be stopped.

Who has emerged from the Ashtanga crisis to model transparent power sharing and engaged ethics within the community and the larger yoga world?

There are many names and pathways, because activism is also prismatic. In the Ashtanga world, its various colors point to how sharply or softly each reformer has to reframe their relationship to the organizational and devotional center, to their colleagues, and to their students.

Coming to grips with Jois's abuse and the institutional betrayal that enabled it and covered it over means so many things. In the public sphere, current and former members can apologize, admit complicity, make policy statements about how they will distance themselves from the Jois legacy and promote new teaching protocols to help empower students and safeguard against abuse.

Consider Greg Nardi's transparent disillusionment with the conventional Ashtanga narrative, and his commitment to the future study of toxic power dynamics.[340] Consider yoga scholar and Ashtanga-authorized teacher Jean Byrne, who is starting to bring consent cards into her Perth studio. Further, with her partner, she is applying for funding to research the prevalence of trauma amongst new yoga students. In New Orleans,

Jessica Blanchard is engaging her students in a conversation about her blind spots over the years. In London, Sarai Harvey-Smith brings her psychotherapeutic understanding of transference and counter-transference into her yoga teaching and training.

None of this is easy. For all of these Ashtanga teachers, modeling a better way has had to unfold while they face the painful challenge of mending their private wounds. Beneath the public confessions and policy statements, reform-oriented teachers typically express sorrow at how the institutional abuse and silence has strained their deepest relationships with colleagues and teachers to the breaking point. Some have had to question whether it's appropriate to muster forgiveness, or whether forgiveness is an act of self-harm. These struggles point back to the work of Alexandra Stein. What happens when you value a relationship in a dysfunctional organization? Is it possible for the insecure or disorganized attachments formed within a high-demand group to be rewired? Or is that network simply scarred, and best avoided?

In my own case, secure rewiring never happened. Cultic love never became real love. There isn't a single person among the hundreds I knew in both of the high-demand groups I was in with whom I'm still friends. Amongst the people in those groups who held power or seniority over me, and who knew that the leader was harmful, I can't think of anyone I would trust reaching out to. If I'm honest, I have to admit that I'm still angry at all of them, despite the fact that intellectually I know we share a history.

But on the other hand, how would I really know unless I *did* reach out, or unless fate had kept us close? Like so many yoga or spiritual high-demand groups, the cults I was in were the products of globalization. We came from all over the world and consumed something. When it was over, for each of us at different times, we each returned to home, scattering back to all over the Unite States, Europe, Australia. Had either of those two groups been based in Toronto where I live today, would I bump into old mates at the café? Would we be able to reconnect under a different sun? What do we have in common with each other, if not the practice we shared?

In the aftermath of Karen Rain's #MeToo post, dozens of Ashtanga practitioner who were really supportive of her would also ask, "Are you still practicing?" It was as if they wanted reassurance that even a person who had suffered so deeply within a community could still find relief and support within it. If Karen was still practicing, it would suggest that Ashtanga practice could help overcome their disillusionment with Ashtanga culture. If Karen still loved the postures and the sequences, current members' relationship to them might feel a little less hollow or doubtful.

For Karen, however, this was an awkward question. She could feel what her preferred answer should be, but couldn't give it. She had left Ashtanga practice forever, but she also found other practices that helped her on her way. In comment threads and blogs, she would describe her non-yoga activities clearly.

Karen is not likely to go back to a yoga shala. To Ashtanga devotees who have been moved by her story, her absence might feel haunting. As if every room contains an empty mat, or several, abandoned by the women who had to leave. Instead of feeling diminished by this, however, perhaps practitioners can use that absence to dig deeper into their meditations on suffering, change, and that old adage that there are many pathways to God. As Ashtanga yogis stretch and sweat, somewhere Karen is riding her unicycle or dancing. These actions may have something in common.

***

Modeling engaged ethics as a cultural project cannot be simply be a matter of leaving individuals to make the best choices they can. Practitioners need institutional and organizational support. If they have left high-demand groups, this will involve the additional challenge of finding new communities and social resources. As we'll see in the following sections, organizations like the US Yoga Alliance may be able to play an influential role in providing this support, despite the fact that they have historically lobbied against the single industry change that some believe would make all the difference: government regulation of yoga teaching, centered on revocable licensing. The forthcoming data from Professor Cunningham and her colleagues may shed light on other concrete mechanisms of institutional support. And progressing from her path-breaking work on institutional betrayal, psychologist Jennifer Freyd is beginning to theorize aspects of what she calls "Institutional Courage", which might be useful for yoga, and other spiritual organizations who wish to be proactive about creating safer spaces, and responsive when safety is breached. Freyd notes that institutions should:

1. Comply with criminal laws and civil rights codes.
2. Respond sensitively to victim disclosures.
3. Bear witness, be accountable, and apologize.

4. Cherish the whistleblower.
5. Engage in self-study.
6. Conduct anonymous surveys.
7. Make sure leadership is educated about research on sexual violence and related trauma.
8. Be transparent about data and policy.
9. Use the power of your company to address the societal problem.
10. Commit resources to steps 1 through 9.[341]

QUESTIONS FOR REFLECTION: MODELING

M.1 What challenges do you personally face in modeling ethical behavior for your community? What strategies do you have for facing those challenges?

M.2 What organizational tools are you aware of from other disciplines or industries that might support transparent ethics in a yoga or other spiritual community?

M.3 If the group you are involved with conducted an anonymous survey to assess safety, what questions would you like to see on it?

M.4 Are there suggestions you would add to Freyd's points on institutional courage?

M.5 Do you know a whistleblower? How can you support them?

SAFER SPACES: TOOLS AND STRENGTHS IN A POST-LINEAGE WORLD

In studios across North America and Europe, hints of institutional courage and **PRISM**-like initiatives are unconsciously playing out through a quiet but profound sea-change in pedagogical standards. There is a highly visible and ongoing shift away from authoritarian teaching models, led by outspoken mid-to-late career women teachers like Diane Bruni and Donna Farhi, who left behind the Jois and Iyengar methods, respectively, and have hewn independent teaching paths rooted in nurturing student empowerment.

Diane has expanded her teaching repertoire to include functional and developmental movement training, as well as the research from the Berlin-based collective of retired (and formerly injured) dancers known as the Axis Syllabus community.[342] Donna has continued to walk a path more closely related to the simple and self-exploratory yoga she grew up with, before she was drawn into a high-demand Iyengar group in the 1980s. Donna now travels the world teaching students and training teachers in asana practice as a form of agented self-inquiry, with special attention paid to both biomechanics and interoception (sense of the inner state of the body). She spent many years never being asked how she felt in her practice. Now she's making up for all that lost time. Neither Diane nor Donna give adjustments.

Emerging trends support standout teachers. One trend is the increasingly common adoption of "consent cards", by which students can indicate, without even having to speak, whether or not they welcome touch while practicing. This is a positive step, but it takes strong managerial support for real effectiveness. Implicit consent in touch is so entrenched in many parts of the yoga world that studios offering the cards without clear explanation and instruction for students when they check in often find that the cards go unused. Affirmative, participatory consent is not yet a clear enough cultural value for the purpose and use of the cards to be self-evident. But the cards are a start.

Another trend is the growing popularity of the "trauma-aware" or "trauma-sensitive" yoga genre. Clinical trauma studies have exploded over the past decade or so, and this wealth of knowledge has flowed over into somatic psychotherapies. By osmosis, it has slowly begun to become a valued principle in yoga trainings. The leaders here are yoga teachers who are also clinical practitioners in various mental health or social service contexts. But they face obstacles involving the unregulated status of training and teaching yoga in most jurisdictions. As "trauma-aware yoga" trainings pop up in every major yoga market, students and trainees have little criteria for assessing their competence or applicability. Given the decades-long history in global yoga of some charismatic teachers inflating their talents and making unproven claims, the new marketing of trauma-awareness opens up new possibilities for everything from well-intentioned incompetence to cynical opportunism.

Tiffany Rose, a yoga teacher in Alberta, Canada, who lives and teaches with trauma-related Complex PTSD and Dissociative Identity Disorder, describes the challenges in detail: "I think a true trauma-informed lens will find yoga teachers claiming less, not more," she writes.

> Less ability to know what a yoga practitioner needs, less desire to put hands on anyone unless the practitioner asks to be touched in a specific way for a specific purpose. I think it takes a depth of

> listening and observing bodily cues for yoga teachers to provide effective touch with the ongoing and conversational consent from practitioners through both verbal and non-verbal indicators. Safe(r) spaces will see students truly in charge of their practice and what happens physically, emotionally and "spiritually" for them. Yoga teachers will need to work harder to develop these skills. They cannot be taught at a trauma-informed training or transmitted through a guru. They are interpersonal skills. It's certainly important that all yoga teachers receive trauma-informed training. However, without shifting our overall opinions about teaching or authority and power, these ideas are useless and clearly can be manipulated to support the continued projection, power dynamics and abuse that has been the norm in yoga land.[343]

***

Both the growing numbers of independently identified practitioners like Diane Bruni and Donna Farhi and spreading policy initiatives like consent cards and trauma-awareness are elements of a broader sociological shift for which yoga scholar Theodora Wildcroft has coined a term: post-lineage yoga.[344] In her forthcoming doctoral thesis,[345] based on years of fieldwork in non-mainstream yoga communities in the UK, Wildcroft shows that the three central pillars that have been used to authorize the integrity of every modern yoga method—all related to charismatic overreach—are now being fiercely contested.

First, Wildcroft explains, *historical narratives* around the antiquity and origins of postures are being upended. Until the 2010 publication of Mark Singleton's *Yoga Body: A History of Modern Yoga Practice*, it was common for students under the influence of the Jois family to say, to take just one example, that his gymnastic series of postures dated back to the Iron Age, and were commonly practiced by groups of yogis who were also immersed in the metaphysics of the *Yoga Sutras*. Some Jois devotees still believe this, but they will be increasingly marginalized over time.

Secondly, the *medical claims* made by Indian yoga luminaries from the 1920s onwards in their anti-colonialist attempt to present yoga practice as an indigenous and scientifically valid element of public health programming are now coming undone. It's simply not true, for example, that shoulder stand improves thyroid function by compressing and "massaging" it, as has been claimed for over 60 years.[346] The veneer of projected medical wisdom that allowed Pattabhi Jois to convince students to throw away their hepatitis medication or refuse surgery for a torn shoulder has now worn through.

Finally, the authority of someone like Jois, seen as a guru leading a *parampara*, has been occluded by more than his death and a growing skepticism around status claims in general. His case is becoming the norm as the entire category of the "master teacher" loses capital. It's not only happening because so many of these men have disgraced themselves, but also because of the pseudo-democratic rise and proliferation of the social media yoga star. Iyengar's *Light on Yoga* may have sold millions of copies worldwide over a half-century, but any one of an increasing number of scantily clad arm-balancing contortionists on Instagram can connect with millions of followers every few hours. This is more than a battle between quality versus quantity. It represents a paradigm shift—technological, political, and economic—in how cultural power is assigned and monetized.

As historical, scientific, and moral sources of integrity and validation crumble, what fills the vacuum? *Community*, argues Wildcroft.[347] Horizontally resourced, inter-lineage, interdisciplinary, cross-pollinated community. Instead of vertical appeals to authoritarian figures or ancient sources, Wildcroft shows that practitioners are increasingly turning to each other—but also reaching beyond the yoga world into disciplines with different values and ways of knowing—for resources that will help them both define and enrich what they practice and teach. There would be no consent cards without an overlap between the yoga teaching population and those who work to prevent sexual assault. Trauma-sensitive yoga is the innovation of psychotherapists trained in bodywork who have imported their licensed expertise into the practice.

Wildcroft's own comfort in studying the post-lineage zeitgeist has been aided with her long-time commitment to pagan communities and practices in the UK. Contemporary paganism, she says, had its own "Singleton crisis" decades ago. In the 1990s, academically inclined witches discovered that their practices and lineages were more reconstructed than ancient in much the same way that modern yoga scholars have discovered that their object of study is more new than old. They did it by rigorously assessing neo-pagan claims against the actual literary and biographical evidence left by key innovators. "We're over it," Wildcroft told me, referring to the age of mystification in modern witchcraft. "We've fully accepted that we're creatively engaged in a mixture of the old and the new."

As the profession of yoga teaching continues to proliferate as a part-time or flex-time staple of the gig economy, it will become increasingly porous to forms of knowing, training, and licensure that many teachers will be pursuing or maintaining in other fields as they cobble together a living. This interdisciplinary drive will strengthen as yoga continues to spill out of the ashram, retreat center, or studio, and its practitioners begin to echo that early modern Indian agenda of making yoga a feature of public health services.

In the yoga world, this is starting to happen through a combination of factors. There are signs that more people are graduating from teacher training programs than can find work in the studios that tend to define industry standards. Yoga research is slowly improving, attracting the interest of medical insurance companies and corporations looking to help clients prevent illness and stress-related productivity loss. Yoga is now widely believed to help children improve focus and emotional self-regulation in schools, although in some places, it has to be called things like "mindful movement" in order to avoid the scrutiny of Christian parents suspicious of anything that might promote non-Christian messaging. And an affinity between feminist and queer-inflected forms of yoga practice and the trauma-sensitivity movement continues to open up the practice for marginalized populations. In my home city of Toronto, there are yoga classes exclusively dedicated to people of color, trans people, and people living with disabilities.

This wave of public-service yoga efforts is finding organizational channels. In 2009, a non-profit called the Yoga Service Council was founded in New York City to help growing numbers of public-service oriented teachers network, share best practices, learn about government and foundation grants, and discuss local and regional political initiatives that would support their work.[348] The Council has attracted yoga teachers who want to serve in prisons, women's shelters, nursing homes, and Veterans Health Administration hospitals. Their funding opportunities rise in tandem with the evidence they offer that shows the effectiveness of yoga as an intervention for the underserved. They try to show how yoga reduces attentional challenges in inner city schools, helps veterans and refugees manage PTSD symptoms, or helps women with sexual trauma recover their agency.

This research drive may quite naturally open out yoga education, and make it more interdisciplinary. You won't be able to get authorized in Ashtanga in Mysore by Sharath Rangaswamy and head straight into a job teaching in a women's shelter. You'll have to learn and show proficiency in many skills that Jois's yoga didn't teach (nor Iyengar's, nor the yoga of Yogi Bhajan). You'll have to take trainings in sexual trauma and recovery. You'll have to agree to be held accountable to an ethics policy with teeth. You may have to apply for and retain a license. Most importantly, you will be encouraged to remain humble about your skills and capacities. That will mean staying in your lane, or adhering to a scope of practice. Unlike so many prominent teachers of the recent past, you won't be valued for your charisma alone, but also for your willingness to be held accountable.

A SCOPE OF PRACTICE FOR YOGA HUMANITIES

After almost 50 years into the globalization of yoga teaching, there is still no professional consensus on what a yoga teacher actually does, and, more importantly, *doesn't* do. This is not just the result of the often-contentious diversity in values and methods competing for legitimacy and market share. It's also an echo of the fact that the first generation of Indian yoga evangelists became famous in part on the basis of *not* having a defined scope of practice. They were expected to be and were seen as masters of a literally limitless subject.

In 2017, the US-based non-profit Yoga Alliance, a credentialing organization that has set industry training standards since 1999 with a training curriculum that has since had global impact, set out on a mission to research and define a scope of practice. (I served as one of the consultants on that project.) At the time of this writing, a preliminary draft has been finished and will soon be published for discussion and debate. It is unclear what the final form will take. But if widely adopted, it may join the work of the IAYT in providing a powerful structural support against personal and organizational abuse.

Informed by clinical and therapeutic discourse, the notion of a scope of practice directly challenges at least three key features of older ways of teaching.

1. **The notion that yoga practices confer generalized and universally applicable knowledge on a wide range of subjects.** This notion is embedded in countless scriptural promises, from the third chapter of the *Yoga Sutras* ("Meditation on the Pole Star gives perfect knowledge of the physical universe."—3.28) to the refrain in many *Upanishads* that knowing the Self gives access to knowing all things. The ancient premise is that *subjective knowledge provides the only accurate pathway to objective knowledge*. This is and perhaps always will be incompatible with contemporary evidence-based processes.
2. **The resulting "halo" effect.** This is apparent when the expert in one

area of yoga is automatically presumed to be an expert in other areas of the theory or practice. That Iyengar came to be lauded as a yoga philosopher is a good example. That Jois was lauded as an expert in women's reproductive health is a strange example. Mastery over postural forms does not imply mastery, or even competency, in any other aspect of yoga theory or practice. Oddly, the halo effect can extend beyond yoga subjects altogether. For instance, the senior disciples of Jois who issued bargaining-type statements in response to the abuse revelations had obviously not reached out to experts in sexual assault and restorative justice for help in understanding these areas. One factor might be that they—and this is by no means limited to the Ashtanga world—have spent decades being expected to hold forth on every subject under the sun. Their cultural competence has been routinely overestimated. In part, this could be because they have become proxies for teachers like Jois and Iyengar, who authorized themselves as experts in accordance with their student's needs.

3. **The infantilized status of the student.** Pre-modern yoga teaching, in general, presumes that the teacher holds something that the student cannot understand. In its most profound expressions, this is communicated through the bio-spiritual transmission of "downward falling of spiritual energy" (*saktipata*). This is an energy the student cannot know without the grace of the teacher, and before it actually happens. It is difficult to see how this could ever be compatible with the principle of *informed consent*. (Remember that *saktipata* was also alluded to by Steve Dwelley as a justification for Jois's assaults.)[349]

A scope of practice both *limits* the power of the teacher or therapist, and *shares* it with the student or client. When a student or client knows what the scope of practice of the service provider is—in most professions, it is clearly posted, or reviewed with the client before the relationship is engaged—they have the ability to make an educated choice about whether and how much engagement they want. This is the basis for informed consent: the client knows what the service is, and knows what would go beyond the service. They can become clear about and manage their expectations, and also know when those expectations have not been met. They know what the treatment is for, and have some basis in assessing whether it is working as advertised. In most licensed professions, informed consent is considered complete when the client clearly understands what recourse they have if the service provider harms them.

Reflecting back on the analysis of **Part Four**, we might say that informed consent would provide substantial protection against the power imbalance and constant uncertainty of the disorganized attachment scenario. Because it is rooted in the principle of care negotiated through open and verbalized contractual communication, it might also be protective against the potential for the trance or similar states associated with some yoga or spiritual practices to become a barrier to the student being able to articulate needs and boundaries.

***

Speaking of Jois, Peter Sanson said: "You had to surrender to his adjustments, and then you would be safe."[350]

When we go to the dentist, we might also surrender to the anesthetic and the drill. But it's not surrendering itself that would keep us safe, but the dentist's scope of practice, his training, and his code of ethics. All of these are matters of public record and scrutiny. Teachers, therapists, and clinicians who are given grave responsibilities over people's bodies and minds must be held to appropriately grave standards and mechanisms of accountability.

Yoga Alliance is also currently tackling the issues of code of conduct and training standards in its overhaul project. Currently, the projected results are unclear, but equally poised to impact yoga teaching globally for decades to come. One of the biggest challenges the organization faces is the general anti-regulatory attitude held by its mainly US-based membership, which it is currently beholden to promote. The US yoga world is fiercely anti-regulatory, even as yoga teachers and therapists (an emerging field) seek professional legitimacy and pursue public health funding and foundation grants. Nobody wants to be or submit to "the yoga police". This seeming liberality is another post-lineage sign, even if it emerges from a culture in which people like Jois were treated as though they had far more than policing powers.

The reasons for widespread suspicion of regulation in the United States are complex, but in the main seem to involve the intersection of arguments in favor of religious freedom, a broad distrust of governmental intervention, and an antipathy towards biomedical institutions, which are seen as predatory in part because of the untenable medical insurance situation.

The regulatory question is not going away any time soon, but in some fields of concern, the problems it would legally address are being considered and worked on in the open market. Yoga safety activists like Diane Bruni and Michaelle Edwards have spearheaded conversations about injury prevention in physical yoga classes, as well as crackling debates on what and how much anatomical and biomechanics training a person should have in order to not injure people with misinformed posture instructions. Meanwhile, the present exposition of Jois's sexual assaults and similar incidents is already beginning to provoke conversations about the appropriateness and even legality of *any* touch in a profession that typically offers a fraction of the training undertaken by licensed manual therapists.

In terms of the bodily safety and agency of the typical yoga practitioner, then, conditions and resources seem to be improving, regardless of whether there's any agreed scope of practice or actionable code of conduct governing the global industry. Competitive educational platforms alone are making a maturing industry aware of the limitations of earlier forms of yoga learning and teaching. Practitioners today have an endless new supply of diverse content to consume, coming from beyond the siloes of more narrowly defined brands like Iyengar and Ashtanga. As teaching becomes more competitive, training standards for obvious goals like safer posture teaching and avoiding assaulting your students will clearly rise on their own.

But there's a subtler aspect of scope of practice that the free market will not even begin to address. Theodora Wildcroft, who also consulted on the scope of practice research for Yoga Alliance, illustrated it with an analogy over a Skype call.

> Let's say you go to your local yoga studio for a drop-in class. It's a regular Tuesday morning, and you're one of 10 students who showed up.
>
> Now, imagine that the teacher announced that if anyone was taking anti-depressant medication, they should immediately throw away their pills and do a special breathing technique that was guaranteed to cure all mood disorders?
>
> Or let's say that one of the students had diabetes, and she told them they could cut down on their insulin by doing shoulder stand everyday.
>
> How many people would walk out of the room?

In 1970—when yoga was still countercultural—maybe two. In 1990—Six? But in 2018, the number who stay might correlate with the number of parents who are anti-vaccine. They're there, and they can be loud, but they're few.

> Now imagine instead that the teacher tells those 10 Tuesday students that she is connected to a lineage of yoga that is 10,000 years old and is based on the principle of non-duality found in the *Yoga Sutras*?

Some would believe what she said, despite there being three falsehoods in that one sentence. Others wouldn't care. But nobody would walk out of the room.

Wildcroft's point is clear. Incompetence and neglect in physical disciplines is getting easier to spot and culturally marginalize. But incompetence, neglect, and even active manipulation of a student's thoughts, intellectual processes, and emotional loyalties is harder to detect. Why is this an important issue to address? *Because every pathway towards the center of toxic group dynamics opens through a door of deception.*

One takeaway of **Part Three** is that gaining a firm grasp on how we know what we know, how we assess who's telling us what, and how we tell fact from fiction is key to developing a more transparent and student-centered yoga literature.

This clarity is a vaccine against the deception of propaganda. It begins with understanding that a substantial proportion of information about the origins, purposes, and authenticity of yoga techniques has been produced by people trying to market those techniques. *Much of the literature is, therefore, burdened by an inherent conflict of interest.* If we understand that a certain amount of writing on yoga is motivated, and this motivation may be complicated by marketing and self-validation, we'll start to look more closely at content producers. We'll get better at picking apart the various categories of yoga information, and using them consciously, according to their benefits.

So who produces the various categories of yoga information?

At the top of the "tradition" hierarchy, we have initiated teachers coming from within an Indian *parampara*. For the vast majority of non-Indian yoga enthusiasts, the opportunity to learn from within this system would be extremely rare, depending on geographical location of the teacher and the student.

A second category of yoga-knowledge producers is made up of those who have published peer-reviewed scholarship in the disciplines of Religious Studies, Indology, Sanskrit, or the philology of yoga texts. *Parampara* students will often grumble that academic work on yoga is not informed by practice, and can be stained by its colonialist legacy. The latter point is serious, but great strides have been made by an increasingly globalized yoga academic community in examining and mitigating the ways in which the Orientalism of 19th -and early 20th-century yoga scholarship othered, misunderstood, and often demeaned its sources. A good example of this progress can be found in the work and cross-cultural faculty composition of the Hatha Yoga Project, based at the University of London.[351] The project's rigorous textual analysis and translation of medieval yoga texts is balanced by ethnographic fieldwork that studies itinerant yoga communities in India with roots dating back to the Middle Ages. Also, the idea that today's yoga scholars are not also practitioners is simply misinformed. Many of the most highly regarded yoga scholars in the world today—among them James Mallinson, Mark Singleton, Jason Birch, Christopher Wallis, Theodora Wildcroft, Roopa Singh, and Suzanne Newcombe—are all practitioners of various forms.

A third category of information-producer would be the "legacy asana yogi" of the modern era. Pattabhi Jois, B.K.S. Iyengar, Swami Sivananda, Swami Vishnudevananda (1927–93), and others are popular not by virtue of their *parampara* credentials or their peer-reviewed scholarship, but through their visibility as asana practitioners or evangelists. Their books in English, which are mostly instructional, are inseparable from the broader marketing efforts that pushed their techniques into the public sphere. In these best sellers, they are not telling you about what their ancestors thought, nor about what "yoga traditions" say, in any objective sense. They are delivering highly subjective slices of content. A subset of this category would be those who produce popular literature that serves to elevate the content and position of legacy yogis. Donahaye's and Stern's *Guruji* would fall here.

Fourth would be the category to which I belong: that of a lay practitioner and teacher who also produces cultural commentary or journalism. My colleagues here would be people like Susanna Barkataki, J. Brown, Jennilyn Carson, Roseanne Harvey, Carol Horton, Be Scofield, and many others. None of us strongly advocate for particular methods or communities. But we all have our angles and passions, and unique ways of translating these into cultural value. Together, we contribute to a vibrant but often contentious online discourse that has exponentially accelerated and intensifie old yoga tradition: the use of debate to foster clarity. Occasionally, it works.

The last category of yoga-information producer is the newest, and perhaps most influential: the "yogalebrity" social media star. When Kino MacGregor took to Instagram on June 14, 2015, with the statement "I always say that pain and injury are the true teachers on the spiritual path", she created a powerful impact upon yoga culture and even philosophy. That mini-sermon went out to a list of over a million followers.[352] What impact will it have on followers who have no context in which to interpret it? How will it influence the student in an abusive relationship, or the student who is prone to self-harm?

The first step is to simply be able to tell these sources apart. Who's telling you what, and why, and what are they getting out of it? Are they speaking about yoga as a distinct spirituality and cultural art form supported by literature and tradition? Or are they speaking more about themselves? Such questions begin to level out sources of knowledge. The idea is to put the student at the center of the learning process. To make it eventually unthinkable that they would ever take something on faith alone.

A SCOPE OF PRACTICE PLEDGE

Here is a scope of practice pledge I offer when I lead training modules in history, culture, and philosophy for aspiring yoga teachers.

> I understand that as a student of yoga traditions, it is my responsibility to communicate the context of the yoga practices I share. I also know that my access to knowledge will be limited by language, time, geography, cultural difference, and unconscious bias.
>
> I pledge to acknowledge my historical and cultural position in relation to an evolving practice.
>
> I pledge to understand the difference between and uses of popular literature on yoga, teachings established by *parampara*, and peer-reviewed scholarship on yoga texts, culture, and history.
>
> I pledge to offer insights from scholarship or established *parampara* not as final truths, but as tools for self-inquiry.
>
> I pledge to be transparent about when I am referring to the work of experts, versus when I am offering my own observations based upon personal practice.

Given the deeply stained history of the modern yoga movement, I personally believe that teacher training programs would benefit from a dedicated module on the mechanisms of undue influence that govern high-demand groups. I think everyone would benefit from formal exposure to the ideas of researchers like Stein, for instance.

But in the absence of dedicated anti-high-demand-group lessons, I believe that basic training in informed consent and trauma-awareness are fundamental. Also, these basic pledges to information integrity and intellectual humility can be very supportive, especially when coming from teachers of privilege like myself. If it becomes a cultural value to protect students of yoga and other spiritualities from the manipulation of their thoughts and beliefs, we'll be well down the road to protecting them from the manipulation of their bodies and hearts.

APPENDIX 1
A Transcript

This book opened with a section from the following interview with T.M. She has asked to remain anonymous, and that details about where she comes from in the United States and what she went on to do after her life in Mysore remain obscure. She wanted to give this testimony, but wants no part of any dialogue that emerges from its publication.

I'll limit the identification to saying that she was a student at Jois's shala for an extended amount of time in the 1990s. She wasn't there for as long as Karen Rain, but she was there for longer than any of the other victims who have offered their voices to this book. I have corroborated with two other students that she was there, the year she was there, and key details of her story.

T.M. spoke with relaxed confidence. Rich descriptions of her experience with Jois, its aftermath, and how she recovered flowed out in full paragraphs. Here is the transcript of our conversation, picked up from where I left off at the beginning of this book. It's been lightly edited for continuity.

[M.R.] *You said that the actions were immediately interpreted by those around you as being not sexual. Was that offered in response to you asking, or did it come out of the blue? Was it preemptive, that explanation?*

[T.M.] There'd always be talk over the morning chai or whatever the breakfast was, and in some cases it was preemptive.

I might make some kind of snide comment or confused comment about it. Then there would be the table talk about how this ... literally, "It isn't sexual." I just remember that over and over. Now, it just kills me. It was both preemptive and on a call-and-response basis.

[M.R.] *I have a sense from other interview subjects how many volumes lie underneath words like "confusing". I'm very aware of the victim-blaming tack that wants to ask "Why did you stay, or why did you keep going back?" I just want to assure you that I'm not ...*

[T.M.] I get that.

[M.R.] *I'm not asking in blame mode—but do you have any insight into how you were able to tolerate or to return day after day in the midst of the confusion?*

[T.M]. As I said I tend to be a bit of an extreme personality, and when I enter something, I did take the instructions to their limit. When you're told that this is part of the path, that has some power if the path is of importance to you. When you're told that this is a master, and why would you come all the way to the other side of the world to argue and debate and not even, quote-unquote, fully take him in?

When your understanding of women and sexism in any of this is not like top-of-mind, and when you're quite young, it's the thing you do to realize the path. I really had two parts fighting inside of me. The part—which ultimately won out—that was confused and didn't think that this could be right, and thought that it was perverted and sexual. And the other part that was dedicated to the path—that was told that this was not sexual.

Keep in mind: the sexual assault is already a boundary violation, and once you experience boundary violation, there's also psychological boundaries that erode. Not just physical ones. Not knowing what you think as opposed to what others think. And when you're told to continually open to the path—and that you may not know what's going on—adds to that inner doubt and confusion. It just gets all laid up on top of each other in some kind of weird tiramisu. Just stacks and layers of denial and then confirmation, meaning that your denial is right next to your impulse that this is wrong is right next to your denial, which is right next to the layer that tells you that you're wrong.

[M.R.] *It's like the way sexual assault boundary leads to psychological boundary violations seems to be a toxic mimic of how practice is described. The outer, physical asanas are going to get inside you somehow. They're going to change your inner landscape. I wonder whether that's an added unconscious or subconscious confusion: that, well, yeah, actually I am being internally transformed.*

[T.M.] At that age, [you] don't know your head from your ass. Now, maybe some other young women were more self-possessed and clearer than I was, but when you add on to the fact that you're in a foreign country with weak social ties. You could say that you had the ties of the community there, but they're a source of confusion and they're not strong social ties. You didn't grow up with them. They don't know anything about your former life.

[M.R.] *In fact, they're not interested in any of those things. They're interested in the way in which you can confirm their identity and their choices.*

[T.M.] Yeah, exactly. What's so interesting about a cult is that members of a cult deny a cult exists. But then they need to defend something that doesn't exist. It's very confusing. I don't want to suggest that I wasn't participating in this, but agency is also a very interesting concept. The idea of personal will. We don't even know how life arrived on this planet. Did it hitch a ride from somewhere else on a rock, or was it homegrown? Yet we have very strong concepts about free will or no free will, some sort of strange dichotomy. The more you look into the behavior of other forms of sentience, the more it becomes clear that humans are pack animals, and the identity is shaped in the social setting.

It would not seem crazy to me to imagine a young woman with weak social ties in a new pack pursuing the thing that she thought was an answer at the time. I didn't think it was *the* answer. I thought it was *an* answer at the time. It's no mystery that I'd continue to participate in something like this, particularly if rationalized as part of the path.

I know that lots of people like to shame victims with 'Why didn't you say no?' And when you're in court, some of that makes sense because they're trying to establish culpability. But outside of court, I see it as another way to defend the mental boundary of the cult.

Many of us were there for life-affirming impulses, connection, spiritual seeking, fulfillment, and yet in that kind of cult environment, you have to narrow what kind of connection and whom. There's a film or a layer of cheesecloth that develops around the sense of connection. You only are allowed to connect from the inside, and members need to affirm their sunk costs. They don't see their sunk costs. They still see Jois as an answer, and they can't move into the gray area around their answers.

Connection is all around them, but they have a pretty strong filter on it. If the aim really is some sort of boundarylessness—and one *should* have a clear understanding of healthy emotional and psychological boundaries—their filters are so strong that they've limited a lot of the connection they could potentially have with the world and sentient beings."

It's not pity. I'm not superior to them in any way. It's just so limited that I don't get super triggered by the fundamentalists. I'm not a fragile victim in that sense. I don't deny the victim status, but if someone disagrees or comes up with some elaborate way to shame me, they always use this really interesting faux logic. Like they're so logical, that it just cracks me up, but it's where they are. It's what they need to do to keep it together, and I can understand that. I can understand that sometimes you need to do things to keep yourself together.

[M.R.] *So about the bodily experience every day of going as far as you can go, and you finish up at seven or eight or nine in the morning or something like that, do you have a sense now looking back on it what the effort did to your capacity to think, to socialize?*

[T.M.] For sure. It wears it down. You've got nothing left at the end of the day with Jois. Mounting psychological defenses and gaining clarity are a little rough to come by. It takes so much psychic energy to unpack that and get clear about it. You don't have a lot, especially because the vegetarian diet is you don't have a lot of protein for your forebrain to just go, "Huh, this a little bit weird."

[M.R.] *What about pain?*

[T.M.] I had a very important injury. I was in a pose where I'm lying my back doing the splits, and Jois of course came over to do his manly duties and also push on my leg.

I had the flexibility to support a full split. The pose was finished. He was starting to get up, and I was moving out of the pose. I was probably, I don't know, 25% out of the pose, and in that position he used my leg as a lever to stand up, and it sounded like a branch ripping off a tree.

[M.R.] *Oh, fuck.*

[T.M.] Yeah, it was bad. Probably only last year I've successfully gotten out the distortion in my pelvis from that. It starts there. It moves into your lower back. It shortens your ribcage on one side. Your frontal muscles, your psoas, your iliacus goes short. Second and third layer defense.

I stayed in Mysore after that because Jois said it was an "opening". Everybody said it was an opening.

[M.R.] *So it was a full rupture of the hamstring tendon?*

[T.M.] It was still attached to the bone obviously, or I would have been in the hospital, but it was bad. I [had] trouble walking.

[M.R.] *Was this close to the end of your eight months?*

[T.M.] Unfortunately, no. It was probably midway, and I cried through practice and stayed. That part, I do still have a little anger at myself for, as you can imagine. Doing so much damage to myself, and yet humans are these social beings that go along to get along in a lot of ways. Individual agency is a tough thing to claim in a lot of ways.

By that, I'm not trying to skirt out on my own responsibility. I know myself now. This kind of shit would never happen to me again. Never. Not in a million years. I'd walk in, take one look at the guy, wouldn't even put down my mat. I would know right away. My Spidey sense relative to these things is so refined.

Some people say, "Well, you have him to thank for that." I'm like, he didn't do the fucking work. He doesn't get the thanks for that. That wisdom's on me. I did stay and practice, and it did do extreme further damage. I did cry every day, in fact, so much so that one day [a senior student said], "You should take a couple Advil." He was right next to me, as a funny thing. I didn't need to be persistent.

I've had lots of body work over the years. I tried everything at one point, and finally found a good Rolfer two separate times in my life that got me back to normal, but keep in mind in that process, my pelvis was wrapped in layers of barbed wire.

[M.R.] *Oh, man. Were you able to get medical treatment while you were there?*

[T.M.] You wouldn't do that. This isn't a medical issue, according to them. I just felt like Jois was out to lunch. I think he also had maybe some cataracts or something on his eyes. His eye contact was just like distant and unconnected.

[M.R.] *I never met him, but I've wondered while looking at photographs and video clips what the quality of his eye contact was like. There's a couple of moments where you can see him basically mounting women in Yoga Nidrasana (see* Figure 2, p. 47*), and he looks like he's ...*

[T.M.] Yeah, he loved that. I used to call him the Big Kahuna in that one. He would just mount people. That's the one with your two feet behind your head?

[M.R.] *Right.*

[T.M.] Yeah, he loved that.

[M.R.] *Okay, different topic. I don't believe I've heard anybody who has conveyed as much certainty and clarity about having recovered/moved on as you have. I don't know if there's any way that you could answer this, but what did that take? What do you attribute it to?*

[T.M.] I wasn't part of a strong US community. So when I came back, I was not hit with a wave of second-level bullshit. I was dropped out of the sky on my own. I had formed a community of practitioners, who then began practicing together, who then went over, some of who are deeply involved. None of those people would retaliate against me. They know how I feel about that, and that's why I lost all ties because you couldn't really coexist with this perspective in any kind of community that was hell-bent on idolizing and reinterpreting this predatory behavior.

I'm thankful for the ostracization because I wasn't an advanced practitioner. The physical limitations of what had happened to me meant that the kind of pain that I was facing was not insubstantial. Once you're ostracized and alone with yourself, rationalizing that kind of self-inflicted pain is quite difficult to do.

A lot of the arguments that started coming back at me at the early days just were not very bright. At a certain point, you just see through it. I embraced the aloneness of the time. I was angry. I fought. I got into a lot of mental debates. But it'd be like debating Trump. It just goes nowhere.

Understanding that being with myself and that anger and frustration and feeling the worsening of it come about... Okay: to get really "out there": if you're one with your life and your inner life is a piece of shit every day, filled with debates and frustrations and getting nowhere and feeling deeply infuriated... I made a decision that I didn't want my life to be like that. I didn't want to become that.

Those moments, those phases aren't separate from your life. They are your life. They talk these days [about] the neurons that fire together, wire together. I can see who I was going to be, and didn't want to be that person. It was the antithesis of what I originally got into the practice for.

Again: individual agency and will are hard things to claim. I know I came into this life preloaded with some shit. It's called biology, and I've always been very strong-willed in the weirdest kinds of way or very determined whether it's like I'm going to take this thing to the end, and I did. I saw that it was empty, and not in Buddhist kind of way. Let's be clear. It's that nobody was home.

I think some probably did a very good job of "don't throw the baby out with the bathwater." For me, that couldn't work. Every time I encountered my ... To this day, I cannot do five [sun salutation] As and five [sun salutation] Bs, because I just feel the entrainment of it all.

[M.R.] *Do you feel the socialization of the shala at that time as well? In other words, do the postures, do they carry that memory? The memory of those interactions?*

[T.M.] Oh, yeah, for sure. For sure, for me. It's like why else would you do five As and five Bs in a row if you didn't believe this formula is the gateway to something? You just feel the formula come over you. It's the formula. I still practice asana. But the formula of Ashtanga, I just can't go there because it's just so laden with certain variables that add up to, "Fuck this."

[M.R.] *So one thing that I'm hearing very strongly is that having loose or thin social connections during that time exacerbates that kind of dependency or an entrenchment within that. I'm imagining that re-establishing outside relationships while being ostracized from the community was helpful.*

[T.M.] Yes.

[M.R.] *You undertook physical therapy to repair your hamstring. What about for the other impacts?*

[T.M.] I went headlong into alternative forms of psychotherapy, interpersonal mindfulness within a system that specifically had non-violence as one of its principles. Basically, I think the first five years of that work were about boundaries. I became a therapist in a modality that worked with trauma. I practiced setting my boundaries and finding the places where I couldn't set them. It really helped and being amongst a community of practitioners that looked at interpersonal relationships in such a different way was a godsend. That you *could* have boundaries. It conflicts with the whole, "No boundaries. It's all one." kind of lightweight, California, 1970s, avocado philosophy. It was the opposite of that.

[M.R.] *Did you consider yourself to have been traumatized by the Mysore experience?*

[T.M.] Yes. I had heart palpitations, sweating, nightmares, aggression, collapse, all of those things. Swinging from really strong boundaries to none at all. Back and forth between the two.

[M.R] *And there had been no awareness of boundaries in the Ashtanga world?*

[T.M.] Except that, even before I went to Mysore strangely, I went to a Mysore-style class in the States, and the teacher was actually trying to sense for where the boundary was with me and said so. Like, "Is this too far?" I said, "It might be." He said, "Why aren't you saying anything?" I said, "I don't know."

And he backed off, but no one else anywhere in the adjustment world of Mysore is looking for the edge. They're just looking to move beyond it.

[M.R.] *So was that one of the rare instances in which you actually had an explicit consent conversation with an Ashtanga teacher?*

[T.M.] The only one in a decade. Later, I started having it with all my students. I ended up teaching for a long time and all my practice became about was boundaries. Also, it became about how a lot of times, you would see students really straining and moving in these poses. There was a sense of humor that I had that I'd go up to them and go, "Does that feel good, what you've got going on there? That kind of strain, that kind of push?" They'd start to laugh and realize that it didn't. "Why are you making the pose suck so much for you?"

I said, "Because this pose is your life. This is your life. You make your poses suck, and your life will suck." We had lots of discussions about pain and boundaries and pushing past it, and why? Why would you do that? What's that about? What do you think you're going get from doing that? And not in a condescending tone, like in a real exploratory tone. There was nothing you could do that couldn't be studied.

That's what I turned my attention toward. You're having thoughts about the person next [to] you in the pose? That's practice. You're having thoughts about you being better or worse? That's practice. You're having thoughts that you're going to get somewhere, and what are you willing to do to get there? Including hurt yourself and override your own boundaries? That's practice. You think you shouldn't have any tension there, and by pushing through it, it's going to go away? Just experiment with that and see how it works out. I don't think it will be cool, but if you're going to do what you do, study it.

[M.R] *Is there anything else you'd like to add at this point?*

[T.M.] I do think it would be interesting in portraying these thoughts to others to share the conflict because clearly [Jois's senior students] had them as well. To put it out there, so that they can begin to wrestle with that part of themselves that they have also buried that knows. That's how you get people out of fundamentalism. But it has to be gentle. If you take too hard a stance on it, that's where they kick back into the part of them that doesn't know, that needs to defend. If we're really trying to help people find their way, we don't want to avoid the truth in any moment, but we also don't want to force people back into their rationalized self.

I know that [Jois's senior students are] going to be facing a wave of vilification. I'd like to remember the wonderful experiences that I had with those people, and say that I don't hold them to another kind of standard. I don't begrudge them, they're no different from anyone else. Just because they're supposedly leaders in that community doesn't mean that they weren't caught up in psychological confusion. We were all confused together.

APPENDIX 2

Interviewee Stories

In 1984, at the age of 23, **Kiran Bocquet** traveled from Australia to India to study with Pattabhi Jois. Her trip marked an emergence from a depression that began at the age of 15, and which at times had verged on the suicidal. The year prior, she'd been introduced to Ashtanga practice by one of the first Australian students of Jois to bring the method home. To this day, she says that Ashtanga yoga saved her life. But the version of it she still teaches in a small town 150 kilometers south of Sydney bears little resemblance to what she was subjected to in Mysore.

"I remember him coming at the back of me in *Baddha Konasana* (*see* Figure 4, p. 55)," she says via Facebook video chat. She's describing the "Butterfly" posture, in which the practitioner sits upright with her legs folded outwards and the soles of her feet touching. Jois sat down behind her, wrapped his legs around her and over her thighs to press them down, and then reached around to hold her breasts.

"As he was counting, he was pumping my breasts. It was very confusing. I wasn't expecting it. I was thinking "Is this one of the adjustments?""

She feels that she remembers the assaults continuing for a week. "There was a sense I had to endure it," she says.

Kiran managed to give Jois a boundary only after seeing him assault her friend. The friend had recently arrived from Singapore, where she had been the victim of a drugged date rape.

"She was dealing with a lot. Her mat was behind me. For some reason, I turned around and saw Guruji behind her in *Baddha Konasana*, and he was also pumping her breasts. The tears were running down her face. That was the moment I decided "I'm not tolerating this. This is wrong."

"So the next time he went to adjust me in *Baddha Konasana*, I pulled his hand away and pointed my finger and just yelled 'No.'

"He pulled back a bit, his face shocked. I was never mishandled after that. I stayed on for eight months and felt relieved that after I confronted him in that moment I was spared these dubious adjustments that some of the woman were receiving at that time. I was very clear after that what was dubious and what was a beneficial adjustment.

Kiran followed up by email.

"He continued to adjust me deeply into postures for my stay there," she wrote. "He was known for his intensity in adjusting and I was fine with that. I guess, after the boundary was set, I felt as though I was receiving the same kind of adjustments that the male students were receiving..... So not sexual.

"The *Supta … Padangusthasana* (*see* Figure 1, p. 28) was always a bit of a question mark ..... But he gave this for males as well…

"I never received direct inappropriate adjustments to the pelvic region (that I can remember). I say this because his adjustments were pretty full on, involving his whole body... So there are blurry lines I guess...

"It's not that he ignored me, as he still taught me, adjusted me, there were sweet moments. It just always felt a bit strange after I confronted him... It's a complex situation really... I guess the way it was dealt with was to silence it as myself and the other students loved the yoga and intensity so much.

"As I resolved and laid the boundary with what I wouldn't accept, I then went on to experience the best of Guruji . I have never defined him or held him there for it as the transference of yoga and his teachings become a path for me. I have just made sure that the practice is safe in my hands for others."

***

Nicky Knoff was 48 years old when she arrived in Mysore in 1989 with her husband James to study with Pattabhi Jois. Beginning in 1970, she had studied with Bikram Choudhury for four years, and subsequently with B.K.S.. Iyengar and his senior student, Martyn Jackson. She had lived for 10 years in New Zealand "and together with two men started the New Zealand School of Yoga in Auckland, the first to offer full time classes, several a day," she said.

"We realized Iyengar had stopped teaching the Sun Salutation," Nicky said. "This meant we lacked the strength required by the sequences listed in the back of *Light on Yoga*. Pattabhi Jois taught exactly the way he had been taught by Krishnamacharya."

Nicky said that a fellow Australian Ashtanga teacher phoned Nicky and warned her about Pattabhi Jois's "erotic adjustments".

"I laughed," Nicky said. "He would not have any interest in me. There would be younger, prettier female students for him to give adjustments to."

James and Nicky joined seven others in a group in which she was the only woman. On the first morning, James looked through his legs in downward dog (*Adho Mukha Svanasana; see* Figure 3, p. 47) and saw how Jois was adjusting her, and asked her if she felt they should leave.

"I said: 'No, we have come here to learn and I shall handle him.'

"I would be in *Baddha Konasana* (*see* Figure 4, p. 55)," Nicky said, "and he would sit with his penis/pubis right into my sacrum plate and grab my breasts, I would take his hands away and push him back and say, 'Bad Man', or he would try to put his hands on my pubis. I just pushed him away each time.

"In those days, Jois's English was very poor. When we asked him questions, he would reply in Sanskrit.

"In *Trivikramasana* [a standing split] he would adjust me by putting his pubis against mine and holding me close.

"I would say 'Shall we dance?' which made the guys laugh. But they were getting fed up with his giving me all the attention and I felt bad about that. It was altogether a strange situation and felt very awkward especially as Amma was in the kitchen scrubbing the floors with some terrible poisons just when I was in the middle of *Urdhva Dhanurasana* [backbend]. She must have known about the erotic adjustments and I was sad to think of her suffering."

Nicky describes that one day Jois lay on top of her, pubis to pubis, in *Eka Pada Bharadvajasana,* in which her leg was behind her head. He wound his feet around the ankle of her extended right leg and pushed it to the floor. At the same time he pushed her left foot down, telling her "Touch it your toe."

"My back rounded in that position," said Nicky. "There was no way anatomically I should have been touching both feet to the ground. Then there was a loud 'crack' noise and he jumped off in fright.

"I was warm and finished the practice, Third Series. But after *Savasana* [corpse pose] I could hardly get up. My psoas was pulled, wrenched. It took me a week of therapy at the Kaveri Lodge* before I could get back to his shala, and three months of therapy practice to heal the psoas."

James remained uninjured from the adjustments, because, as Nicky said,

* Kaveri Lodge was a popular hotel for Jois students.

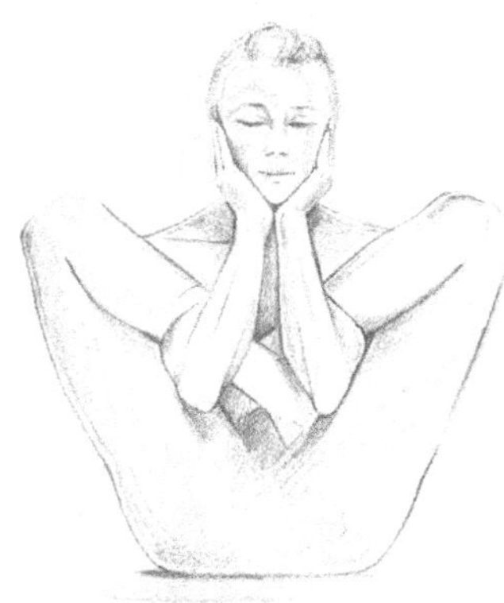

Figure 8: Garbha Pindasana

"He would just let go, relax, and wait for the end of the adjustment before he would do the asana again by himself.

"I listened to many of the female and male Ashtanga practitioners all over the world and I was amazed how many were in complete denial. They would say 'Pattabhi knows just what you need and the adjustments are just fine.'

"To be fair," said Nicky, "we have to remember, we from other countries, wore leotards in those days and the Indian women wore Punjabi suits or even saris and were completely covered up. Perhaps we should have been more sensitive to that. Perhaps we were partly to blame with hindsight. For me for yoga practice, a leotard is perfect, it is very uncomfortable to wear more clothes, but having said that I have done *Mayurasana* [peacock pose] in a ball gown, so it is possible!"

***

In 2009, Jennilyn Carson, the writer behind the popular *YogaDork* blog, posted a photograph that had till then only been circulating through dark corners of the internet. It shows Jois teaching in a large gymnasium, leaning over to fondle the genitals of two women immobilized in inverted *Garbha Pindasana* (*see* Figure 8, above). They are upside-down with their vulvas exposed. The pose name translates to "embryo".

Responses to the posting were polarized, predicting the later conflict over the Jois adjustment video,[353] and the urge to suppress. Amongst the back and forth between accusers and defenders, Ashtanga blogger Angela Jamison, writing under her internet moniker OvO, lamented the publication. The photo was "extremely inflammatory", she wrote, and caused "outrage, disillusionment, confusion, denunciation, and even internecine battling." It condemned a "brilliant, just-deceased teacher at his most confusing, offensive and difficult to understand."

Several sources say that that photo is a still from a VHS tape of Jois teaching an intensive in Kauai in 2002, but I have not been able to find the tape. One senior Jois student who didn't want to be named said that it was watching that video, shortly after it was released, that made it clear to him what he had always suspected.

But Jois's assaults in Hawaii began at least a decade before that video was shot.

In 1991, **Michaelle Edwards**, a yoga teacher and bodyworker from Kauai, attended a Jois retreat on Maui. Via email, she describes how Jois manhandled her into a version of *Garbha Pindasana* (*see* Figure 8, p. 306)—the pose of the two women in the viral image. The contact made her feel claustrophobic.

"The next day I said NO to Jois when he came by for the *Garbha Pindasana* pose in the series," she writes. "He tried to make me and I said NO again and so he called me a 'Bad Lady', then repeated, 'Bad Bad Lady'.

"The next day or so after that, I was in *Paschimottanasana* (a seated forward fold: *see* Figure 7, p. 124) when he leaned the weight of his body (and laid down on top of me.) He then reached around underneath my upper legs and hips with both arms on either side of my torso and began to use his fingers to grope my vagina. I was shocked and thought maybe he was confused about what he was doing and then I really felt molested and very uncomfortable to have his weight on me too. I said NO several times."

At some point in that class, she then remembers Jois's American assistant intervening to tell Jois that he would be assisting her from that point on. "I do not know if the assistant witnessed Jois on top of me in the forward bend, but he did sense that I needed help and he began to work with me on the Ashtanga practice."

"Jois backed off and I was very nervous around him after that. I felt and heard nothing 'spiritual' from Jois as he could not even speak English other than calling me 'Bad Lady' and counting to 10 slowly. Other people were kissing his feet as though he was some kind of deity or enlightened being."

Edwards has gone on to become a tireless advocate against abuse in yoga teaching, and for a more sound understanding of biomechanics safety in yoga practice through her innovated yoga for posture realignment method, called YogAlign.

***

"I remember my first thought being: 'What the fuck is going on here?' From day one. I was pissed off."

I'm talking to **Marisa Sullivan** from Manhattan via Skype. She's describing meeting Pattabhi Jois in Mysore in 1997, and watching him assault a woman on the first day she attended class in Lakshmipuram.

Jois's old shala, built as an extension to his family home in 1964, could accommodate only 12 mats at a time. This meant that students came in several morning shifts to work through their 90-minute sequences. The day began at 4am. Jois would be in the room until noon or beyond, counting out the breaths, adjusting students. On breaks, he would sit on a little stool in the corner sipping thick black coffee prepared by his wife and reading the newspaper. In later years, he would sometimes doze off.

People waited their turn for mat space in the room by sitting obediently on the stairs going up to the second floor "finishing room", where students who had completed their main practice went to do their finishing (or cool-down) postures and then lie down in corpse pose. From the stairs connecting the two rooms, one could look through the open doorway onto the mats below.

Sullivan sat on the stairs on the first day and watched Jois put his hand on a woman's buttock and stare off blankly into space. She watched, aghast, as he kept pawing the women. As the days stretched into weeks, she commiserated with two other American students who were a couple. They were also outraged.

"We watched like hawks and were asking—'Is he really doing that?' We were beside ourselves."

When it was her turn to practice in the room, she was hypervigilant.

"I'd pace myself to not get an adjustment. I'd rush things so that I was never in a position that he would touch me in."

She described the adjustments she saw applied to other students as rough, as well as inappropriate. When he did touch her, she froze.

"I would think 'Okay, his hand is there, now there. Is that okay?' I couldn't even breathe."

Sullivan and her compatriots talked with others about what was happening. It was common knowledge. Couples were separating over it. In one couple, the man left, disgusted with Jois, but his partner stayed and tolerated it. In another couple, the woman left in disgust, but her partner stayed and continued to attend classes.

"We were talking about it constantly," Sullivan said. "It was like: 'We traveled all the way here… we spent all this money… this is bullshit… we really want to just be doing this practice… what does this mean? We hate this.'"

Sullivan heard all the standard rationalizations from the seasoned students.

"'He's lifting their *kundalini*,' they would say. Or 'Some of these people have sexual issues, and he's healing them.' Or: '*You* bring this on. *You* create this. *You* sexualize this. Because *you're* sexually traumatized, this is bothering *you*. It's just a touch, just part of the assist. Get over it.'"

When objectors would point out that Jois wasn't touching the men that way, devotees would default to the presumed homophobia of the culture.

"'That's because he's Indian,' they would say. 'So touching men would be scarier for him. He can do this work with women.'"

The American couple left. Sullivan was alone, with no one to talk to about it. She made a radical decision.

"One day I said 'I'm here, I came here to do Ashtanga practice. I'm just going to dive in. Enough with this questioning.'

"I'd always been on the outside of communities. And I have a huge sexual abuse history. And incest in my family. So I just said, 'I'm going in.' I made a commitment.

"That day, Pattabhi suddenly saw me. And he gave me tons of attention. I blossomed. I was kissing his feet at the end. Loving him. I just let go of the whole thing. The attention was physical and involved adjustments, and I let go of the questioning."

Sullivan's blissful immersion, however, was cut short.

"One day I was in the standing forward bend with my legs spread wide and my arms raised up and over with my hands reaching towards the floor (*Prasarita Padottanasana C*). He pushed my hands to the floor. That was physically agonizing. I was immobilized. Then he put his hand on my sacrum, and walked it over my sacrum, walked over my butt crack, over to my vulva, and moved his fingers back and forth over my leotard.

"At that moment, I was out of there. I can't remember whether I left after that pose or whether I finished the poses for that morning and then left."

"Do you think not remembering might come from dissociating in that moment?" I asked.

"Well, I dissociate in a horrible way. I can't drive because of that. I have been trying off and on for years to learn how to stay in my body so that I can drive but haven't fully managed it. Now I have a handle on it in the rest of my life. Like I'm not dissociating now while I'm telling you this. But back then it was horrible."

Sullivan fully owns what she calls the "honeymoon" period, from before the assault.

"That was totally mine. I did it. I wanted to manage the intrusions. I had spent all that money to get there. I had a personal goal to learn this practice, and I committed myself to it. Attaining my personal goal of committing to this yoga practice meant giving my will over to this teacher. I made a conscious decision to do that."

I asked Sullivan how she thought, in hindsight, she'd been able to execute such a sharp turn in her attitude towards Jois and the whole scene.

"When I was 16," she said, "I was raped at home by a foster brother for over a year. I told my mother. She didn't pay attention. I thought she told my father. Turns out she didn't. So it went on until I found a way to stop it.

"So for me, this experience of my truth being denied—this complete inability to trust my own truth—meant that I shut down that I was raped for years. Then it came back in a flashback in my early twenties. But there was a period where I pretended that it never really happened."

In Mysore, not only pretending that it wasn't happening, but reframing it as positive, meant that Sullivan could hold on to her community, just as she'd held on to her family.

"I thought, 'I always do this to myself. I always put myself on the edges of communities. I never let myself be fully inside.'"

When the illusion snapped, Sullivan's attempts to remain inside felt like prison.

"I didn't want to tell anybody. There was no way, in that community. That's when I knew that I didn't trust anybody with my story. This was my story. This fucking happened, and I'm not going to let anybody take this away from me. I saw them reframe other people's stories consistently. They were going to say that he was raising my *kundalini*! I was not up for more abuse."

Sullivan did manage to share her story with one other woman who'd experienced something similar at Jois's hands. **Maya Hammer** was 22 at the time, and a student of Diane Bruni's in Toronto. Sullivan and Hammer commiserated over a meal in Mysore before traveling together for a few days.

When Sullivan returned to New York, she practiced with Guy Donahaye for a short while, and also at the Ashtanga shala run by Eddie Stern. Eventually, Sullivan injured her foot dancing. She tried to continue Ashtanga practice with Donahaye, but the pain, plus the burden of self-silencing, slowly turned her cold on the scene.

Three years after Sullivan was assaulted in Mysore, Stern hosted Jois for a week-long intensive. They rented the ballroom of the old Puck building in SoHo, which can hold hundreds. She decided to go to one of the packed class.

"I went," she said. "And when class was over, I lined up to hug him. I thought 'I don't need to hold onto the crap.' This man is so imperfect. We're all so imperfect. The system is imperfect. We're pedestalizing him in this power play. I felt compassion for him. I'd been carrying a lot, and I was going to stop. I forgave him on some level. I thought 'I can see you're good, and the system is at fault that we give you so much power. And—I can't be here.'"

I asked Sullivan why she thought the male students in particular didn't confront the behavior.

"Nobody wanted to shatter this beautiful lifestyle. Imagine it: you could come to India and throw yourself into practice. In the afternoons, you could study music, and scriptures, and pranayama. All for very little money with your big US dollars. And stay in these nice apartments, and go to the spa and hang out at the pool.

"You had this beautiful practice, and you had a job. If you were going to say something, there was a lot to lose."

***

Before leaving Mysore to return to New York, Sullivan met up with **Maya Hammer,** then 22 years old, from Toronto. They shared stories.

On the first morning of practice, Jois groped Maya's breast. She thought it might have been an accident. By the third morning, he was leaning his crotch into her buttocks and vulva.

Maya was shocked. That afternoon she called her father. He asked how the trip was going, and she told him what had happened. Moshe Hammer was steady and supportive.

Did she need to leave? He asked.

She did. But she'd paid Jois US$400, and wasn't about to let a sex abuser keep her money as well. Her father asked her if she felt she could go and demand her money back. His simple question gave her the feeling that she could.

But what if he denied what he did? She asked.

He knows what he did, said Moshe. *He was there.*

Twenty years ago, making a long distance call in India meant going to a telephone center with open cubicles. After Maya hung up, an American woman approached her and said that she'd overheard her call. The woman acknowledged that these incidents with Jois happened regularly, but asked that Maya keep quiet about it. If Maya made a fuss, the woman said, it would ruin the experience for all of the other foreign students. She said that Jois would stop adjusting them, and that's what they were there for.

Nonetheless, Maya went to Jois's office to confront him.

"I said to him, 'I'm leaving, and I'd like my money back.' He said 'Oh, no, no,' and then 'Why?'

"I told him I didn't want to be touched by him. He said 'I won't adjust you anymore.' I said 'No: I'm leaving and I want my money back.'"

Jois got out his ledger book where he kept handwritten student accounts. He found her name and the classes she had taken, but then said that he had no money to refund. She reminded him she'd given him US$400 five days before. He conceded, closed the book, went into a back room and returned with US$200 cash in his hand.

Maya had the impression that he'd been through such negotiations before. "He clearly had money back there," she says.

***

At 27 years old, **Charlotte Clews** felt she'd found a home in the silent discipline of Richard Freeman's Ashtanga community in Boulder. Three years earlier, she'd packed up her life and driven all the way from Maine after someone told her about Richard in the local burrito shop. She appreciated the seriousness and austerity of the people and the practice.

"The practice served me tremendously," she told me by phone. "It held me in the world."

That world was solitary. One thing that stood out for Charlotte was the lack of social interaction. There was nowhere for people to hang out, no nearby café. Conversations were limited to the theory and practice of Ashtanga yoga with little or no room for questioning or critique. Quietly, she progressed towards the most demanding postures. Many years later, she would turn to physical therapy to help manage the debilitating pain caused by her yoga practice. When her therapist advised that she stop putting her leg behind her head, she felt almost instant relief.

"After some time in Ashtanga yoga," she tells me, "you know that injuries are part of the deal. It's a badge of honor."

Pain notwithstanding, Charlotte was excited to meet Jois on his Boulder stop in 2002.

During one practice, Jois tore her hamstring as he approached her from behind, stood on her thighs, and pushed her torso forward into a deep forward fold while she sat in a wide-angled posture (*Upavistha Konasana*). She persisted through the pain.

Later, Jois approached her to hold her steady as she bent over backwards into a series of dropbacks. He pressed his groin directly against hers to support her as she arched up and down. She had never been touched in that way in that posture before. He was supporting her lumbar spine, which made resistance nearly physically impossible.

Clews tells me that she was trained to believe that pain in practice was irrelevant, and that injury was inevitable in Ashtanga. But part of her also believed that a "good" student —who properly submitted to the teacher —would not get hurt.

Being assisted by Jois was a considered a special honor by the group. She remembers no impulse to tell Freeman or her friends about the pain she was in, nor to resist Jois when he aggressively assisted her, or later when Sharath Rangaswamy insisted she fold her right leg first in lotus position despite her ankle being sprained. When she didn't comply, he aggressively torqued her legs into position and badly re-injured the ankle. It didn't occur to her at the time to blame the teachers for the pain, she says. She felt she was choosing the experience.

Many of the women I spoke to suggested that their sense of self-worth and agency was confused in Jois's presence, not only by his stature within the group dynamic, but by a gendered and metaphysical hierarchy. Charlotte recalls a woman student asking Jois whether Ashtanga practice was meant for women at all.

"He chuckled," she tells me. "He said that if a woman is lucky, she might be reborn as a man. Luckier still, as an Indian man. Or ultimately, as a Brahmin priest. What I took away was that women could play at yoga all we wanted, because we were, in this lifetime, irrelevant."

When she isn't running 100-mile wilderness races, Charlotte still teaches yoga. She still believes in the power of cultivating a steady, easy presence in one's life, but feels ambivalent about the role of modern postural yoga. And she doesn't adjust anyone anymore.

***

Katchie Ananda was 35 when she encountered Jois at that same 2000 event in Boulder. She posted her account to Facebook early in 2018.[354]

"In the early 90s," she wrote, "while I was studying and teaching at Jivamukti yoga, most of us teachers were practicing Ashtanga yoga. Many of my peers were traveling to Mysore on a regular basis. I couldn't, because I was an illegal immigrant at the time and was afraid I wouldn't get back into the country if I left.

"I was also concerned, as I heard of many people who had gotten injured. I remember one of the other Jivamukti teachers who came back from Mysore with a torn hamstring, the next year she went back and got her other hamstring torn too.'

But when Jois came to Boulder, Katchie took a chance and went.

She described being both physically and sexually assaulted by Jois over the span of several days. In one encounter, Jois wrestled her into a deeper standing backbend than she was ready for. Her hands were on her ankles—already a strong position. Jois moved her hands sharply up to behind her knees until she heard an internal pop. Later, an MRI showed a disc herniation. She has maintained her yoga practice despite suffering from back pain ever since.

During that same event, Jois leaned into her and pressed his penis directly onto her vagina while she was on her back with both legs behind her head in *Yoga Nidrasana* (*see* Figure 2, p. 47).

"I remember registering that this was wrong," she writes, "but I was also completely absorbed in the sensation of having my hips opened, probably past what they could handle."

Katchie told me by Facetime from Europe that at the time she didn't consider the assault sexual, given that Jois wasn't erect. She understands it differently now. "I really never thought it such a big deal," she writes, "but I too have been internalizing patriarchy."

***

***Content warning**: childhood sexual abuse*

In 2001, Jois sexually assaulted **Anneke Lucas** during an intensive in Manhattan that was hosted by Eddie Stern. It happened in the same room where Marisa Sullivan had forgiven him the previous year. On December 7, 2010, Lucas, a writer from Belgium, published a matter-of-fact account of the encounter on a website that is now offline. It was the first written testimony about Jois published. For years, it remained the only one.

"A few days into the workshop," she wrote, "with four hundred or so students curled up into *Halasana*, I was suddenly groped by the guru."

Halasana (plow pose: *see* Figure 9, below) is a less intense variation of *Karnapidasana*, which opens the postures on display in the infamous video montage. Lucas was in a shoulder stand with her hips flexed so that her straightened legs reached down towards the floor.

"In absolute shock," she wrote, "I rolled to sitting and found myself staring across the room at Sharath, Pattabhi Jois's grandson, who stared back looking as horrified as I felt."

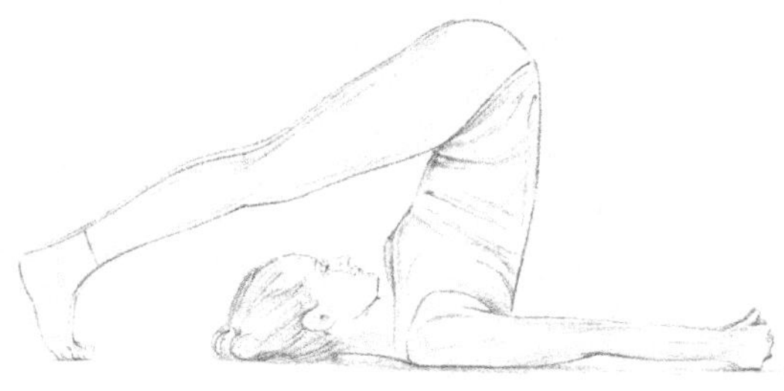

Figure 9: Halasana

Lucas continues.

"I heard Pattabhi Jois remonstrating: 'Bad Lady!' and the mild laughter of the crowd at the guru's old joke. In disbelief, I crouched on all fours to look into Pattabhi Jois's eyes. He smiled as if he had no idea what had just transpired, and said: 'You no come out of pose.'

In the moment, Anneke held her tongue, afraid of making Jois angry and being shunned by her fellows. After class, she privately confronted Jois, asking him why he didn't respect women. Jois first feigned confusion, but then agreed to not touch anyone the next day. "I hoped that I could make a difference," she told me, "that he would stop."

Amongst the Ashtanga friends she had at the time, Anneke's post of her blog received a mere five "likes" and three comments. One comment was from the yoga teacher Leslie Kaminoff: "I'm sure many people will relate to your experience, and will wish they had had the courage to speak up."

In general, the lack of response to Anneke's original post is a good example of what Theodora Wildcroft means when she says that victims and their stories are contagious.

For Jois students intent on protecting his reputation, Anneke is a powerful threat. Her yoga cred is rock-solid. She's practiced for over 20 years and now heads a non-profit organization that brings yoga classes to incarcerated populations. She's well-connected. And her life-story leading up to her meeting with Jois guaranteed that she would see right through the culture's rationalizations. A horrific childhood experience, and the years of therapy that followed, equipped her to instantly glean the intersections of violence, sex, patriarchy, and longing—and to name it frankly. She seems to have an almost shamanic power to thread the needle between light and shadow in the yoga world.

Via Skype from her Brooklyn flat, Anneke says that she's recorded her childhood experiences in a book that's taken 10 years to write. Now, she says, the task is to let the healing part of her journey shine through.

"It was too difficult," she says of the 350-page manuscript. "I can't see how the reader will go there with me. It was the most concise way I could write down the details of what actually happened. But the experiences are too gruesome." She's currently releasing parts of the manuscript on her personal blog, alongside other posts that reflect on the healing process. Hours of interviewing and emailing and a meeting in Manhattan shows that healed voice ringing through.

She describes how, in 1969, at the age of five, her mother and stepfather began to rent her to weekend orgies held by a sex trafficking ring. Her mother was paid, but it wasn't about money: the family had attained a nouveau riche status after emerging from prewar poverty. Lucas's stepfather was the mayor of a small Flemish town and worked as a cameraman for Belgium's first television outlet.

Her mother had herself survived a father who had returned from internment at Bergen Belsen. Later, she spent the chaotic ferment of the postwar decade flitting from partner to partner.

"My mother was always sexually inappropriate," Anneke says. "And she absolutely had her own sexual abuse story. As an adult, whenever I tried to speak to her about what happened to me she would always begin to talk about how much worse it had been for her. But there were never any specifics, even when I asked. She had all of the symptoms of someone who had been extremely sexually abused. But she couldn't remember any of it.

"I and my brother were the only creatures over whom she wielded any power. It was very difficult to be around her because she treated me as an extension of herself, but I had to be a bland and ugly—or powerful and evil—extension. So I couldn't have anything that was of myself in her presence. It was desperately hard to carry all her shame and guilt all the time, but that was the only way I could be 'good'.

"As soon as I resisted, I became bad in her eyes. She'd start to act like I was a rich and powerful abuser. She would punish me by taking me to the network. But then sometimes she would act as though she was jealous that I would be getting sexual attention."

"This was from the time you were six?"

"She was crazy."

"Mentally ill?"

"Not diagnosed, but…"

"So she would flip reality any which way," I offered.

"All abusers have to do that."

There's something unbearably frank about Anneke's voice and manner. It's more highly charged material than I've ever encountered, and she's speaking with a mixture of fatigue, nonchalance, and spiritual zeal. She's digested her story down to a smooth bone of resistance.

Anneke says her mother brought her to weekend orgies where she was raped and tortured. She claims she witnessed children being murdered. Some details she shared with me are unspeakable, and for her to tell one day. Suffice it to say, Anneke says her slavery ended in a zero-sum night of horror and deadly violence so abject that she resorted to complete dissociation to survive. It was that radiant moment, she explained, that would later drive her towards yoga.

One of her captors felt compelled to help her escape. Driving her home from a villa near Brussels, he gave her what she feels to this day were almost messianic instructions: She should leave home as soon as she was able. She should try to live in London, Paris, or maybe New York. She should never prostitute herself or trade sex for drugs.

By 1986, Anneke was in Los Angeles, where five years later she entered an MFA screenwriting program at the American Film Institute, and met her future husband. She discovered yoga through the Self-Realization Fellowship, founded by the late Paramahansa Yogananda, whom she considers to be her posthumous guru. She plunged into postural yoga practice as a form of recovery from her torture injuries—she had been repeatedly cut and stabbed in the backs of the knees. She also went into psychotherapeutic care. In 1997, she moved back to New York and began practicing at the Ashtanga Yoga Center of New York. Eddie Stern was her teacher. She became well-connected in the local community, and wrote regular yoga news columns for *yogacitynyc.com*. In 2001, Anneke gave birth to a daughter.

I refilled my glass of water and reset myself to ask about the blog piece.

"Can you describe Jois's sexual harassment of you a little beyond using the word 'grope'?" I asked. "Was there any other feeling you got from it? Did you get any sense of his intention?"

"Absolutely I did. But that sense is related to my past. When I was a child I learned to attune to my abusers, so that I could give them what they wanted.

"When the men were abusing me, I often received visions of their own abused childhood self, which was coming out in the present, in need. A self that wasn't nurtured or heard. It was showing itself in this perverted way of searching for something, perhaps a completion of the trauma. So I often had visions of what happened to my abusers."

"You're saying that at six years old, you learned to empathize with your abusers?"

"I was made to. I felt that my role was to be a little mother for all of these men. You have to understand that the reptilian survival state of the brain is very different from you and I talking here, over Skype. It's a very different world. My actions were rooted in the intuitions of survival. It consisted of feelings and sensuality. I could hear things from far away. The higher brain centers are not online. It's important to know that the victim and abuser are together in that state.

"The vision I got from Pattabhi Jois in the moment he touched me was the image of a little boy very happy to be getting away with something. But it came from a place of feeling very gross, very disgusted."

"With himself?" I asked.

"Yes. Very dirty. And for a moment, he was able to put it out of himself, to get it out, and as a little boy, have fun getting it out. It was very gross. Very old-world gross."

"Did you feel it was cathartic?"

"Cathartic means you don't have to go back. This was unconscious."

"Did you feel in that moment that your body was anything more than an object for that touch?"

"No. I felt totally violated. I was treated as inhuman. That was my experience in childhood as well."

"So you were powerfully attuned to that dynamic, because I imagine by that point —"

"I'd done a lot of therapy."

Anneke said that after Jois had returned to India, she went to Eddie Stern to report the groping incident. He was Jois's host, after all, and Stern was her teacher. According to Anneke, Stern's wife—another senior Jois student—was also at the meeting.

"Eddie referred to 'Guruji's unfortunate problem,'" Anneke said, "apologized and told me I had done the right thing. His wife also offered words of sympathy.

"At the time," Anneke said, "I was satisfied with the acknowledgment alone. But Eddie carries his share of responsibility by failing to warn me and others, and by persisting in spreading an image of Pattabhi Jois as though he was an enlightened guru."

Nine years later, Anneke showed Stern a draft of the article she was about to publish.

"Eddie's first question was 'Why do you want to humiliate him like that?' to which I answered: 'He humiliated himself.' Eddie agreed with me.

"Later on in that conversation," Anneke continued, "he brought up Yogananda and that his (alleged) sexual abuse was 'worse than Guruji's.' He explained this by referring to Jois's 'childlike innocence', because he didn't try to hide anything, while the (alleged) sexual abuse by Yogananda all happened behind closed doors.*[355]

"I did not want to stoop so low as to have to defend my guru, Paramahansa Yogananda. The abuse Eddie referred to was that he had allegedly fathered a son. In 2002, the *LA Times* reported that DNA tests performed with family members of Yogananda in India had confirmed that Yogananda was not the father.[356] But I did not want to get into a guru-contest with Eddie in that moment, and demean my own experience of sexual assault."

Stern insisted that our Skype call about Anneke's statements be off-record, but nothing in our tense exchange contradicted what Anneke described.

* The report of Brazilian-born, London-based Ashtanga teacher Luiz Veiga suggests it was possible that not everything happened out in the open with Jois. "I witnessed [Jois sexually assaulting women] at least 8 times, with 4 different students," Veiga wrote on Facebook. "Sadly, some of them were invited to practice with him privately at the old shala in Gokulam in the afternoon, sadly they all accepted his invitation. One of them got authorised straight after her first visit to Mysore." In an interview, Veiga clarified that the year was 2004, and that two of the women he saw being assaulted at the new Gokulam shala in the mornings would travel to the old *Lakshmipuram* shala residence in the afternoons to meet with Jois for private classes. In our interview, he protected their anonymity, knowing that at least one of them did not want the meetings disclosed.

Later, by email, Stern attempted to discredit Anneke. "She is using her past to publicize her current 501c3,'" he wrote, referring to Lucas's non-profit that brings yoga classes to prisons.

"[She] feels the need to exert power over Pattabhi Jois as part of her story.... She very well could have told the same story without having to use his name, but she probably feels that she is speaking up for anyone else who was 'abused' by him."

Stern is actually correct about that last bit. From our first communications, Anneke expressed the hope that other women would come forward about Jois.

Eighteen years later, Anneke is not surprised that Stern did not step in to protect her or other women.

"He could not oppose the father-figure," she says.

***

By 2002, the whisper network that warned of Jois's physical "corrections" was in full operation in Hawaii and elsewhere. **Micki Evslin** was 55 years old when she attended a week-long event with Jois on Kauai as part of his American tour that year. Micki remembers being excited by the prospect of meeting the master, but was also wary, having been warned of his behavior.

Micki was in a standing forward fold when she saw Jois's feet approach from behind. He hooked his finger under her tailbone and yanked upwards, ostensibly to help better position it. Micki felt that this was a strange but possibly useful correction, and continued with the class.

Minutes later, she was in an another forward fold, but with her legs at a wide angle.

"Suddenly, he forcefully jammed his fingers into my vagina, through my tights. He had to use a lot of force," in order to stretch the fabric of her clothing.

Before Micki could react, Jois moved on down the line of bent-over practitioners. After the class, Micki spoke with two other friends who reported that he'd done the same to them. They were shocked. They noted with confusion that they were the three oldest women in the class, presumably unlikely targets for sexual assault. The two other friends are now deceased.

Sexual assault experts know that what Micki describes meets the technical definition of rape in many jurisdictions. This brings into question the validity of Richard Freeman's statement to Kathryn Bruni that Jois "never raped the students."[357]

Jois's host for that Hawaii event wishes to remain anonymous. Evslin and two other women—not the friends she spoke to after the class—came to the host with their stories. One of them threatened to call the police. The host intervened by calling a meeting with Jois, his daughter Saraswati, his grandson Sharath, and long-time Jois chaperone, Joseph Dunham. Dunham died in 2010. Saraswati and Sharath often traveled with Jois, and are now the lead teachers in the growing Jois business. The inner circle now calls Sharath *Paramaguru*, which translates as "the highest (*parama*) dispeller of darkness (*guru*)", and implies that he now holds his grandfather's "lineage"— a putative combination of ancient techniques, spiritual realizations, and inherited authority.

Via email, the host confirms the details of the meeting. "It was not my intention to shame him," she writes. "But to delicately inform him that in the West, such behavior could result in a law suit."

She writes that Saraswati interjected: "'Not just the West, but anywhere!'

"Sharath then said that if he continued such behavior, he would not teach with his grandfather anymore."

The lore among those senior students who are able to acknowledge that Jois had a "problem" is that Jois stopped assaulting women after that confrontation. But throughout the rest of his teaching career, it remained an acknowledged practice for Jois to squeeze the buttocks of women who lined up to greet him after every class, and kiss them on the lips.

***

After my feature on Jois was published in *The Walrus*, I received an email from a 72-year-old woman in Seattle named **Kathy Elder**.

"I felt both sickened and vindicated by your article," she wrote. "I was so over the moon to have an opportunity to practice with the guru of Ashtanga yoga. At his 2002 retreat on Kauai he sexually assaulted me. I went to his people and told them but they just made excuses for him. At last your article has freed me from years of trying to make sense of what happened."

Kathy was at the same retreat as Micki Evslin and her two friends, but she did not know them. She'd come to Kauai from the Big Island where she had been taking care of her elderly father.

"The very first day at the end of the practice I was in *Urdhva Padmasana*," she told me by phone. The posture involves folding your legs into lotus above you while in a shoulder stand.

"It was beyond groping. We all wore those little thin tights. It was so hard and quick and fast and deep, it hurt. It hurt me. I gasped, and by the time I untied myself from the posture, he had toddled off.

"I was devastated. I was staying at the YMCA camp down the road, the workshop was in Kīlauea. So I went back and I was staying in one of the cabins, and I was so upset. I called my husband up and he said, 'Well, what should you do?.' and I said, 'I don't know.' And he said, 'Well, you can come back. Just leave.' He said, 'Or think it out and see what you can get, see what you can do about it.' So I decided to stick it out, and then that night everybody was sitting on the beach.

"There was a woman there, I don't remember her name, but she was in charge of his entourage. I told her what happened, and she said to me, 'Oh, well, he was just trying to show you where your *mulabandha* was.'

"'This is so outrageous!' I said, 'I'm so angry, I don't know what to do about this.' But I couldn't confront him. I'm not a shrinking violet, believe me.

"I remember the next day I went to practice, and I was standing in the line. There must have been 120, 30 people in there. It was filled to the rafters, and we were all very close to each other. We were just maybe going to start the standing poses, and he sees me, and I make eye contact with him. And he starts to waddle towards me. He's in those stupid Calvin Klein underpants. I put my finger in the air and pointed at him. And I mouthed, 'Stay the *fuck* away from me.' And he was just veered off to the side, and that was the last he bothered me.

"But I stood there at the end of class when people were lining up to touch his feet. He'd come back in his white robes and sit there, and people were lining up to touch his feet. And I kept saying, 'Kathy, say something, say something, say something.' But I never did.

"It's very cathartic to describe all this. It's something that I've talked to other female yoga teachers about, and I've told my other students about it."

Kathy's description reminded me of the famous groping photograph published by *YogaDork* in 2009. I asked if I could send it to her on the off chance that she would recognize herself in it. She hadn't seen or heard of the photograph. She consented for me to send it and I waited over the phone as she opened the link in her email.

She wasn't in the photo. She'd been almost 60 at the time, and these women were younger, she noted. "He just didn't press on me," she added. "He tried to get his fingers in there, you know?"

"Now why aren't they screaming?" she asked, her voice rising. "Why didn't I scream? Why did we let this happen? I've been a woman long time, and that's the worst that's ever happened to me. But I grew up in that age when men would pat you on the rear, or pinch your rear, or say inappropriate things. But this whole #MeToo thing has changed everybody.

"I thought, 'Did that really happen? What did I do?' 'Maybe I shouldn't have worn those pants ...' They were kind of a wine-colored Suki pants. When I got them, I thought, 'Boy, that's pretty show-off to wear something like that at that your age."' I went through all of that.

"I adored him. I didn't know him, but I adored what I'd heard about him, I adored the practice. I never got hurt, I wasn't injured. Yeah, and I always used his teachings and my teachings, and I still did. Even after that happened, I still used the Iyengar, the Jois, and the Sivananda practice, the three practices that I had studied. And I kind of mixed them together, and took the best of all of them. Because you don't want to throw the baby out with the bathwater. I mean there was some great things that came about from bringing yoga into America. It saved my life.

"It's like being assaulted in church or something. You go some place you think is safe, and that you're going for spiritual solace, and mental and physical well-being, and somebody does that to you. It's hard to believe. I didn't tell anybody about it except my husband for a long time."

***

Nicola Tiburzi was in her early twenties when she drove down with a friend from Roberts Creek, on the Sunshine Coast, north of Vancouver to attend a day-long workshop with Jois in Seattle in 2002. His hosts were David Garrigues and Catherine Tisseront, the teachers of Tracy Hodgeman. They rented out a gymnasium, and 225 people came.

"It was an incredible experience to host the man who has helped us transform our lives," wrote Garrigues in an article published a year later, "and doubly so as we watched so many of our students practicing with him—many for the first time."[358]

Nicola had been practicing in the Vancouver Ashtanga community for a few years. She had taken courses with David and Doug Swenson, and Mysore-style classes with some second-generation teachers. She'd also studied with Jois disciples Lucy Martorella (partner of Brad Ramsey), Larry Schultz, and a woman whom she remembers warning her that "when Jois likes you, he touches." Up until meeting Jois, she'd only had positive experiences.

By phone, she described being in the morning class. Jois paced the room, called out the postures, and counted off the breaths.

"I remember being in downward facing dog [*Adho Mukha Svanasana, see* Figure 3, p. 47] and seeing his feet behind me," she said,

> and then having his hand come right into my groin and almost a feeling he's gonna lift me up a bit. Quite a strong touch. It wasn't a light brush. It was like, "Oh! Okay."'And it was a confident touch. I'm a very intuitive person and I haven't had any big trauma that way, I just knew in my body it was not a healthy feeling. But, even though it wasn't a good feeling, it wasn't healthy, it also wasn't making sure the tone of my pelvic floor was in good standing for the sake of my spine or anything.... I just knew that it wasn't right. I did some self-reflection, like "was there a need, was my pelvic floor really misaligned?" But, I just felt like, "Oh, I need to get out of here," it just didn't feel right at all.

The assault wasn't entirely unexpected. Rumours of Jois's behavior were so common that they had trickled down even to the Vancouver tier.

"I had already had, in the back of my head, a warning that perhaps this man was once in a while inappropriate with his touch of students. I don't have a history of any big trauma, so I was shocked but not shocked to the point where it was debilitating in any way.

"I was lucky. Because I could imagine if I had been there for years and in different context, it would have been really disturbing being a young person. I guess I was open-minded to the idea that maybe there was more of an esoteric need for him to touch in some way. I had heard he checks to see if *mulabandha* is engaged. So, I think I wasn't shocked, but when it happened I was like, Oh well maybe, 'Is my *mulabandha* engaged, or...' I kind of took it as a self-reflection moment, and then instantly was like..."

After speaking with Nicola, reading Garrigues's blog about the event is like staring through Alice's looking glass. He's writing approximately five years after Karen remembers how Jois would repeatedly and intensely assault his partner Catherine:

> Guruji imparts an entire approach to life in his teaching. He is not merely counting out numbers in a strange language. As he takes you through the sequence, there is a poignancy, a weight, a feeling

> that something important is transpiring. Yet he retains his sense of humor. There exists a feeling of adventure and fun along with the seriousness of the endeavor.
>
> Guruji has been teaching this system for more than 65 years. His body, his family, his life have been molded and shaped by this practice. He has watched hundreds and hundreds of people unlock the gate into the garden of themselves. He knows the magic, the potency of this practice.
>
> The class is a little slice of heaven, a culmination of his life's work, like a master chef creating his favorite dish. So many woderful ingredients combined with consummate artistry and skill, such care and love. The list of ingredients: tempo, rhythm, breath, silence, space and devotion, all combined in the hands of the master with one purpose in mind—to set you free![359]

Nicola's read on Jois's purpose was different.

"He was just, feeling like into me basically, for no reason for my own purpose. More just for him to… have that experience."

The incident didn't dampen her enthusiasm for yoga practice, however. Back in Vancouver, she began studying with a group of women who taught Iyengar yoga. She immersed herself in the method, and after several trips to the Iyengar Institute in India, became certified in the method. She credits her practice with healing her ovarian cysts. As we speak by phone I can hear her two-year old babbling happily in the background.

***

Michelle Bouvier studied Ashtanga yoga with one of Jois's senior American students, Tim Miller, from 1997 to 2004. She never got to Mysore to study directly with Jois; injury had held her back twice.

Miller was a co-demonstrator with Karen Rain in that 1993 video. By email, Miller tells me that he hosted Pattabhi Jois 10 times over the years at the Ashtanga Yoga Nilayam—the first Ashtanga studio outside of India—which he took over after its founders, Brad Ramsey and Gary Lopedota, left for Maui. When Jois came on tour, Miller would rent a local gym.

Michelle went to Jois intensives in 2000 and 2002. At the first one, she remembers being a neophyte amongst a large cohort. She wasn't comfortable with the bowing, kneeling, and wide-eyed devotion, but she mostly enjoyed the event.

By the 2002, she had advanced substantially in her practice. The intensive that year was focused on a more advanced series, and there were fewer people in attendance. Jois groped her genitals every day for three days as she was in forward folds, and he stood behind her. At one point, he also pressed his genitals onto hers in the *Yoga Nidrasana* posture (*see* Figure 2, p. 47) described by Katchie Ananda.

Michelle remembers at first being confused, and then trying to ignore him by syncing up her energy with that of the older woman beside her.

Afterwards, she overheard discussions amongst senior practitioners. They were minimizing and rationalizing his behavior, saying that he was "working on energy".

"I thought: this is not really real anymore," Bouvier tells me. "If I had thought there was anything spiritual about this scene, that feeling was gone."

APPENDIX 3

Request to KPJAYI for an Apology

Dear Sharath,

I'm writing to you both as a long-term student of the lineage you are the leader of and as a brother and friend to the various sisters who were students of your grandfather and who suffered his abuse. I realize that this is an abrupt way to start this letter, but I can think of no other way to communicate my concern for our tradition.

I debated writing you because I wondered whether my words would hold a great deal of standing in your eyes, especially given the fact that I have not visited Mysore in many years, nor do I still teach. Nevertheless, I continue to practice what you and your grandfather taught me almost daily and have been dedicated to these teachings for twenty-five years. I hope that my dedication in itself would be enough to lend credibility to my words. Besides, I have and continue to care genuinely about this practice and how the tradition of Ashtanga is perceived in the world.

You would know better being at the helm of the ship, but from where I stand, I cannot help but see that the tradition is at a very significant crossroads. The primary crisis I see that we're in is that your grandfather touched women inappropriately. In the West, we would consider that sexual abuse. I know that neither you or your mother condoned this behavior. In fact, it is public knowledge that you tried to stop him. I also remember how close you were to your grandmother, so I can only imagine how disturbing this was to you.

I also heard that you announced this in a public forum, which is helpful, but I'm afraid you haven't gone far enough. It would be good if you sent out a public statement denouncing these acts, of naming them as sexual abuse. It would be healing if you could apologize as the lineage holder on behalf of the tradition. At the moment, it appears that you are silent on the matter, and, as such, it seems that you are sweeping the whole thing under the rug.

I share this with you because I don't believe that this is good for the tradition; in fact, it demonstrates an insensitivity to the women who suffered your grandfather's abuse. Many, in effect, continue to suffer the painful repercussions of his predation: lack of self-worth, physical fatigue, and depression. These and many more varied and negative symptoms result from being subject to the abuse of power your grandfather inflicted on many women within the community.

As far as I am concerned, these women are my sisters—in fact, many were your sisters, too—sisters within the family of Ashtanga yoga. The truth of the matter is that none of us did anything to protect our sisters. We denied your grandfather's abuse and swept it under the rug by couching his behavior in pseudo-spiritual terms. There's nothing spiritual about grinding your genitals into your students' genitals or inappropriately grabbing their breasts and buttocks. Nobody deserves that kind of treatment, especially people who come to yoga with a pure aspiration.

To have that purity sullied is a disgrace and is a blight on the tradition. Not only are these women still suffering as a result of those experiences at his hands, but also in the communit[y]'s lack of apology. Aside from Mary Taylor and Kino McGregor, no senior students have come out on public record to denounce the behavior or make a public apology. In fact, we recently heard of a movement afoot to defame the journalist who brought … your grandfather's abuses to light on a public stage. This attempt to slander him is an even more profound shame than not saying anything. To do so would be to deepen the denial and to discredit these students' experiences.

I believe these senior students wanting to defame the journalist are waiting for your leadership, maybe they're even attempting to protect it. But honestly, this sort of behavior will undermine it more. You are in an unusual position. I cannot imagine how tough it may be. Nothing trained you to have to deal with such a situation.

If you do or say nothing, not only am I concerned that these women will continue to suffer, I'm also worried that this will stigmatize the tradition you lead. People will see you and the tradition you represent as insensitive and worse, abusive.

Without a doubt, it will create more divisiveness than may be needed. Some will leave altogether. Many will avoid you and Mysore. The students who will remain loyal will likely be sycophants, telling you only what you want to hear, hiding the truth from you. I doubt that this is something you would want. It's nice to have people around us that care about us, but its horrible to have people around who protect us from the truth. It leads to a situation known in the West as an "emperor with no clothes." You start to believe that you're more perfect than you are by believing lies.

I guess that this is what this letter is attempting to be, a wakeup call from someone who cares about you and the tradition. No, I'm not nor have I ever been one of your "poster child" students, but I have cared for the tradition and spoken out where I think that the tradition has gone awry. That may not be the kind of student that makes you feel comfortable or at ease, but please know that my intention is not to undermine you or your leadership. It's to hold up a mirror and to ask you, "Is this where you want to steer the ship?"

Best,

Chad Herst[360]

NOTES

All eBook references are to Kindle editions. Due to the nature and size of the references and notes, they are held in full online at https://embodiedwisdom.pub/paaic/resources.

FRONT MATTER, INTRODUCTION

1 G Donahaye and E Stern. *Guruji*. 2010: p. xiii.
2 A Stein. *Terror, Love and Brainwashing*. 2017.
3 J Lalich and ML Tobias. *Take Back Your Life*. 2006: loc. 206 (emphasis added).
4 G Donahaye. 'Pattabhi Jois and #MeToo'. 8/31/2018. https://yogamindmedicine.blogspot.com/.
5 RJ Lifton. *Thought Reform and the Psychology of Totalism*. 1961: 429–30.
6 Statement from Greg Nardi and Scott Johnson. Email to author, 10/5/2018 (emphasis added.).
7 M Singer. 'Coming Out of the Cults'. *Psychology Today*. January 1979: 72–82.
8 HL Rosedale and MD Langone. 'On Using the Term "Cult"'. https://www.icsahome.com/.
9 J Lalich and ML Tobias. *Take Back Your Life*. 2006: loc. 226.
10 J Lalich and ML Tobias. *Take Back Your Life*. 2006: loc. 665.
11 C Mann. 'The MIND Model of Cult. Dynamics'. https://cultexpert.weebly.com/.
12 LJ West and M Langone. 'Cultism'. *Cultic Studies Journal* 3. 1986: 119–20.
13 I wrote about this personal exchange here: M Remski. 'That Time When I Was in a Cult…'. 7/12/2017. http://matthewremski.com/wordpress/.
14 K MacGregor. 'Ashtanga Yoga—Accountability, Acceptance and Action…'. 12/26/2017. https://www.kinoyoga.com/.
15 'Teachers': https://sharathjois.com; http://www.ashtanga.com/.
16 E Stern. '100 Years'. July 2015. http://ayny.org/100-years/.
17 G Donahaye and E Stern. *Guruji*. 2010: 265. Also RA Medin (inter) and D Summerbell (ed). '3 gurus, 48 questions'. *Namarupa*. Fall 2004: 7.
18 M Singleton and T Fraser. 'T. Krishnamacharya'. In M Singleton and E Goldberg (eds). *Gurus of Modern Yoga*. 2014: loc. 2274, citing S Dars. 'Entretiens'. *Viniyoga* 24. 1989: 61–2.
19 M Singleton. *Yoga Body*. 2010.
20 BKS Iyengar. *Astadala Yogamala, vol. 1*. 2000: 16–61.
21 Shaw's unpublished article is a notable exception: EJ Shaw. 'Seizing the Whip'. http://www.academia.edu/.
22 Singleton's groundbreaking work is essential reading here: M Singleton. *Yoga Body*. 2010.
23 S Binkley. *Getting Loose*. 2007: 32.
24 For an example of the "keep practicing" strategy during an institutional abuse crisis, see M Remski. 'Judith Simmer-Brown to Distraught Shambhala Members'. 8/6/2018. http://matthewremski.com/wordpress/.
25 Rain's first professional writing credit appears in Medium.com's *Power Trip* online magazine: K Rain. 'Yoga Guru Pattabhi Jois Sexually Assaulted Me for Years'. *Power Trip*. 10/6/2018. https://medium.com/s/powertrip/.
26 Yoga and Movement Research Community. [Facebook page]. https://www.facebook.com/groups/1648029625458814/.
27 A Lucas. 12/7/2010. The original article was posted to Facebook on on the now-defunct version of the yogacitynyc.com site. Facebook link: https://www.facebook.com/anneke.lucas.2/. YogaDork posted an excerpt. YD. 'Good Touch, Bad Touch'. 12/9/2010. http://yogadork.com/. Lucas posted an updated version in 2016: 'Why The Abused Don't Speak Up'. 3/7/2016. https://www.yogacitynyc.com/. The article was posted a third time in 2018: '#MeToo Rouses a Yoga Community'. 6/8/2018. https://theshiftnetwork.com/blog/2018-07-09/metoo-rouses-yoga-community.
28 J Cooke. 'Why Didn't Somebody Warn Me?" 7/11/2018. http://www.decolonizingyoga.com/.
29 J Cooke. Email to author, 11/16/2018.

30 From a personal conversation, explored in M Remski. 'Why We Don't Listen To Trauma Survivors'. 4/7/2018. http://matthewremski.com/wordpress/.
31 A Stein. *Terror, Love and Brainwashing*. 2017: 91.
32 CP Smith and JJ Freyd.'Institutional Betrayal'. *American Psychologist*. 69(6). 2014: 575–87.
33 b hooks. *The Will to Change*. 2005.

PART ONE

34 'Genny Wilkinson Priest'. [podcast]. 11/19/2018. https://www.jbrownyoga.com/. The post by Mary Taylor to which she refers was published on 12/8/2017: M Taylor. 'Can Difficulties Give Us Insight?' 12/8/2017. https:// www.richardfreemanyoga.com/musings/.
35 *Primary Series Ashtanga with Sri K. Pattabhi Jois*. [online video]. 1993. https://www.youtube.com/.
36 Now visible on the private server of the *Decolonizing Yoga* website, under the title of *Pattabhi Jois Yoga Adjustments*. [online video]. http://www.decolonizingyoga.com/.
37 Examples include S Desai and A Wise. *Yoga Sadhana for Mothers*. 2014; S Griffyn and M Clarke. *Ashtanga Yoga for Women*. 2003; and A Beale and D Yu (Coord); S Marino and T Jeng (eds). *Strength & Grace*. 2015.
38 G Donahaye and E Stern. *Guruji*. 2010: 164.
39 *Pattabhi Jois Yoga Adjustments*. [online video]. http://www.decolonizingyoga.com/.
40 G Donahaye and E Stern. *Guruji*. 2010: 29–30.
41 A Stein. *Terror, Love and Brainwashing*. 2017: 180–9.
42 L Gallagher. 'Lotus 1, 2, 3'. *Details* Magazine. September 1995: 198–241.

PART TWO

43 A Stein. *Terror, Love and Brainwashing*. 2017: 21.
44 See M Stone. 'What's that Yoga breath?' 4/ 30/2014. http://www.theyogimovement.com/.
45 According to a personal conversation with my late friend, Michael Stone, in about 2015.
46 M Taylor. Email to author, 8/19/2017.
47 'Richard Freeman on the Evolution of Yoga'. [podcast]. 1/11/2018. https://kathrynbruniyoung.com/.
48 N McInerny. 'Terrible, Thanks for Asking'. [podcast]. https://www.apmpodcasts.org/ttfa/.
49 K Rain. 'Yoga Guru Pattabhi Jois Sexually Assaulted Me for Years'. *Power Trip*. 10/6/2018. https://medium.com/s/powertrip/.
50 K Rain. 'My Full Testimony'. 7/30/2018. https://karenrainashtangayogaandmetoo.wordpress.com/.
51 *Inside Owl*, the blog of certified Ashtanga teacher Angela Jamison, provides consistent examples of positive stereotyping, such as here: A Jamison. 'Autonomy, Moral Codes + Naked Beer Goats'. [web blog]. 3/1/2018. http://www.insideowl.com/.
52 M Hawley. 'The Privatization of Religion and Personal Identity'. *Sikh Formations*. 11(1–2). 2015: 210–22, Also see E De Michelis. 'Modern Yoga: History and Forms'. In M Singleton and J Byrne (eds). *Yoga in the Modern World*. 2009: 17–35.
53 C Lavrence and K Lozanski. '"This Is Not Your Practice Life"'. *Canadian Review of Sociology/Revue Canadienne De Sociologie*. 51(1). 2014: 76–94.
54 K Felt. 'Katherine Felt on Yogi Bhajan and friends'. http://yogibhajan.tripod.com/.
55 C Mann. 'The MIND model of Cult. Dynamics'. https://cultexpert.weebly.com/.
56 K Rain. 'Yoga and #MeToo'. 1/1/2018. http://www.decolonizingyoga.com/.
57 Karen Rain. [Facebook page]. 11/11/2017. https://www.facebook.com/karen.rain.9615/.
58 K Rain. 'Clear Witness Testimony'. 2/27/2018. https://karenrainashtangayogaandmetoo.wordpress.com/.
59 *Tracyogini*. https://sites.google.com/site/tracyogini/.
60 Dimi Currey. [Facebook page]. 1/14/2018. https://www.facebook.com/dimi.currey/.

PART THREE

61 KP Jois. *Yoga Mala*. 2010: loc. 1871.
62 'Beryl Bender Birch'. [podcast]. 7/2/2018. https://www.jbrownyoga.com/.
63 MD Langone. *Recovery from Cults*. 1995.
64 C Mann. 'The MIND model of Cult. Dynamics'. https://cultexpert.weebly.com/.
65 J Lalich and ML Tobias. *Take Back Your Life*. 2006: loc. 651–89.

66 BKS Iyengar. *Light on Yoga*. 1996.
67 *Medical class, BKS Iyengar in Australia 92*. [online video]. https://www.youtube.com/.
68 J Birch and J Hargreaves. 'Yoganidrā'. 1/8/2015. https://theluminescent.blogspot.com/. For more, see also M Singleton. 'Salvation through Relaxation'. *Journal of Contemporary Religion*. 20(3). 2005: 289–304.
69 The more accurate backstory of Bhajan's group 3HO is recounted here: P Deslippe. 'From Maharaj To Mahan Tantric'. *Sikh Formations*.8(3). 2012: 369–87.
70 Described here: 'Universal Principles of Alignment'. *Anusara School of Hatha Yoga*. https://www. anusarayoga.com/teacher-support/.
71 C Mann. 'The MIND model of Cult. Dynamics'. https://cultexpert.weebly.com/.
72 According to my Jyotisha and Sanskrit mentor Davis Batson, based upon his *gurukulum* studies with Krishan Lal Mantri (d 2017) in Toronto, early 2000s.
73 TM Krishnamacharya. *Yoga Makaranda or Yoga Saram (The Essence of Yoga) First Part*. L Ranganathan and N Ranganathan (trans). 2006: 10, 40, 42, 49, 75, 81, 103.
74 Svātmārāma and BD Akers. *The Hatha Yoga Pradipika*. 2002: 44.
75 DE Moerman. *Meaning, Medicine, and the "Placebo Effect"*. 2002: 127–13.
76 KP Jois. *Yoga Mala*. 2010: loc. 116.
77 J Russell. 'Yoga Korunta'. 11/11/2015. http://www.jamesrussellyoga.co.uk/.
78 The most thorough research on this topic comes from J Birch. 'The Proliferation of Āsanās in Late-Medieval Yoga Texts'. In K Baier, PA Maas and K Preisendanz (eds). *Yoga in Transformation*. 2018: 101–80.
79 DG White. *The Yoga Sutra of Patanjali*. 2014: 197–224.
80 J Birch. 'The Proliferation of Āsanās in Late-Medieval Yoga Texts'. In K Baier, PA Maas and K Preisendanz (eds). *Yoga in Transformation*. 2018: 141.
81 J Birch. Email to author, 10/14/2018.
82 M Singleton. *Yoga Body*. 2010: 185.
83 G Donahaye and E Stern. *Guruji*. 2010: loc. 198.
84 J Birch. Email to author, 10/14/2018.
85 M Singleton. *Yoga Body*. 2010: 186.
86 More on this controversy is found in M Remski. 'Mark Singleton Responds to Critics …'. 11/1/2015. http://matthewremski.com/wordpress/.
87 AG Mohan and G Mohan. *Krishnamacharya*. 2010: 138.
88 G Maehle. *Ashtanga Yoga Practice and Philosophy*. 2013: 16.
89 J Birch and J Hargreaves. 'Vinyāsa'. 7/14/2016. http://www.theluminescent.org/.
90 AG Mohan and G Mohan. *Krishnamacharya*. 2010: 29.
91 J Birch. Email to author, 10/14/2018.
92 G Donahaye and E Stern. *Guruji*. 2010: 417.
93 G Donahaye and E Stern. *Guruji*. 2010: 20.
94 A Hall. 'Updated: Yoga's Loss of Purpose'. *Krishnamacharya's Mysore yoga… at home*. [web blog]. 3/20/2015.https://grimmly2007.blogspot.com/.
95 'The Practice > Parampara'. http://sharathjois.com/.
96 http://www.ashtangaparampara.org/.
97 YJ Editors. 'Practice and All is Coming'. *Yoga Journal*. 6/22/2009. https://www.yogajournal.com/.
98 L Kaminoff. 'I teach Viniyoga®. So, sue me'. [Facebook page]. 1/24/2018. https://www.facebook.com/notes/leslie-kaminoff/.
99 YJ Editors. 'Kausthaub Desikachar Faces Abuse Allegations'. 10/3/2012. https://www.yogajournal.com/blog/.
100 YD. 'Update: Sad Details of Kaustaub Deiskachar's Psychopathic Abuse …'. 10/17/2012. http://yogadork.com/.
101 'Legal Closure | September 2014'. http://kausthub.com/legalclosure.
102 'Testimonials> Yoga Therapy In Trauma Care'. 7/31/2015. http:// kausthub.com/testimonial/.
103 G Donahaye and E Stern. *Guruji*. 2010: 250.
104 'Literature > Sri K. Pattabhi Jois: A Tribute'. http://yogashala.ru/en/.
105 G Donahaye and E Stern. *Guruji*. 2010: 115.
106 G Donahaye and E Stern. *Guruji*. 2010: 124.
107 TK Sribhashyam. Correspondence with author, 2/12/2016.

108 *Kino Speaks on Pattabhi Jois*. [online video]. https://www.youtube.com/.
109 K MacGregor. 'Ashtanga Yoga—Accountability, Acceptance and Action...'. 12/26/2017. https://www.kinoyoga.com/.
110 J Birch. Email to author, 10/14/2018.
111 J Birch. Email to author, 4/17/2018.
112 BR Smith. 'With Heat Even Iron Will Bend'. In M Singleton and J Byrne (eds). *Yoga in the Modern World*. 2008: 140–60.
113 J Birch. Meaning of *hatha* in Early Hathayoga. *Journal of American Oriental Society*. 131(4). 2011: 527–54. https://www.academia.edu/.
114 J Birch. Email to author, 10/14/2018.
115 J Birch. Email to author, 10/14/2018.
116 A Cushman, 'Power Yoga' *Yoga Journal*. February 1995: 144.
117 'Richard Freeman on the Evolution of Yoga'. [podcast]. 1/11/2018. https://kathrynbruniyoung.com/.
118 Mallinson's essay on *vajroli mudra*, including a personal description of his experience with it, is instructive here: J Mallinson. 'Yoga and Sex'. Paper. Yoga in Transformation conference. University of Vienna. September 2013. https://www.academia.edu/.
119 WD O'Flaherty. *Siva*. 1981.
120 K MacGregor. *Sacred Fire*. 2012.
121 K MacGregor. *Sacred Fire*. 2012: 29.
122 K MacGregor. *Sacred Fire*. 2012: 34.
123 K MacGregor. *Sacred Fire*. 2012: 35.
124 M Remski. 'Karen Rain Responds to Mary Taylor's Post ...'. 12/11/2017. http://www.decolonizingyoga.com/. Dwelley in Comments.
125 *Ask Richard and Mary*: 'Is there any fundamental difference between trantric [sp] yoga and ashtanga yoga? [online video]. https://www.facebook.com/richardfreemanyoga/.
126 Via Sanskritist and Tantric scholar Christopher Wallis. [However, lineages start from someone and often their practices are amended in the process of creating a lineage].
127 K Rain. Email to author, 9/16/2018.
128 J Pankhania and J Hargreaves. 'Culture of Silence: Satyananda Yoga'. 12/22/2017. http://theluminescent.blogspot.com/.
129 J Hargreaves. Email to author, 11/11/2018.
130 M Taylor. 'Can Difficulties Give Us Insight?' 12/8/2017. https://www.richardfreemanyoga.com/musings/.
131 J Hargreaves. Email to author, 11/11/2018.
132 Photos can be seen at M Remski. 'Pattabhi Jois Sexually Assaulted Men'. 11/11/2018. http://matthewremski.com/wordpress/.
133 K Rain. 'Yoga Guru Pattabhi Jois Sexually Assaulted Me for Years'. 10/6/2018. https://medium.com/s/powertrip/.
134 Monica Gauci [Facebook page]. https://www.facebook.com/monica.gauci/.
135 E Goldberg. *The Path of Modern Yoga*. 2016: 223–33.
136 BKS Iyengar, JJ Evans, and D Adams. *Light on Life*. 2008: xix.
137 DG White. *The Alchemical Body*. 2012: 279.
138 G Donahaye and E Stern. *Guruji*. 2010: 28.
139 G Donahaye and E Stern. *Guruji*. 2010: 43.
140 G Donahaye and E Stern. *Guruji*. 2010: 373.
141 G Donahaye and E Stern. *Guruji*: 259.
142 KP Jois. *Yoga Mala*. 2010: loc. 1034.
143 KP Jois. *Yoga Mala*. 2010: loc. 1871.
144 G Donahaye and E Stern. *Guruji*. 2010: 53.
145 G Donahaye and E Stern. *Guruji*. 2010: 255.
146 G Donahaye and E Stern. *Guruji*. 2010: 252.
147 A Hall. 'Updated: Sharath's NEW KPJAYI Authorisation/Certification Code of Conduct'. *Krishnamacharya's Mysore Yoga... at home*. [web blog]. 1/27/2018. http://grimmly2007.blogspot.com/.
148 T Hodgeman. 'Summer 2007'. [web blog]. 11/5/2010. http://tracyhodgeman.blogspot.com/.

149 J Kramer. 'A New Look at Yoga: Playing the Edge of Mind & Body'. *Yoga Journal*. Jan 1977. http://joeldiana.com/.
150 'Final Questions. Sri K. Pattabhi Jois Public Talks on Ashtanga Yoga — France 1991'. http://www.aysnyc.org/.
151 BKS Iyengar and N Perez-Christiaens (comp and ed). *Sparks of Divinity*. 2012: loc. 2044. Here *prakriti* refers to material, biological nature. Iyengar is suggesting that asana practice brings the body into a purifying relationship with the soul.
152 BKS Iyengar and N Perez-Christiaens (comp and ed). *Sparks of Divinity*. 2012: loc. 1993.
153 BKS Iyengar and N Perez-Christiaens (comp and ed). *Sparks of Divinity*. 2012: loc. 1544.
154 BKS Iyengar and N Perez-Christiaens (comp and ed). *Sparks of Divinity*. 2012: loc. 2060.
155 Jules Mitchell's *Yoga Biomechanics*. 2018 Provides an excellent analysis on the current science of stretching.
156 L Cohen. "The Window". *Field Commander Cohen: Tour of 1979*. Columbia Records. 2001.
157 K MacGregor. *The Power of Ashtanga Yoga*. 2013: 4
158 KP Jois. *Yoga Mala*. 2010: loc. 533.
159 G Donahaye and E Stern. *Guruji*. 2010: 62.
160 G Donahaye and E Stern. *Guruji*. 2010: 63.
161 Along with M Singleton. *Yoga Body*. 2010 and E Goldberg. *The Path of Modern Yoga*. 2016, the work of Joseph Alter provides excellent background for this historical shift, especially JS Alter. *Yoga in Modern India*. 2004.
162 J Birch. 'Premodern Yoga Traditions and Ayurveda'. *History of Science in South Asia* 6. 2018: 1-83. https://www.academia.edu/.
163 J Mallinson and M Singleton. *Roots of Yoga*. 2017: 133.
164 RP Brown and PL Gerbarg. *The Healing Power of the Breath*. 2012.
165 G Donahaye and E Stern. *Guruji*. 2010: 409–10.
166 G Donahaye. 'Pattabhi Jois and #Metoo'. 8/31/2018. https://yogamindmedicine.blogspot.com/.
167 'Books>Guruji . . . ' https://shop.ashtanga.com/.
168 'Angela's Reviews > Guruji'. 7/ 19/2014. https://www.goodreads.com/review/show/1000656714.
169 'Angela's Reviews > Guruji'. 7/19/2014. https://www.goodreads.com/review/show/1000656714.
170 See, for example, customer reviews for *Guruji* on https://www.amazon.com/.
171 H Arendt. *The Origins of Totalitarianism*. 2017.
172 A Stein. *Terror, Love and Brainwashing*. 2017: 57.
173 A Stein. *Terror, Love and Brainwashing*. 2017: 54.
174 A Stein. *Terror, Love and Brainwashing*. 2017: 54.
175 G Donahaye. Email to author, 10/25/2016.
176 G Donahaye. Email to author, 10/26/2016.
177 G Donahaye and E Stern. *Guruji*. 2010: 400.
178 'Beryl Bender Birch'. [podcast]. 7/2/2018. https://www.jbrownyoga.com/.

PART FOUR

179 A Stein. *Terror, Love and Brainwashing*. 2017: loc. 894 (emphasis added).
180 Langone's thesis has been extracted here: M Remski. "'Deception, Dependance, and Dread…'" 5/14/2018.http://matthewremski.com/wordpress/.
181 C Mann. 'The MIND model of Cult Dynamics'. https://cultexpert.weebly.com/.
182 S Hassan. *Combating Cult Mind Control*. 3rd edition. 2016.
183 Lis Harris's investigative report provides excellent coverage of Muktananda and his community Siddha Yoga Dham America (SYDA): L Harris. 'O Guru, Guru, Guru'. *New Yorker*. 11/14/1994: 92. Also available at http://www.leavingsiddhayoga.net/o_guru_english.htm.
184 D Shaw. *Traumatic Narcissism*. 2014.
185 L Oakes. *Prophetic Charisma*. 1997.
186 H Arendt. *The Origins of Totalitarianism*. 2017.
187 A Stein. *Terror, Love and Brainwashing*. 2017: loc. 801.
188 "Sweet is the lore which Nature brings; / Our meddling intellect / Mis-shapes the beauteous forms of things:— / We murder to dissect." W Wordsworth. 1798. *Lyrical Ballads*.

189 DW Winnicott. The Theory of the Parent-Infant Relationship: Further Remarks. *International Journal of Psychoanalysis* 43. 1962: 238–9. Online at *Oxford Clinical Psychology* http://www.oxfordclinicalpsych.com/.
190 LJ Kaplan. *Oneness and Separateness*. 1978.
191 MD Ainsworth et al. *Patterns of Attachment*. 1978.
192 DN Stern. *The Motherhood Constellation*. 1995.
193 A Stein. *Terror, Love and Brainwashing*. 2017: 32.
194 A Stein. *Terror, Love and Brainwashing*. 2017: 33.
195 A Stein. *Terror, Love and Brainwashing*. 2017: 38.
196 *Wild Wild Country*. 2018. https://www.netflix.com.
197 A Stein. *Terror, Love and Brainwashing*. 2017: 68.
198 A Stein. *Terror, Love and Brainwashing*. 2017: 68.
199 A Stein. *Terror, Love and Brainwashing*. 2017: 28.
200 G Donahaye and E Stern. *Guruji*. 2010: 156.
201 G Donahaye and E Stern. *Guruji*. 2010: 356.
202 G Donahaye and E Stern. *Guruji*. 2010: 282.
203 G Donahaye and E Stern. *Guruji*. 2010: 312.
204 G Donahaye and E Stern. *Guruji*. 2010: 250.
205 G Donahaye and E Stern. *Guruji*. 2010: 186.
206 G Donahaye and E Stern. *Guruji*. 2010: 408.
207 R Lauer-Manenti. *An Offering of Leaves*. 2009.
208 R Lauer-Manenti. *Sweeping the Dust*. 2010.
209 R Lauer-Manenti. 'My Teachers'. https://www.ruthlauermanentiyoga.com/.
210 R Lauer-Manenti. *An Offering of Leaves*. 2009: loc. 1065.
211 R Lauer-Manenti. *An Offering of Leaves*. 2009: loc. 1069.
212 R Lauer-Manenti. *An Offering of Leaves*. 2009: loc. 1045.
213 R Lauer-Manenti. *An Offering of Leaves*. 2009: loc. 1048.
214 R Lauer-Manenti. *Sweeping the Dust*. 2010: loc. 822.
215 Holly Faurot—v.—Jivamukti Yoga Center, Inc. et al. 150790/2016. New York County Supreme Court. Exhibit A. https://iapps.courts.state.ny.us/.
216 A Slater and PC Quinn. Face recognition in the newborn infant. *Infant and Child Development*. 10(1–2). 2001: 21–4.
217 E Goldberg. 'Swami Krpalvananda'. In M Singleton and E Goldberg (eds). *Gurus of Modern Yoga*. 2014: loc. 4527.
218 G Donahaye and E Stern. *Guruji*. 2010: loc. 262.
219 G Donahaye and E Stern. *Guruji*. 2010: loc. 3299.
220 G Donahaye and E Stern. *Guruji*. 2010: loc. 4310.
221 G Donahaye and E Stern. *Guruji*. 2010: loc. 6710.
222 G Donahaye and E Stern. *Guruji*. 2010: loc. 6773.
223 K Rain. 'Actionable Steps Towards Restorative Justice'. 1/24/2018. https://karenrainashtangayogaandme-too.wordpress.com/.
224 G Donahaye and E Stern. *Guruji*. 2010: 68.
225 G Donahaye and E Stern. *Guruji*. 2010: 69.
226 Name not disclosed. Email to author, 6/19/2018.
227 *Remembering Guruji Shri Pattabhi Jois II — Gretchen Sanchez*. [online video]. https://www.youtube.com/.
228 *The American Yoga Revolution with Iyengar disciples Manouso Manos and Patricia Walden*. [online video]. 2015. https://www.youtube.com/.
229 A Stein. *Terror, Love and Brainwashing*. 2017: loc. 1039.
230 G Donahaye and E Stern. *Guruji*. 2010: loc. 271.
231 G Donahaye and E Stern. *Guruji*. 2010: loc. 271.
232 G Donahaye and E Stern. *Guruji*. 2010: 29–30.
233 'Angela's Reviews> Guruji'. 7/19/2014. https://www.goodreads.com/review/show/1000656714.
234 G Donahaye and E Stern. *Guruji*. 2010: 29.

235 'Teaching with the Hands'. *Yoga Workshop*. 2018. https://yogaworkshop.com/ (emphasis added). While this page is no longer available, the same text appears on 'Assisting Intensive'. https://yogaworkshop.com/assisting-intensive/, with the singular amendment noted in brackets.
236 G Donahaye and E Stern. *Guruji*. 2010: 160.
237 G Donahaye and E Stern. *Guruji*. 2010:164.
238 G Donahaye and E Stern. *Guruji*. 2010: 316.
239 PL Brown. 'At home with: Dr Robert M Sapolsky'. 4/19/2001. http://www.nytimes.com/.
240 *Dopamine Jackpot!* [online video]. https://www.youtube.com/.
241 G Donahaye and E Stern. *Guruji*. 2010: 350.
242 G Donahaye and E Stern. *Guruji*. 2010: 373.
243 *Warning*: sexual assault is depicted in this photo. *Ashtanga Yoga Therapy*. http://ashtangayogatherapy.com/ es/node/128. (accessed 10/5/2018).
244 T Miller. 'A Brief History of Ashtanga Yoga in Encinitas'. http://ashtangayogacenter.com/.
245 G Donahaye and E Stern. *Guruji*. 2010: 43–4.
246 *Advanced A Ashtanga Yoga Practice, Kealakekua, HI with Sri K. Pattabhi Jois. 1985.* [online video]. Parts 1–5. https://www.youtube.com/.
247 G Donahaye and E Stern. *Guruji*. 2010: 47.
248 Ie Catherine Tisseront.
249 davidgarriguesyoga. [Instagram feed]. 2/1/ 018. https://www.instagram.com/.

PART FIVE

250 G Wilkinson Priest. 'Sexual abuse in yoga'. *Healthista*. 12/18/2017. https://www.healthista.com/.
251 S Gannon and D Life. *Jivamukti Yoga*. 2002: 82.
252 R Worth. *Elisabeth Kübler-Ross*. 2005. For more on this topic, see M Stroebe et al. 'Cautioning Health-Care Professionals'. *OMEGA* 74(4). 2017: 455–73.
253 Freyd's excellent DARVO resource page is here: JJ Freyd. 'What is DARVO?'. 2018. https://dynamic.uoregon.edu.
254 K MacGregor. 'Ashtanga Yoga—Accountability, Acceptance and Action…'. 12/26/2017. https://www.kinoyoga.com/.
255 'Kino MacGregor'. [podcast]. 4/23/2018. https://www.jbrownyoga.com/.
256 K MacGregor. 'Ashtanga Yoga—Accountability, Acceptance and Action…'. 12/26/2017. https://www.kinoyoga.com/.
257 G Wilkinson Priest. 'Sexual abuse in yoga'. *Healthista*. 12/18/ 2017. https://www.healthista.com/.
258 The name and prior conviction is found on the sex offender registry of the State of Hawaii. Prior conviction is registered with the State of Michigan Judicial District, 21st Judicial Circuit, Case No. 99-008788-FH, June 15, 1999. The practitioner provided screenshots of the UCLA event via email.
259 The Facebook comment was made in a private group. The practitioner needs to maintain anonymity, but has confirmed the quote by email to the author, 10/9/2018.
260 Holly Faurot—v.—Jivamukti Yoga Center, Inc. et al. 150790/2016. New York County Supreme Court. https://iapps.courts.state.ny.us.
261 'A Message to the Jivamukti Yoga Community'. *Jivamukti Yoga*. Archived at https://tinyurl.com/ycxw7gl9.
262 Holly Faurot—v.—Jivamukti Yoga Center, Inc. et al. 150790/2016. New York County Supreme Court. https://iapps.courts.state.ny.us/.
263 S Gannon and D Life. *Jivamukti Yoga*. 2002: loc. 1617.
264 E Stern. Email to author, 7/23/2016.
265 M Remski. 'Jivamukti Light and Dark'. 4/24/2016. http://www.decolonizingyoga.com/.
266 S Gannon and D Life. *Jivamukti Yoga*. 2002: loc. 1573.
267 S Gannon and D Life. *Jivamukti Yoga*. 2002: loc. 1588.
268 S Gannon and D Life. *Jivamukti Yoga*. 2002: loc. 1597.
269 Jivamukti Yoga 300-hour training manual. 2007: 89.
270 From Darkness to Light. [Facebook page]. https://www.facebook.com/.
271 Name not disclosed. Email to author, 6/15/2018.

272 S Gannon and D Life. *Yoga Assists*. 2014.
273 S Gannon and D Life. *Yoga Assists*. 2014: loc. 227.
274 S Gannon and D Life. *Yoga Assists*. 2014: loc. 320.
275 S Gannon and D Life. *Yoga Assists*. 2014: loc. 406.
276 S Gannon and D Life. *Yoga Assists*. 2014: loc. 346.
277 B Frost. 'Betrayal of Trust'. *West (San Jose Mercury News)*. May 26, 1991: 6-11. Available at http://matthewremski.com/wordpress/.
278 M Leitsinger. '#MeToo Unmasks the Open Secret of Sexual Abuse in Yoga'. 9/7/2018. https://www.kqed.org/.
279 Ethics Committee notes from the complaint brought by Ann West: Ethics Committee, Iyengar Yoga National Association of the United States. Reference notes and Report on MM-MM case. 9/13–18/2018. https://iynaus.org/sites/default/files/ethics-committee-reports/fInal-report-ethics-comm-case-MM-AW.pdf.
280 R Brathen. '#MeToo — The Yoga Stories'. 12/6/2017. Archived at https://tinyurl.com/y73ewmkv.
281 *Yoga and Body Image Coalition*. http://ybicoalition.com/.
282 Such as B Berila et al. *Yoga, the Body, and Embodied Social Change*. 2016.
283 L Mulvey. Visual Pleasure and Narrative Cinema. *Screen* 16(3). 1975: 6–18.
284 *Mysore Style with Tim Miller*. [online video]. https://www.youtube.com/.
285 ifilmyoga. [Instagram page]. https://www.instagram.com/.
286 See note 235.
287 T Landrum. 'Yoga and Sexual Fantasy'. 12/31/2017. https://www.tylandrum.com/ .
288 "Sanskrit and vernacular poems of the Gorakhnāthī and other north Indian ascetic traditions are highly misogynistic, and other Gorakhnāthī legends, as well as current ethnography, suggest that like other male ascetic traditions, the Gorakhnāthīs have always shunned the company of women. Women are never explicitly prohibited from practising yoga, although hatha texts commonly insist that male yogis should avoid the company of women." J Mallinson and M Singleton. *Roots of Yoga*. 2017: loc. 1758.
289 Ashtanga Yoga Confluence. March 1–4, 2018. http://ashtangayogaconfluence.com/schedule/. The panel was recorded by an attendee.
290 T Feldman. 'Sexual Misconduct, Pattabhi Jois, Ashtanga Yoga & Me'. 1/22/2018. https://www.elephantjournal.com/.
291 M Taylor. 'Can Difficulties Give Us Insight?' 12/8/2017. https://www.richardfreemanyoga.com/musings/.
292 The talk is preserved here: *Pushpam Magazine*. Dec 18, 2017. https://tinyurl.com/yaenw3ey.
293 G [Wilkinson] Priest. 'A KPJAYI Statement on Pattabhi Jois'. 2018. https://www.change.org/.
294 Chad Herst. [Facebook page]. 9/18/2018. https://www.facebook.com/chad.herst/.
295 'LG38 — Genny Wilkinson Priest and Sarai Harvey-Smith'. [podcast]. 4/21/2018. http://www.trueryan.com/.
296 A Hall. 'Update: Ashtanga Yoga: Inappropriate Adjustments/Sexual Abuse'. *Krishnamacarya's Mysore Yoga... at home*. [web blog]. Jan 2018. http://grimmly2007.blogspot.com/.
297 Anthony Hall discusses the code issuance and list controversy: A Hall. 'Updated. Sharath's NEW KPJAYI Authorisation/Certification Code of Conduct'. *Krishnamacharya's Mysore Yoga... at home*. [web blog]. 1/27/ 2018. http://grimmly2007.blogspot.com/..
298 'LG38 — Genny Wilkinson Priest and Sarai Harvey-Smith'. [podcast]. 4/21/2018. http://www.trueryan.com/.
299 'Richard Freeman — "Still Looking"'. [podcast]. 2/5/2018. https://www.jbrownyoga.com/.
300 M Taylor. 'Pulling Things Apart'. 7/7/2018. https://www.richardfreemanyoga.com/musings/.
301 Greg Nardi. [Facebook page]. 12/18/2017. https://www.facebook.com/greg.nardi/.
302 S Harvey-Smith. 'The Sexual Misconduct of Pattabhi Jois'. *Directions in Yoga*. 3/17/2018. https://saraiyoga.wordpress.com/.
303 G Maehle. 'My Initial Response to Karen Rain's Interview About Sexual Abuse'. 5/17/2018. https://chintamaniyoga.com/.
304 M Gauci. 'Why I Left the Mysore Community in 1999'. 5/17/2018. http://chintamaniyoga.com/.
305 M Gauci. 'Why Did She Let It Happen?' 5/23/2018. https://chintamaniyoga.com/.
306 G Maehle. 'My Initial Response to Karen Rain's Interview About Sexual Abuse'. 5/17/ 2018. https://chintamaniyoga.com/.

307 J Blanchard. 'Why We Need To Talk About The Sexual Abuse Committed By Pattabhi Jois'. *Balance Yoga & Wellness*. 2018. http://www.balanceyogawellness.com/.
308 S Johnson. Email to author, 10/12/2018.

PART SIX

309 'Shannon Roche, COO, Addresses Sexual Misconduct'. *Yoga Alliance*. 1/5/2018. https://www.yogaalliance.org/.
310 'Gregor Maehle'. [podcast]. 11/12/2018. https://www.jbrownyoga.com/.
311 P Cunningham, M Drumwright and B Foster. "Networks of Complicity and Networks of Empowerment," presentation at La Trobe University, Melbourne, Australia, Jul 2, 2018. Professor Cunningham can be reached at PeggyC@dal.ca for more information.
312 J Lalich and ML Tobias. *Take Back Your Life*. 2006: loc. 59.
313 'Adult tobacco use>Smoking in Canada'. https://uwaterloo.ca/tobacco-use-canada/.
314 The IAYT's scope of practice can be found on their website www.iayt.org.
315 D Farhi. *Teaching Yoga*. 2006.
316 J Lalich and ML Tobias. *Take Back Your Life*. 2006: loc. 1437.
317 S Hassan. *Combating Cult Mind Control*. 3rd edition. 2016: 319.
318 J Lalich and ML Tobias. *Take Back Your Life*. 2006: loc. 1434.
319 RJ Lifton. *Thought Reform and the Psychology of Totalism*. 1961: 429–30.
320 J Lalich and ML Tobias. *Take Back Your Life*. 2006: loc. 1429.
321 H Frankfurt. *"On Bullshit." The Importance of What We Care About*. 1988.
322 K MacGregor. 'Ashtanga Yoga—Accountability, Acceptance and Action…'. 12/26/2017. https://www.kinoyoga.com/.
323 The CYTA was the first English-language yoga organization to publish a Code of Conduct for its members in 1995. J Hanson Lasater. 'A Special Message from the California Yoga Teachers Association'. *Yoga Journal*, Nov/Dec 1995: 136-137. Archived at https://tinyurl.com/ycqotdm3. *Yoga Journal*, originally founded by CAYT Director Judith Hanson Lasater and others, was its publishing arm until it was sold in 1998.
324 M Leitsinger. '#MeToo Unmasks the Open Secret of Sexual Abuse in Yoga'. 9/7/2018. https://www.kqed.org/.
325 Ethics Committee, Iyengar Yoga National Association of the United States. Reference notes and Report on MM-MM case. 9/13–18/2018. https://iynaus.org/sites/default/files/ ethics-committee-reports/fInal-report-ethics-comm-case-MM-AW.pdf.
326 Ethics Committee, Iyengar Yoga National Association of the United States. Reference notes and Report on MM-MM case. 9/13–18/2018. https://iynaus.org/sites/default/files/ ethics-committee-reports/fInal-report-ethics-comm-case-MM-AW.pdf.
327 M Remski. 'Manos Disciple to Manos Accuser'. 9/24/2018. http://matthewremski.com/wordpress/.
328 IYNAUS President David Carpenter addresses the issue and its history in this letter: D Carpenter. Letter to IYNAUS members. 9/12/2018. Available at https://tinyurl.com/y739z7e7.
329 For more on IGM, see M Remski. 'The Unbearable Smugness of "I Got Mine-ism"…'. 4/6/2018. http://matthewremski.com/wordpress/. (Thank you to Joseph Teskey for introducing me to the phrase.)
330 M Remski. "Feminist-Informed" Ashtanga and "Trauma-Informed" Kundalini'. 11/15/2018. http://matthewremski.com/wordpress/.
331 B Berila et al. *Yoga, the Body, and Embodied Social Change*. 2016: 267.
332 P Deslippe. 'From Maharaj To Mahan Tantric'. *Sikh Formations*. 8(3). 2012: 369–87. See also note 54.
333 Karen answers many of these questions and more in this interview: M Remski. 'Karen Rain Speaks About Pattabhi Jois and Recovering from Sexual and Spiritual Abuse'. [video interview]. 5/15/2018. http://matthewremski.com/wordpress/.
334 L Greenblatt. 'Independent investigation confirms "physical, sexual, emotional abuse" by Sogyal Rinpoche'. 9/6/2018. https://www.lionsroar.com/. The Lewis Silkin investigation into allegations against Sogyal Lokar, a Rigpa teacher, is available here: 'Independent Investigation'. https://www.rigpa.org/.
335 S Domet. 'Unanswered questions about Shambhala investigation'. 9/16/2018. https://www.thecoast.ca/.

336 Two other pre-internet investigative pieces are not well-known. One is Lis Harris's 1994 coverage of the allegations against SYDA's Swami Muktananda (see note 183). There is also Katherine Webster's 1990 *Yoga Journal* investigative report on Swami Rama is not available in its original form but is available here: K Webster. 1990. 'The Case against Swami Rama of the Himalayas'. http://www.prem-rawat-bio.org/nrms/info/rama1.htm.

337 Nowhere on his website does it mention formal training in this context. http://kausthub.com/testimonial/.

338 M Remski. 'Jivamukti Yoga Claims Position "At the Forefront" of the Consent Card Movement'. 8/1/2018. http://matthewremski.com/wordpress/.

339 Jill Miller's lecture "Lights, Camera, Yoga"(unpublished) at the April 2016 Yoga Education Series talks, hosted by Yoga Alliance in Toronto, provided a unique view into this industry reality. She described how her earlier career in Hollywood gave her the stagecraft skills that have helped her engage workshop audiences around the world. Miller's insights are worth careful study, given how many workshop-circuit yoga teachers — Sean Corne, Kathryn Budig, Rod Stryker, David Life, and Sharon Gannon, to name but a few — are former actors or performers.

340 Greg Nardi. [Facebook page]. 12/18/2017. https://www.facebook.com/greg.nardi/.

341 JJ Freyd. 'When sexual assault victims speak out, their institutions often betray them'. 1/11/2018. https://theconversation.com/.

342 *Axis Syllabus*. http://www.axissyllabus.org/.

343 T Rose. Email to author, 10/9/2018.

344 T Wildcroft. 'Post-lineage yoga'. *Wild Yoga*. 4/20/2018. https://www.wildyoga.co.uk/2018/04/post-lineage-yoga/.

345 T Wildcroft. Private message to author, 11/21/2018.

346 E Goldberg. *The Path of Modern Yoga*. 2016: 101–8.

347 T Wildcroft. 'Post-lineage yoga'. *Wild Yoga* 4/20/2018. https://www.wildyoga.co.uk/.

348 *Yoga Service Council*. https://yogaservicecouncil.org/.

349 M Remski. 'Karen Rain Responds to Mary Taylor's Post About the Sexual Misconduct of Pattabhi Jois'. 12/11/2017.http://www.decolonizingyoga.com/.

350 G Donahaye and E Stern. *Guruji*. 2010: 373.

351 *Hatha Yoga Project*. http://hyp.soas.ac.uk/.

352 When this project was mainly focused on injuries, I covered this statement in this article: M Remski. 'Kino's Hip'. 7/12/2015. http://matthewremski.com/wordpress/.

353 *Pattabhi Jois Yoga Adjustments*. [online video]. http://www.decolonizingyoga.com/.

354 Katchie Ananda. [Facebook page]. 2/2/2018. https://www.facebook.com/katchie.ananda/.

355 Luis Veiga. [Facebook page]. 11/15/2018. https://tinyurl.com/y8vzvlmu.

356 T Watanabe. 'DNA Clear Yoga Guru in Seven-Year Paternity Suit'. 7/11/2002. http://articles.latimes.com/.

357 'Richard Freeman on the Evolution of Yoga'. [podcast]. 1/11/ 2018. https://kathrynbruniyoung.com/.

358 D Garrigues. 'The One-Year Anniversary: Pattabhi Joie in Seattle, Seattle Yoga 1. 2003. https://www.ashtanga.com/html/article_garrigues.html.

359 D Garrigues. 'The One-Year Anniversary: Pattabhi Joie in Seattle, Seattle Yoga 1. 2003. https://www.ashtanga.com/html/article_garrigues.html.

360 Chad Herst. [Facebook page]. 9/18/2018. https:www.facebook.com/chad.herst/.

INDEX

CPSIA information can be obtained
at www.ICGtesting.com
Printed in the USA
BVHW061253080419
544915BV00010B/386/P

9 780473 472078